PRAISE FOR DR. PATRICK WILSON AND *The Athlete's Gut*

"Ultrarunners drop out of 100-mile races due to gut distress more than any other reason. *The Athlete's Gut* is a godsend. It presents practical, efficacious, and immediately applicable advice that any ultrarunner can benefit from. It's a resource I will use with every single one of my athletes as well as with our entire coaching staff. It's that valuable."
—Jason Koop, Head Coach of Ultrarunning at CTS and author of *Training Essentials for Ultrarunning*

"Races aren't won at the dinner table, but they can be lost there, and nutrition science is becoming increasingly important to athletes. We're unique beings, however, and the science is not always one-size-fits-all. With *The Athlete's Gut*, Wilson addresses the workings (and malfunctions) of our guts to better understand how to make nutrition science work for us, as individuals with peculiar innards."
—Chad Haga, WorldTour cyclist, stage winner in the 2019 Giro d'Italia

"Dr. Wilson uses anecdotes and humor to explain and simplify complex anatomy and physiology in a way that any athlete will be able to relate to. Causes of, and prevention strategies for, gut issues are at your fingertips, as well as a plethora of 'fun facts' and well researched scientific insight."
—Dr. Martyn Beaven, The University of Waikato Adams Centre for High Performance

"For athletes, coaches, and practitioners interested in learning more about the athlete's gut, Dr. Wilson has created a go-to, science-based resource. It is comprehensive, funny, and packed with useful information glued together with easy-to-understand stories and analogies!"
—Jeff Rothschild, MS, RD, sports dietitian

"Dr. Wilson marries his brains about the gut with his witty humor to produce *The Athlete's Gut*. You will eat this book up fast! It is an easily digestible, science-backed read that will educate and entertain at the same time. If you are a weekend warrior or a professional athlete that has some crappy issues to deal with, this is a must-read. Be ready to laugh out loud a few times while learning something new along the way."
—Tommy Jensen, MS, RD, Director of Sports Nutrition at University of Minnesota

"Dr. Wilson takes a well-thought-out approach to explaining the intricacies of the athlete's gut—specifically, expanding on topics such as how stress and anxiety influence gut symptoms in relation to performance. His use of wit and humor, blended through relevant anecdotes and peer-reviewed research, make the concepts interesting and enjoyable. The summaries at the end of each chapter were a great way to wrap up essential material in an easy-to-understand format that may be useful to students, athletes, and practitioners."
—Dr. Leilani Madrigal, PhD, CMPC, Assistant Professor at California State University, Long Beach

"Patrick Wilson is one of a handful of people in the world qualified to write this book. Writing in an accessible but still highly informative style, he takes us from the biological 'desert' that is the stomach to the jungle of the colon and everything in between. Referencing everything from *Wayne's World* to the classical 19th century research of William Beaumont, this book is a must-read for any athlete, coach, or medical professional who wants to optimize performance without compromising wellness."

—Dr. Robert Fearn, Medical Director and gastroenterologist

"*The Athlete's Gut* has the information that coaches and athletes have been waiting for about performance fueling, GI distress, and its impact on sports performance. Dr. Wilson has meticulously researched the topics that plague all athletes at some point in their careers. This book provides the latest research—no fads—in an informative and entertaining read."

—Jason Kask, Head Coach and President, Superior Performance Endurance Coaching

"*The Athlete's Gut* takes us along a fascinating journey from the moment we put something in our mouth to the moment it exits stage right and everything in between. In the first chapter alone I learned things that, as an athlete, I've been doing wrong for years, and as a coach, I can use to improve my clients' performance. We often overlook the importance of understanding the digestive system in our performance and life, but *The Athlete's Gut* helps us realize just how vital it is!"

—J.P. Caudill, running coach and ultrarunner

"*The Athlete's Gut* is a comprehensive yet easy-to-read guide to the endurance athlete's engine. Coaches and athletes: Here are the fundamentals for developing the nutrition plan that will fuel your best performance ever."

—Dan Netzer, National Champion Masters cyclist

"A remarkable compendium in a still-overlooked topic in sports nutrition. Dr. Wilson does an outstanding job using funny, everyday analogies to present solid, scientific data with excellent graphical support, making it easy to read and quite comprehensible. The research experience and nutrition background from Dr. Wilson make this a reliable source of information and possibly the most complete go-to book to date when looking to understand and minimize gut distress in endurance athletes."

—Gabriel Baltazar-Martins, cycling nutritionist and founder of *Fuel the Pedal* podcast

"Digestion isn't the sexiest topic in our sport—we'd rather discuss springy shoes and training hacks. Yet *The Athlete's Gut* will convince you to prioritize gut health for performance gains. All the weird GI questions you're afraid to ask your doctor—and endurance athletes have so many weird GI questions—are answered in this clear and complete guide from a bona fide expert."

—Susan Lacke, author of *Life's Too Short to Go So F*cking Slow*

THE ATHLETE'S GUT

PATRICK WILSON, PHD, RD

The inside science of digestion, nutrition, and stomach distress

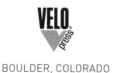

BOULDER, COLORADO

▼velopress

4745 Walnut Street, Unit A
Boulder, CO 80301-2587 USA

VeloPress is the leading publisher of books on endurance sports and is a division of Pocket Outdoor Media. Focused on cycling, triathlon, running, swimming, and nutrition/diet, VeloPress books help athletes achieve their goals of going faster and farther. Preview books and contact us at velopress.com.

Distributed in the United States and Canada by Ingram Publisher Services

Library of Congress Cataloging-in-Publication Data
Names: Wilson, Patrick B. (Professor of exercise science), author.
Title: The athlete's gut: the inside science of digestion, nutrition, and
    stomach distress / Patrick B. Wilson.
Description: Boulder, Colorado: VeloPress, 2020. | Includes
    bibliographical references and index.
Identifiers: LCCN 2019053526 (print) | LCCN 2019053527 (ebook) | ISBN
    9781948007108 (paperback) | ISBN 9781948006217 (ebook)
Subjects: LCSH: Digestion. | Gastrointestinal system—Diseases. |
    Athletes—Nutrition. | Physical fitness—Nutritional aspects.
Classification: LCC QP145 .W55 2020 (print) | LCC QP145 (ebook) | DDC
    612.3—dc23
LC record available at https://lccn.loc.gov/2019053526
LC ebook record available at https://lccn.loc.gov/2019053527

This paper meets the requirements of ANSI/NISO Z39.48-1992 (Permanence of Paper).

Art direction by Vicki Hopewell
Cover and interior illustrations by Andrew J. Nilsen
Cover design by Corey Hollister
Interior design by Erin Farrell / Factor E Creative
Author photo by Mark Winterstein

20 21 22 / 10 9 8 7 6 5 4 3 2 1

To Cecilia, for your love and support,
and Oscar, for the joy you bring to my life.

CONTENTS

Introduction   ix

Part 1

GUT FUNCTION AND THE EFFECTS OF EXERCISE

01 Gut Anatomy and Physiology   3
02 The Origins of Gut Symptoms   29

Part 2

NUTRITION AND THE ATHLETE'S GUT

03 Energy   77
04 Carbohydrate   89
05 Fat   111
06 Protein   123
07 Fluid and Hydration   133
08 Sodium   147
09 Training the Gut   155
10 Dietary Supplements   167

Part 3

PSYCHOLOGY AND THE ATHLETE'S GUT

11 Stress and Anxiety   191
12 Managing Stress and Anxiety   213

Appendix A: Gastrointestinal Disorders   227
Appendix B: Medications Affecting the Gut   253
Acknowledgments   263
Notes   265
Index   297
About the Author   305

INTRODUCTION

If members of the public were polled to name the most important anatomical and physi-

ological features that make a great athlete, several answers would likely come up over and over again—powerful muscles, a big heart, efficient lungs, nerves of steel. References to the digestive tract would almost certainly fail to make it to the top of people's lists. To be sure, all of us are aware that the gastrointestinal tract—or the gut, as I'll also call it—breaks down and absorbs the foods we eat, but many of the other indispensable duties of this roughly 30-foot-long fleshy tube remain opaque to the average Joe or Jane.

Even though most of the public doesn't consider the gut to be a key part of sporting success, countless athletes know all too well how crucial it can be to making the winners' podium or even simply finishing a race, for that matter. For many, their guts have betrayed them in the midst of competition or during a critical training session. Indeed, it's safe to assume that almost every athlete has—at some time or another—been stricken with gut distress. If you're reading this book, it's fair to assume you've experienced gut dysfunction yourself, or at least know of an athlete who has. Maybe you had to duck into roadside greenery to assuage an angry bowel. Maybe you were overcome by an excruciating side stitch that stopped you dead in your tracks. Maybe you tossed your déjeuner in the locker room because of pre-game nerves. Or perhaps you're one of those unfortunate souls who suffers from nearly every conceivable form of digestive torment known to man. Rest assured, you're not alone.

Although it's difficult to generalize about the prevalence of gut distress during exercise (it depends on exercise intensity, duration, and a survey's methods), the great majority of endurance athletes and even many team-sport athletes at least occasionally struggle with unpleasant symptoms.[1, 2] Even the elite of the elite aren't immune to these digestive disturbances. Bill Russell (Boston Celtic and 11-time NBA champion), Steve Young (San Francisco 49er and three-time Super Bowl winner), Jim Ryun (1960s running phenom), Paula Radcliffe (former world record–holding marathoner): these names represent just a smattering of notable athletes who have had encounters with severe or reoccurring gut troubles before or during competition.

This book—organized into three parts—addresses the causes of and solutions to athletes' alimentary afflictions. In Part 1, I answer the question of why so many athletes develop unpleasant gut symptoms, particularly in the midst of their most important contests. As you'll learn, there's not a singular answer to this question. Instead, each symptom—whether it is nausea, reflux, flatulence, or diarrhea—often has its own unique underlying origins, and that is precisely why I take a symptom-by-symptom approach to understanding and managing gut disturbances. For example, a strategy that alleviates nausea may be of little value for managing abdominal cramps. Likewise, tips for preventing reflux may do nothing to ease urges to defecate. Further, the ideal tactic for managing a given symptom can differ depending on the situation. Take for example nausea, a vexing ailment that often rears its ugly head not only during intense exercise like sprinting, but also during extremely prolonged exercise. Although nausea may feel the same in both situations, the underlying causes do differ. Consequently, the strategies I discuss for dealing with a particular symptom often vary depending on the circumstances.

Part 2 of *The Athlete's Gut* is devoted exclusively to diet-gut interactions, and it is easily the largest section of the book. This shouldn't be surprising given that the main job of your gut is to digest and absorb the variety of victuals you consume day in, day out. I take a nutrient-by-nutrient approach to illuminate how various components of your diet can trigger—or, in some cases, relieve—gut woes. Energy, carbohydrate, fat, protein, fluid, sodium, and a variety of supplements are discussed in detail. I also review what the science says about your gut's capacity to morph and change in response to stimuli. Simply asked, is it possible to train your gut over time to tolerate greater intakes of food and fluid during exercise? As you'll come to find out, the evidence tells us that—just as with your muscles, lungs, and heart—your gut is a highly malleable organ that is capable of adapting to the various exposures it encounters, whether that be avocado toast or Twinkies.

There's another reason such a sizeable chunk of *The Athlete's Gut* is devoted to diet: it's been the focus of my professional training for the past 15 years. The first five years of this journey was spent becoming a registered dietitian, which included obtaining a bachelor's degree in dietetics and completing a nearly yearlong internship at the Mayo Clinic. Over the next five years, I obtained master of science and doctorate degrees in exercise physiology from the University of Minnesota. It was during this time that my attention shifted toward studying gut function in athletes; my PhD research evaluated the use of a carbohydrate feeding strategy in runners that was previously utilized with success in cyclists. Although I won't go into the specifics now (they're covered in Chapter 4), this tactic involves consuming multiple types of sugars as a way to maximize carbohydrate burning while also minimizing unpleasant bowel symptoms. For one of my studies, I spent roughly one hundred hours measuring physiological responses and gut symptoms in 20 runners who slogged away on a treadmill in two-and-a-half-hour blocks of time. After finishing my PhD in 2014 and working for a year as a postdoctoral researcher in Nebraska, I moved to Virginia to take a faculty position at Old Dominion University. During my time at Old Dominion, I've continued to perform studies on gut function in athletes, some of which are detailed in the pages that follow.

Telling you about the extent of my training isn't an attempt to impress you. In reality, I have a strong aversion to talking about myself. (Perhaps it's the aw-shucks-Minnesotan in me.) Nevertheless, it's incumbent on me to be transparent in terms of my expertise. To use the parlance of baseball, nutrition science is most definitely in my wheelhouse. In contrast, there are some topics covered within the pages of *The Athlete's Gut* that I haven't received formal training in. Part 3 covers one of these subjects, the connections between the mind and gut dysfunction. Even though I don't have formal psychological training to draw on, I rely extensively on the research and wisdom of scientists who have spent their careers trying to understand the connections between the gut and the brain. Still, you'll find caveats strewn throughout *The Athlete's Gut*, because, in my experience, anyone claiming to be an expert in everything while also offering simple solutions for complex problems are, to put it mildly, usually full of equine crap.

After reading Parts 1, 2, and 3 of *The Athlete's Gut*, you should have a much-improved understanding of how exercise affects your gut, how your nutritional choices impact gut symptoms, and how the connections between your mind and gut contribute to digestive misfortunes. Along the way, you'll read anecdotes of gut mishaps that have befallen prominent athletes throughout the years; these stories serve as powerful reminders that enteral problems can strike any athlete, even those in the upper echelon of their sport. Much of this book, though, is devoted to reviewing the scientific investigations that have shed light on the mysteries of the gut over the past two centuries, from a case study of a fur trapper with a fist-sized hole in his stomach to studies that employ million-dollar functional brain scanners. In fact, I rely on roughly seven hundred references, most of which come from the esoteric pages of scientific journals. As a scientist, I've been trained to substantiate nearly every claim I put forward, and while this makes for a laborious writing process (to the annoyance of my wife, I probably could have finished this book in half the time if I had used a less scrutinizing writing style), it allows you, the reader—if you so desire—to evaluate the veracity of my claims. This style of writing is so important today given the voluminous quantity of dubious health and performance claims found on the internet and social media.

Most of the material in this text pertains to "normal" functional changes that come about during training and competition. Obviously, millions of athletes across the world live with medical illnesses that affect the gut. While *The Athlete's Gut* is mainly concerned with the changes that occur before and during exercise and competition, I would be remiss if I didn't also review some of the ailments that directly or indirectly impact the digestive system. Likewise, medications that target gut functioning and symptoms have obvious implications for athletes. Consequently, Appendix A provides an overview of disorders that can be a source of gut problems, while Appendix B provides a summary of medications commonly used to manage gut symptoms or that are known to induce gastrointestinal side effects. One point I need to make clear is that the material covered in this book—including in Appendixes A and B—is for informational purposes and isn't intended to diagnose, treat, or cure any gastrointestinal (or other) medical condition. I can appreciate that it's not fun to tell someone else about problems like chronic explosive diarrhea or straining on the loo, but you should seek the counsel of a trusted healthcare provider if you're personally suffering from persistent or bothersome gut problems.

With each passing year, we learn more about how the gut functions in response to stressors like exercise and athletic competition, and although there are questions we still don't have the answers to, *The Athlete's Gut* should serve as a go-to, science-based resource when dealing with digestive difficulties in athletes. Athletes spend countless hours training to improve their fitness and refine their skills. Some even spend thousands of dollars on the latest and greatest pieces of equipment or technology that, in many cases, end up having no lasting impact on performance. For many athletes, the alimentary canal is an afterthought, akin to the plumbing in their home in that they take it for granted until something goes horribly awry.

Marathon legend Bill Rodgers, who won a combined eight Boston and New York City Marathons, is reported to have told a group of runners that "more marathons are won or lost in the porta-toilets than at the dinner table."[1] While maybe not accurate in an absolute sense, this statement rings true for an awful lot of athletes around the world. My hope is that by reading *The Athlete's Gut* you'll gain a better grasp of the inner workings of your gut and, by applying this newfound knowledge, reduce the chances that your next contest will be ruined by a petulant bowel.

1

GUT
FUNCTION

AND THE EFFECTS OF EXERCISE

GUT ANATOMY AND PHYSIOLOGY

Before we dive into the science on exercise and the gut, it will be helpful to establish a base of knowledge on the anatomy and function of the digestive system. Thus, we begin by taking a stepwise journey through the gut, from the mouth to (you guessed it!) the anus. As you'll come to see, the alimentary canal is not 30 feet of tubular uniformity. Rather, each section of the gut was designed (or, more precisely, has evolved) to carry out distinct aspects of the digestive process. To put it another way, the gut is sort of like an automobile assembly line, in that each section carries out a unique task and all of these sections need to function properly for a car to come out right. A Ferrari that has no wheels won't be able to hit 200 miles per hour no matter how well the rest of the car is put together. Similarly, a malfunction occurring in any part of your gut can dramatically change what gets digested and absorbed and how your body functions, usually for the worse.

The purpose of this chapter isn't to detail every function of the gut. Instead, my goal is to strike a balance of providing enough information so that you understand how nutritional and other choices impact your gut's function while also avoiding so much detail that you're bored to tears. Even with this simplified overview of the digestive system, some of the information gets technical, though hopefully not pedantic. Don't fret if you find it challenging to follow each and every detail; the most important takeaway is a general sense of how your gut is structured (in terms of order; see Figure 1.1) and how the basic processes of digestion and absorption work.

nasal cavity

salivary glands

mouth

esophagus

4

figure 1.1. **ANATOMY OF THE GUT**

This roughly 30-foot-long system is responsible for digesting and absorbing the foods you eat.

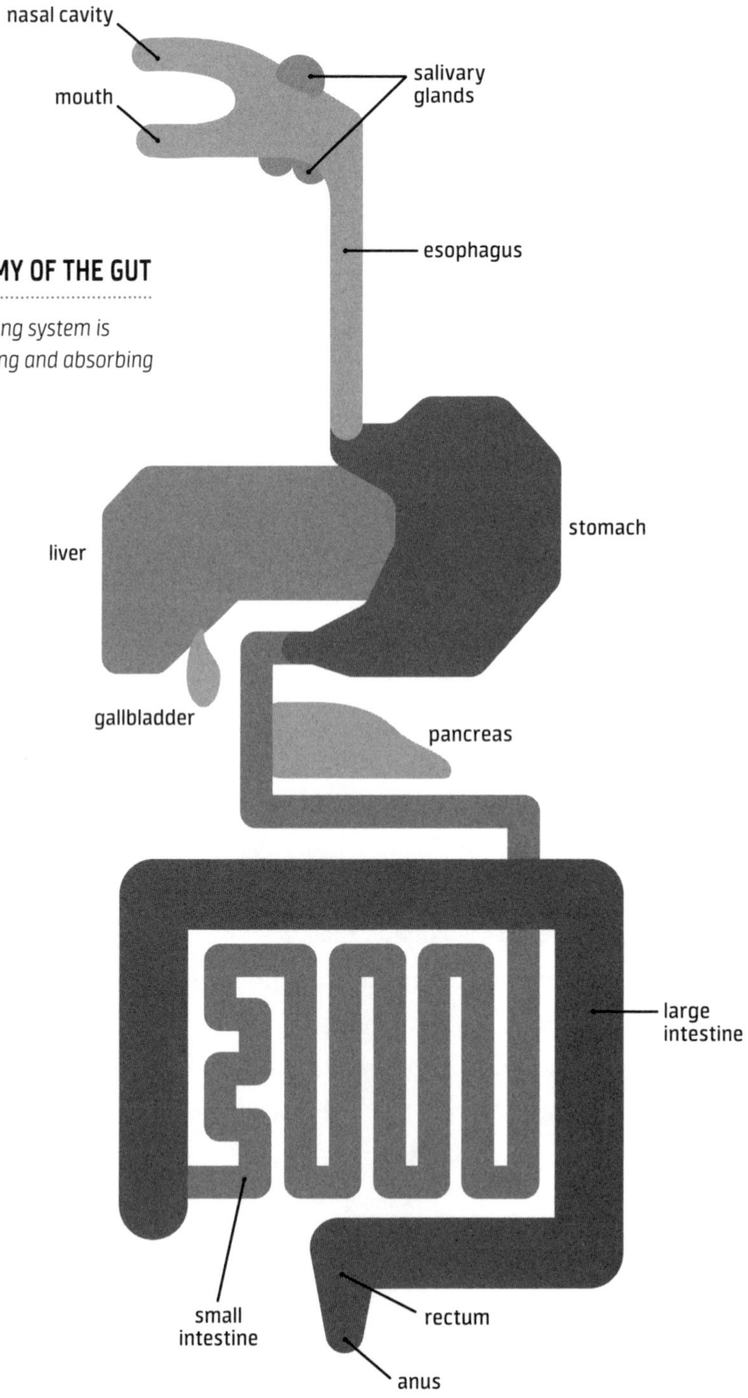

liver

stomach

gallbladder

pancreas

large intestine

small intestine

rectum

anus

If facts about digestion really aren't your jam, you could consider skipping ahead to subsequent chapters, as the majority of the practical information presented later on isn't dependent on having an in-depth knowledge of digestive processes. However, if you do jump ahead, bear in mind that you'll be missing out on references to Mick Jagger, Shaquille O'Neal, Muggsy Bogues, blue whales, a shark movie, anacondas, hot dog eating contests, Sir Michael Caine, and Meryl Streep!

THE MOUTH

The first stop on our alimentary journey is the mouth. Although there are several techniques for quantifying mouth size, one way is to have people suck as much fluid into their mouths as humanly possible without swallowing, which is precisely what one 2012 study asked volunteers to do.[1] The average adult was able to hold approximately 2 ounces of fluid in their mouth, which is about the size of a chicken egg, though the best of the best were able to hold more than 3 ounces. Interestingly, researchers found a correlation between external facial measurements and volumes that participants could keep in their mouths. To put that in layman's terms, Mick Jagger and Steven Tyler (of the Rolling Stones and Aerosmith, respectively, for my non-rock 'n roll-literate readers) probably have larger capacities for holding grub in their pieholes than most other front men, though you probably didn't need a scientific study to tell you that.

When it comes to function, the most important job of your mouth is to mechanically break apart solid foods you eat, from fruits and vegetables to head-sized burritos (no judgment here . . .). The grinding and chewing that occurs in your mouth is a bit like the process of crushing grapes before they're made into wine, and this physical breakdown of food makes the process of chemical digestion easier by increasing the surface area where enzymes work their magic. Amylase is one of the first enzymes your body deploys to get this process of chemical digestion rolling. It's released from your salivary glands into your lumen, which is just jargon for the hollow space by which food passes through you. Salivary amylase's job is to attack the bonds that hold large carbohydrate molecules together, breaking them apart into shorter chains. Another enzyme, lingual lipase, is also secreted in the mouth and initiates fat digestion. While lingual lipase is an important enzyme in animals such as mice (and human babies), adult humans secrete it in only small amounts, and, consequently, little fat digestion takes place in your mouth.

Once you've finished masticating (chewing), the next step in the digestive process is swallowing. While a seemingly simple task, swallowing requires all the precision and coordination of a championship-caliber dance team. Most of us take for granted that this intricate feat of physiology occurs almost flawlessly five hundred to a thousand times every day, including several dozen times while we sleep.[2] In the first step, your tongue holds and presses the semispherical mass of food (called a bolus) against the roof of your mouth, at which point it sends the bolus to your oropharynx, the section of throat behind your oral cavity. Sensory receptors detect this bolus, triggering the base of your tongue to drop and your uvula—that punching bag of flesh at the back of your mouth—to elevate, opening a path for the bolus to travel through. To prevent choking, several automatic actions kick in, including the covering of your airway by your epiglottis, a stiff flap of tissue at the base of your tongue. These and other steps need to occur in a coordinated, sequential manner for a successful swallow to occur. Aberrations in swallowing contribute to a multitude of health issues, including several thousand cases of death by choking every year in the US alone.[3]

THE ESOPHAGUS

The next stop on our enteral voyage is the esophagus, or as our vowel-happy Brit friends like to spell it, the oesophagus. Your esophagus serves chiefly as a transport tube between your mouth and your stomach.

An average adult's esophagus is roughly 41 centimeters long (measuring from the incisors to the esophagogastric junction),[4] although lengths vary based on a number of factors, most importantly one's vertical prowess. At 7'1", Shaquille O'Neal's esophagus is expected to be 54 centimeters long, while at just 5'3", Muggsy Bogues (the shortest basketball player in NBA history) is estimated to have an esophagus right around the average of 41 centimeters. And coming in at staggering 8'11", the tallest human in recorded history, Robert Pershing Wadlow, would have had an esophageal length of 68 centimeters, which, if you're curious, is about the length of an alligator snapping turtle or a smallish bobcat.

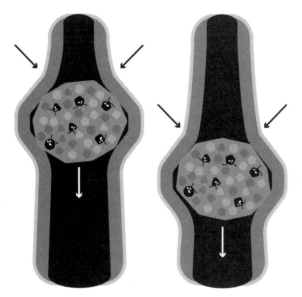

figure 1.2. **PERISTALSIS**

This wavelike motion propels foodstuffs forward through the constriction and relaxation of your gut's walls.

Regardless of whether your esophagus is like Shaquille O'Neal's or more like that of Muggsy Bogues, its ability to regulate the movement of foodstuffs is impressive. In fact, the passage of a bolus through your esophagus is so well coordinated that you could, in Count Dracula–style, swallow blood (or any non-vampire sustenance of your choice) while hanging upside down from the ceiling. This also explains why astronauts are able to eat and drink in zero-gravity environments. Your esophagus achieves these gravity-defying feats via a process called peristalsis, which is a wavelike motion in your gut's walls created by the constricting and relaxing of smooth muscles. In very simplistic terms, peristalsis is a better-coordinated version of squeezing toothpaste out of its tubing or squeezing ketchup out of a packet. Once the swallowing process is initiated, it takes about 5 to 10 seconds for peristaltic waves to transport a bolus through the entirety of a normally functioning esophagus[5] (see Figure 1.2).

The entry and exit of a bolus into and out of your esophagus is regulated by sphincters, your gut's security gates. Sphincters are specialized rings of muscle that open and close based on input from your nervous system; thankfully, most of your sphincters open and close without conscious input. (For those of us inept at multitasking, having to consciously regulate our sphincters would spell disaster for general life productivity.)

Entry of a food bolus into your esophagus is controlled by your upper esophageal sphincter, while at the bottom end of your esophagus, your lower esophageal sphincter controls entry into your stomach. Dysfunction of these sphincters—particularly the lower sphincter—contributes to disorders such as gastroesophageal reflux disease (GERD), which is discussed in subsequent chapters.

THE STOMACH

Compared to the other portions of your gut, your stomach has an enormous capacity for expansion. The stomach is kind of like the puffer fish of the gut; it's about the size of a fist when empty, but at max capacity it can hold 2 to 4 liters of foodstuffs, representing a 50-to-75-fold increase in volume. While that may seem like a lot of chow, it's by no means anywhere close to the largest capacity for mammals, as it's been estimated that it takes over a ton of krill to fill a blue whale's stomach.[6]

Interestingly, the maximum volume of food that people can tolerate in their stomachs depends on their typical eating behaviors. In essence, if you're a regular at Old Country Buffet, you can almost certainly tolerate greater volumes of foodstuffs before feeling uncomfortably full. In one illustrative study, three groups of women had balloons placed into their stomachs that were gradually inflated to the point of maximum discomfort.[7] The first to sense discomfort were women with normal body weights, who were only able to tolerate about 0.75 liter of inflation before tapping out. As you might expect from people who habitually eat enough food to gain excess body weight, the obese women tolerated a higher volume (about 0.9 liter), but this was almost entirely driven by a subset of women who binge ate. Specifically, obese women who regularly binged were able to tolerate close to 1.0 liter of inflation, while obese women who didn't regularly binge responded on par with the women with normal body weights. Finally, the most impressive tolerance to stomach distension, coming in at a whopping 1.2 liters of balloon inflation, was found in women with bulimia (a hallmark of bulimia is recurrent binge eating).

Obviously, inflating a balloon in the stomach isn't eating, but these results suggest that the stomach can be trained to hold large volumes of stuff, including food. The most extreme example of this stomach trainability concept comes from the world of competitive eating. The world record (set in 2018) in hot dog eating, for example, is 74 franks in 10 minutes, which is held by Joey Chestnut, the LeBron James of the competitive eating world. (If you're curious, 74 hot dogs and buns adds up to over 20,000 kilocalories, which is about 7 to 10 days' worth of food for us mere mortals.)

Unfortunately, there's scant research on how competitive eating changes the structure and function of the stomach over time, but fascinatingly, researchers at the University of Pennsylvania did get an opportunity to evaluate a competitive eater during a simulated hot dog eating contest. For the study, the eater (later reported to be first-class eater Tim Janus) and a control subject the researchers reported as having "a hearty appetite" consumed hot dogs along with barium, a substance that, when mixed with water, coats the gut and allows the size and shape of components of the digestive tract to be visualized with fluoroscopy, a sort of X-ray movie. What happened to Janus's stomach was described in the researchers' 2007 article:

> **❝** *Intermittent fluoroscopy revealed progressive accumulation of an ever-increasing volume of hot dog pieces outlined by residual barium in the stomach. . . . At 6 minutes, the stomach had become a dilated, flaccid sac. . . . At 10 minutes, the speed eater had eaten a total of 36 hot dogs. His stomach now appeared as a massively distended, food-filled sac occupying most of the upper abdomen.*[8]

Images of Janus's stomach shown in the article are almost unrecognizable, looking more like a fireball explosion than a portion of a human being's alimentary canal. Bear in mind that he ate "only" 36 hot dogs without buns, which is roughly half of the current world record of 74 red-hots with buns. In case you're wondering, the fellow with the "hearty appetite" that served as the control subject managed to down a measly seven dogs before saying he was about to be sick.

Undeniably, competitive eaters and individuals with bulimia prove the stomach is more than capable of accommodating sizeable quantities of food. You would think that these extreme binging episodes would rupture the stomach on occasion, but that sort of catastrophic injury is very rare. Still, there are a few case reports of individuals dying or experiencing major harm from gorging themselves. In one report published in *The Lancet*, a 23-year-old model with bulimia perished after eating 19 pounds of food in one sitting— among a host of items, she ate two pounds *each* of carrots, plums, grapes, and kidneys.[9] In another case, a woman died after overindulging on two loaves of bread, three sweet buns, two packs of instant noodles, 4.3 liters of carbonated water, and 1.4 liters of beer.[10] Somehow her stomach withstood this onslaught of carby goodness without bursting, but her luck ran out when her distended stomach compressed her inferior vena cava (a large vein) and heart as she lay on a hospital examination table. Remarkably, the occlusion of major blood vessels after extreme binges has been documented in similar cases, including a man whose aorta was blocked after reportedly scarfing down 10 meals' worth of food at lunch[11] and a woman whose aorta was obstructed after gorging on an unknown quantity of food (though 15 liters of gastric contents were emptied from her stomach).[12]

Now that we've established some facts (including a few macabre ones) about the stomach's capacity to act as a food depot, let's return to the actual process of digestion. Mechanical digestion continues via peristalsis and strong, coordinated muscle contractions that churn and mix food boluses. However, churning and mixing only go so far, so your body turns loose its chemical warriors, acid and enzymes. Gastric lipase is one of these chemical warriors, and in contrast to the low amounts of lingual lipase in your mouth, the stomach version contributes substantially to fat digestion. Carbohydrate digestion continues as salivary amylase accompanies food boluses into your stomach, but with time, it's deactivated in the stomach's acidic environment, leaving a substantial proportion of carbohydrate digestion to be handled in your small intestine.

Protein is also a target of digestion in your stomach, perhaps more so than fat and carbohydrate. The stomach is a hostile place for proteins, thanks in large part to the secretion of caustic hydrochloric acid from so-called parietal cells (see Figure 1.3). Hydrochloric acid has a couple of jobs as it relates to breaking down protein. First, it unravels the three-dimensional structure of proteins through a process called denaturation. This unraveling allows enzymes to attack the peptide bonds that keep proteins together. Denaturing a protein is sort of like removing your clothes on a cold winter's day, in that it leaves you entirely vulnerable to the elements. In the case of proteins, denaturation leaves them defenseless against enzymes. The second thing that hydrochloric

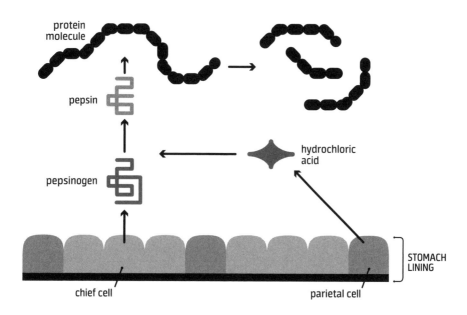

figure 1.3. **PROTEIN DIGESTION**

The stomach is a major site of protein digestion, which is facilitated through the release of hydrochloric acid and activation of pepsinogen to pepsin.

acid does is activate a protein-digesting enzyme, pepsin. The inactive version of this enzyme (pepsinogen) is secreted from a different set of specialized cells known as chief cells. Pepsinogen itself doesn't digest protein, but in the presence of hydrochloric acid, pepsinogen transforms to pepsin. (Pepsinogen is like the hapless Clark Kent while pepsin is like Superman.) Activated pepsin then splits apart proteins into smaller molecules such as peptones and polypeptides, which are chains of amino acids, the basic building blocks of proteins.

The fact that your stomach is a hot spot of protein digestion has several implications. Logically, upping the protein in a meal should increase the time required for hydrochloric acid and pepsin to break down that protein. Indeed, including a substantial amount of protein in a meal—say, from a half-pound burger or an entire turkey leg—is known to lengthen the time it takes for a meal to empty from the stomach, which is one reason high-protein diets seem to blunt hunger more than other diets.[13] In addition, the slowed emptying that accompanies a protein-rich meal means it isn't a wise choice to eat a thick, juicy steak an hour before commencing intense exercise.

Another vital job of your stomach is to regulate the flow of substances into your small intestine. If semidigested food—referred to as chyme—passes from your stomach to your small intestine too quickly, it can overwhelm your small intestine, which, in turn, can trigger symptoms like abdominal cramping, flatulence, and diarrhea. To prevent this, your gut has evolved an elegant feedback system that tells your stomach to step on the metaphorical brake pedal if your small intestine detects too much of certain substances. This feedback is analogous to engineers reducing the flow of water through a mountain dam after getting reports of heavy water flows down in the valley below.

There are a variety of substances that, when detected in your small intestine, inhibit stomach emptying. For example, when hydrochloric acid, polypeptides (products of protein digestion), sugars (particularly glucose), or free fatty acids enter your small intestine, contractions in your stomach are curtailed, which ultimately retards the emptying of chyme.[14] Likewise, fluids that are hypertonic or hypotonic (i.e., well above or well below the concentration of your blood) hinder emptying. Sports beverage makers have long known this, which is why most sports drinks are concocted to contain roughly 6 percent carbohydrate (ensuring that the osmolality doesn't deviate extremely from that of your blood). Most drinks markedly above 6 percent carbohydrate hinder fluid emptying from the stomach. You can calculate the carbohydrate concentration of a sports beverage by dividing the grams of carbohydrate in one serving (listed on the Nutrition Facts panel) by the volume of one serving in milliliters. (There are roughly 30 milliliters in 1 ounce, so as an example, a 20-ounce bottle is equivalent to about 600 milliliters.)

The emptying of chyme is also regulated by the opening and closing of your pyloric sphincter, which serves as the gateway between the world of the stomach and the world of the small intestine. (*Pylorus* is from the Greek word for "gatekeeper.") Your pyloric sphincter is essentially a bouncer that works the door at Club Small Intestine, preventing too many partygoers from entering all at once and ruining an otherwise enjoyable evening. A visual representation of these feedback responses (which are regulated through connections between your gut and nervous system) is shown in Figure 1.4.

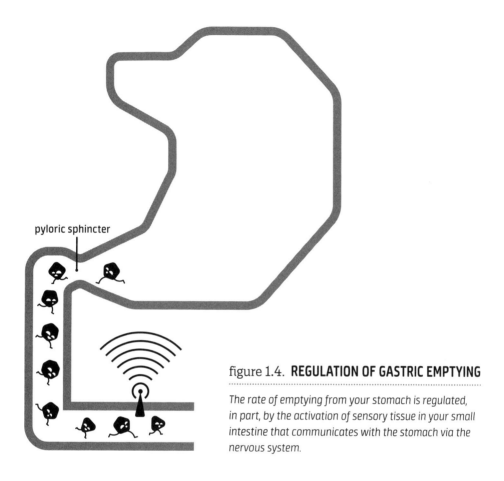

pyloric sphincter

figure 1.4. **REGULATION OF GASTRIC EMPTYING**

The rate of emptying from your stomach is regulated, in part, by the activation of sensory tissue in your small intestine that communicates with the stomach via the nervous system.

THE SMALL INTESTINE

The small intestine is by far the longest portion of the gut, so to be able to fit all of this tissue in your abdominal cavity, your small intestine takes on a coiled orientation. Though lengths vary based on how the measurements are taken (and whether they're taken from a corpse or a living, breathing human), the typical small intestine is 3 to 7 meters long.[15] To give you some perspective, that's the same length as a female green anaconda snake. Yes, you heard that right, there's the equivalent of an anaconda—albeit a skinny, hollow version—residing inside your abdomen.

Your small intestine is made up of three segments with odd-sounding names: in sequential order, they are the duodenum, jejunum, and ileum. The name *duodenum* comes from a Latin translation of an old Greek phrase that meant "12 finger widths." (While conducting autopsies at the Mouseion of Alexandria, the Greek anatomist Herophilos of Chalcedon observed that the first part of the intestine was 12 finger widths in length.)[16] As chyme enters your duodenum, the digestive process for carbohydrates, fats, and proteins is taken over by your pancreas. Putting out an estimated 2.5 liters of juices per day, the pancreas is the workhorse of your digestive system.[17] To use a pop culture reference, I like to think of the pancreas as the Michael Caine of the digestive tract—it just keeps working. According to the website IMDb.com, Sir Caine had 175 acting credits as of 2020, including a role as carefree pilot Hoagie Newcombe in *Jaws: The Revenge*, widely thought of as one of the worst movies of all time. (As awful as the film is, it's worth checking out the ending on YouTube if you're in need of a good laugh.) To be fair to Caine, he also owns two Oscars for Best Supporting Actor.

This flow of pancreatic juices is stimulated by stomach acid (and other substances) coming into contact with the cells lining your duodenum. In turn, this leads to the secretion of hormones (secretin and cholecystokinin, for example) into your bloodstream. These hormones then travel to your pancreas and tell it to dump its juices into your small intestine (see Figure 1.5). One of the most important substances discharged from your pancreas is bicarbonate, an acid buffer. Unlike your stomach (which protects itself by producing a mucus that acts as a defensive barrier), your small intestine isn't equipped to deal with chronic exposure to strong acids, so your pancreas secretes bicarbonate. In addition to acid-squelching bicarbonate, your pancreas releases several enzymes that target fat, protein, and carbohydrate molecules. Pancreatic lipase acts on fat molecules (triglycerides and diglycerides), while pancreatic amylase continues to split apart starch and other carbohydrates. The process of protein digestion is continued through the release of precursor enzymes known as trypsinogen and chymotrypsinogen, which end up being fully activated to trypsin and chymotrypsin. Like other parts of the gut, your small intestine relies on peristalsis to keep chyme and these digestive juices moving forward.

Apart from your pancreas, your liver also plays an instrumental role in the digestion that occurs in your small intestine. Bile is produced in your liver, temporarily stored in your gall bladder, and ultimately released into your small intestine lumen. It acts to emulsify globs of fat, downsizing them into smaller fat droplets. Emulsification of

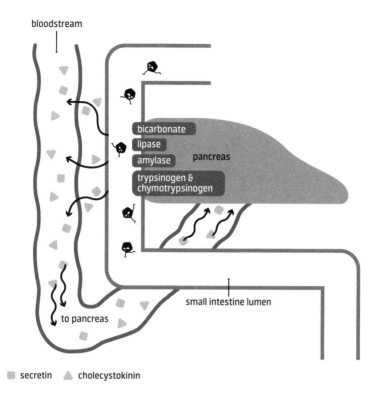

figure 1.5. **DIGESTION IN THE SMALL INTESTINE**

The entry of chyme into the small intestine triggers the secretion of hormones (secretin and cholecystokinin) from specialized gut cells. These hormones travel to the pancreas via the bloodstream and cause pancreatic juices (water, enzymes, and bicarbonate) to be dumped into the small intestine lumen.

fat is necessary because pancreatic lipase is water-soluble, meaning it can't effectively penetrate large globs of fat to do its job. Thus, transforming these fat globs into smaller droplets dramatically increases the area where lipases can work.

In addition to serving as a location for digestion, your small intestine is the alimentary canal's most important site of absorption. Over the course of adulthood (say, from 18 to 80 years of age), people in industrialized societies can consume the equivalent of a female rhinoceros's mass worth of protein, a male hippo's mass worth of fat, an elephant's mass worth of carbohydrate, and 15,000 to 20,000 gallons of water. Even more astonishing are the consumption totals of serious athletes; a runner who trains heavily and runs marathons for 30-plus years might consume a triceratops's mass worth of carbohydrate and 25,000 to 30,000 gallons of water over their adult life. The vast majority of these ingested nutrients get absorbed somewhere in your small bowel. If you need further proof of its importance, keep in mind that surgical removal of large sections of the small intestine leads to severe health consequences in comparison to when other parts of the gut are excised.[18] To return to pop culture analogies, if the pancreas is the Michael Caine of the gut, then the small intestine is the Meryl Streep—always doing vital work. (As of 2020, Streep had received a staggering 21 Oscar nominations.)

Your small intestine's immense capacity for absorption is a product of its anatomy. On a gross level, it has numerous circular folds that increase the area where absorption occurs. If you zoomed in on these folds, you'd see that the epithelial cells lining your small intestine are arranged in such a way that they form small projections called villi. If you zoomed in even closer, you'd see tiny hairlike structures called microvilli protruding from the outer cell membrane of the epithelial cells; this membrane is often referred to as the brush border because it resembles a brush under a microscope (see Figure 1.6).

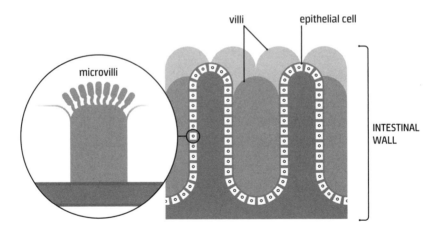

figure 1.6. **INTESTINAL VILLI AND MICROVILLI**

These finger- and hairlike projections dramatically increase the area where absorption occurs in the small intestine.

Just like how bristles of a paintbrush provide a large surface area for applying paint to a wall, the villi and microvilli increase the surface area where absorption of nutrients occurs. Although some references put the surface area of the small intestine at 100 square meters, recent estimates are closer to 30 square meters,[16] which is about the size of the standard American living room.

After your pancreatic enzymes finish attacking carbohydrates, proteins, and fats, the remaining products of digestion still need to cross the cellular barrier that protects you from the nasty outside world. Products of protein digestion—amino acids and small peptides (two to three amino acids joined together)—pass through carriers located at the brush border, and the speed by which they're absorbed depends on their structure and chemical properties. For example, branched-chain and essential amino acids (i.e., the type your body can't make) tend to be absorbed more rapidly than nonessential amino acids.

Before carbohydrates are absorbed, enzymes at your brush border must first split any remaining longer-chain molecules into short chains of glucose or individual glucose molecules. Similarly, disaccharides such as sucrose (table sugar), lactose (milk sugar), and maltose (two glucoses bound together) are enzymatically split into single sugar molecules. The resulting single sugar molecules (glucose, fructose, galactose) are absorbed into your intestinal cells through protein-based transporters, the two most important being SGLT1 and GLUT5. These specific transporters are discussed more in Chapter 4, as they have important implications for how much carbohydrate you can tolerably ingest during exercise. Figure 1.7 presents a simplified overview of carbohydrate digestion.

In contrast to the absorption of carbohydrates and amino acids, fat absorption occurs mostly through simple diffusion. Small emulsified fat droplets made of fatty acids and monoglycerides are carried to the brush border, where they diffuse across the cell membrane, which is fat-soluble itself. Once inside your intestinal cells, fatty acids and monoglycerides get repackaged into triglycerides, and these triglycerides combine with other fat-soluble substances (e.g., cholesterol, fat-soluble vitamins) to form chylomicrons, which are conglomerations of protein, cholesterol, triglycerides, and phospholipids. Chylomicrons are then dumped out of your intestinal cells into your lymphatic system and join up with blood circulating in your chest.

17

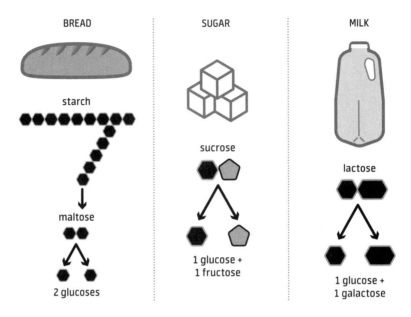

figure 1.7. **CARBOHYDRATE DIGESTION**

In order to absorb carbohydrate, your body must break down chains of carbohydrate into single sugar molecules.

Vitamins and minerals are also readily absorbed in your small intestine, mostly via specialized carriers or transport systems. Your entire small bowel is capable of absorbing vitamins and minerals, but the highest rates of absorption occur in your duodenum and the first half of your jejunum. One notable exception is vitamin B_{12}, which is primarily absorbed near the very end of your small intestine, in your distal ileum.[19]

A final essential nutrient that's absorbed in your small intestine is water. Most couch potatoes living in temperate environments need to consume 2–3 liters of fluid per day to balance water losses from pooping, peeing, and sweating. In contrast, an athlete exercising for multiple hours in sweltering conditions may need to consume two to three times that amount to compensate for sweat loss. Clearly, your gut is part and parcel of maintaining hydration because of its role in absorbing water from the fluids and foods you eat. However, the volume of water you consume doesn't actually represent the total water absorption load of your gut because you also secrete approximately 7 liters—or

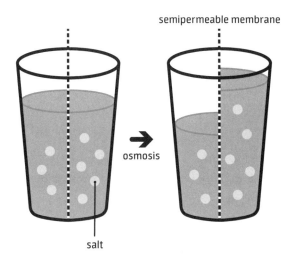

semipermeable membrane

osmosis

salt

figure 1.8. **OSMOSIS**

19

Fluid movement in and out of the gut is largely driven by the concentrations of solutes (sodium, sugar, etc.) in the lumen and in the body.

almost an entire case of beer's worth—of fluid into your lumen each day. This fluid secretion occurs for digestive purposes (e.g., release of gastric and pancreatic juices) as well as to reduce the osmolality of any highly concentrated fluids that enter your intestines (as will be explained shortly). Instead of letting this secreted fluid pass through you as watery stool, your gut reabsorbs more than 95 percent of it—at least when it's functioning normally. This recycling system is a favorable adaptation that dramatically reduces the amount of water you need to consume on a daily basis.

The bulk of water absorption—perhaps up to 80 percent—takes place in your small intestine[20] and occurs via osmosis. If you slept through most of your science schooling as a youth, let me remind you how osmosis works. Osmosis means that water movement is based on the concentration of molecules on each side of a semipermeable membrane. Water passes from the side with a lower concentration to the side with a higher concentration of molecules, ultimately leading to an equilibration on both sides. (The technical jargon used to describe the concentration of molecules in a fluid is osmolality.) A simple experiment you can do to illustrate how osmosis works is to place two slices of a potato into separate dishes that contain different solutions: one with tap water and one with saltwater. After several hours, the slice in the saltwater should weigh less because water from the potato has moved into the saltwater solution. If you're not a fan of home-based potato experiments, you can refer to Figure 1.8, which illustrates the process of osmosis.

What, you might be justifiably wondering, is the practical value of knowing this information? Ultimately, it means that chugging a beverage loaded with carbohydrate and/ or electrolytes will cause a net movement of water from your blood into your small intestine lumen, which is the opposite direction of what you want when exercising. Beverages with osmolalities that are higher than your blood plasma are said to be *hypertonic*, and examples of these sorts of libations include apple juice, soft drinks, and pickle juice. With that in mind, avoiding extremely hypertonic beverages is a prudent choice when you want to optimize the *speed* of fluid absorption in your small intestine, as these hypertonic drinks cause an initial net movement of water into your small intestinal lumen and delay water absorption (see Figure 1.9).

It's worth noting that beverage osmolality is most important to consider *during exercise*, as this is when the speed of hydration is critical. In other situations (throughout the day), there's less need to worry about beverage osmolality because most of the water secreted into the first part of your small intestine eventually gets reabsorbed farther down in the intestinal tract.

If extremely hypertonic beverages aren't the speediest hydration choice during exercise, then consuming *hypotonic* beverages (i.e., those well below the osmolality of blood plasma) like plain water must be, right? Although hypotonic beverages create a large osmotic gradient that drives water absorption, there's actually an advantage to choosing a beverage with a bit more sodium and carbohydrate in it. For example, drinks that contain 10–25 grams of glucose and 1,000 milligrams of sodium per liter are slightly hypotonic (which creates an osmotic drive for water absorption), and as an added benefit, additional water is dragged along for the ride as the sodium and sugar in these beverages get absorbed. Unfortunately, plain water doesn't benefit from this cotransport of water from sodium and glucose absorption, which is precisely why modern-day therapeutic rehydration solutions (e.g., Pedialyte, Hydralyte, Dioralyte) contain modest amounts of carbohydrate and sodium and are often formulated to have an osmolality that's slightly below or right around blood levels.[21]

One thing to keep in mind is that, in contrast to these therapeutic rehydration solutions, sports beverages like Gatorade and Powerade are mildly hypertonic because they contain extra sugar (50–70 grams per liter) for fueling purposes. Even though fluid

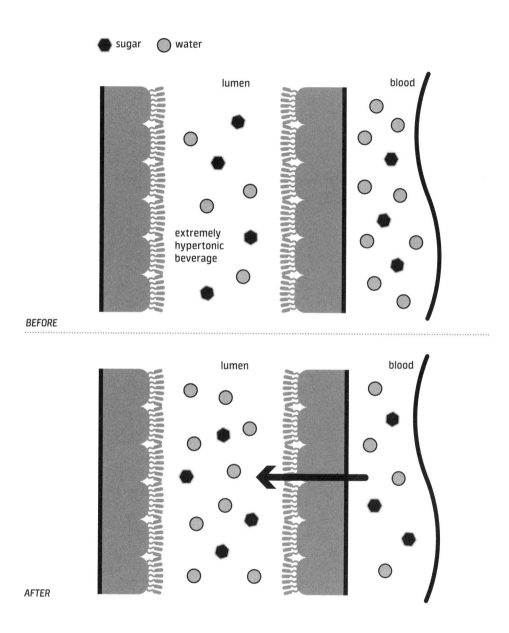

figure 1.9. **EFFECTS OF BEVERAGE OSMOLALITY ON FLUID MOVEMENT IN THE INTESTINES**

A hypertonic beverage can cause fluid to move from your blood to your gut lumen, slowing the overall process of fluid absorption.

absorption may be optimal with carbohydrate concentrations of 10–25 grams per liter, it turns out that carbohydrate absorption and delivery to the muscle is increased at higher concentrations. In essence, sports beverages were designed to find the right balance between fluid and fuel delivery during prolonged exercise.

If all of this sounds a bit convoluted, it's because the dynamics of fluid absorption are fairly complicated. In the end, one simple message you can take from all of this information is that, when you want to prioritize the speed of fluid absorption, beverages with osmolalities on the extreme ends of the spectrum (especially on the high end) are not the quickest to be absorbed. As with many things in life, the Goldilocks principle applies well to the concept of osmolality and fluid absorption.

Almost all of the nutrients absorbed in your small intestine pass into your capillary blood and are transported to your liver. (Long-chain fats are an exception because they must first enter your lymphatic system due to their insolubility in water.) Once in your bloodstream, these nutrients are channeled through various veins that merge to form your portal vein, which ultimately leads to your liver. This gives your liver, the body's chemical processing plant, a first shot at metabolizing most nutrients, and it takes full advantage by extracting significant quantities of sugars, amino acids, and other nutrients. I like to think of the liver as the Paul Giamatti of the gut, a strong character actor who takes on a diverse set of roles. Whatever isn't extracted by your Paul Giamatti (er, I mean liver) travels to other organs, such as your skeletal muscles, heart, and brain, where it can be used for the production of energy or other critical processes. As its journey through your small intestine ends, any unabsorbed chyme ends up at your ileocecal valve, a sphincter controlling passage into the shorter but wider segment of your bowels, the large intestine.

THE LARGE INTESTINE

The 0.5 to 2.5 liters of chyme reaching your large intestine each day is a mixture of undi-gested food residue, fiber, water, and electrolytes, and your 5-foot-long large intestine (also referred to as your colon) is responsible for downsizing that to 100 to 200 grams of stool,[22] or, as it's known in more colloquial language, poo. While 200 grams is on the high end of the daily poo production spectrum for Westerners, daily stool output is up to two times as much in some parts of the world.[23] The differences in production, as you might expect, are primarily due to variances in the intake of fiber, a type of non-digestible carbohydrate.[24]

The primary method your large intestine relies on to turn chyme into fully formed fecal matter is the absorption of water and electrolytes. Although your small intestine is responsible for the lion's share of water absorption, your large bowel is also an important player in this process and ultimately absorbs 90 percent of the fluid that passes into it.[25] Like its smaller sibling, your large intestine absorbs water via osmosis. However, this big brother differs from the small intestine in a couple of ways: (1) the movement of chyme (or stool) is slower, and (2) it consists of saclike pouches that facilitate the absorption of water. Both features allow your large bowel to efficiently absorb water and make poo.

Apart from serving as a crap factory, your colon is home to an almost countless number of microscopic critters, especially bacteria. Your large intestine is essentially the jungle of your gut—everything grows there. In stark contrast, your stomach and small intestine are unwelcoming homes for the microorganisms present in the foods and beverages you eat. If your colon is a jungle, then the environment of your stomach is akin to the hostile conditions of a desert. "Growing conditions" are marginally better in your small intestine, but it's still hard for most microorganisms to thrive there. The reason for this desertlike environment is that gastric acid, bile, and pancreatic secretions all function as antimicrobial agents. On top of that, food passes through these segments relatively expeditiously, limiting the amount of time available for microbes to take up residence there.

To put hard estimates on it, there are perhaps 40 trillion bacterial cells in the average man's colon, vastly outnumbering the few million residing in said average man's stomach.[26] Even if you assume that some people have only half as many bacteria in their large intestine, their colonic bacteria will still far outnumber the bacteria living in any other part of their gut. Because there are so many bacteria in your colon, it means you have at least as many bacterial cells in your body as you have of your own cells. However, because microbial cells are only a fraction of the size of animal cells, the bacteria within the average human weigh only about half a pound despite their enormous numbers. (A commonly cited number is closer to 3 pounds, but that's likely an overestimate.) These gut microorganisms—along with their genes and the metabolites they produce—are referred to collectively as the gut microbiome.

23

As recently as a few decades ago, most people—among the public, anyway—believed that nearly all bacteria were detrimental to health. However, there's been a growing awareness that some of these microbugs keep our bodies in tip-top condition. In terms of the digestive process, colonic bacteria play an important role in breaking down foodstuffs that are otherwise indigestible by humans. Ultimately, foodstuffs that are invulnerable to your body's attempts at digestion go unabsorbed in the small intestine and pass into the colon. At that point, certain species of bacteria metabolize some of these unabsorbed nutrients, the most prominent being fibers and other poorly digested carbohydrates.[27] The end products of this metabolism of carbohydrates are gases (hydrogen, carbon dioxide, methane) and short-chain fatty acids (acetate, propionate, butyrate).

Interestingly, some of these short-chain fatty acids are absorbed in your gut and serve as fuel for your intestinal cells. There's also mounting evidence that the types and amounts of short-chain fatty acids produced in the bowel are linked to health conditions such as obesity, celiac disease, colorectal cancer, and even brain disorders.[28, 29] Specific to athletes, recent research suggests that exercise training may increase butyrate-producing bacteria,[30] which are thought to promote gut health.

THE RECTUM AND ANUS

Technically, your rectum and anus are part of your large intestine, but they have functions that make them unique and noteworthy parts of your gut. Your rectum makes up the final inches of your colon, and its main function is to receive and briefly store stool before it exits your body forever. In contrast to the twisted nature of the rest of your intestines, your rectum is straight, which makes sense when you learn the word comes from the Latin *intestinum rectum* ("straight intestine").

As stool or gas enters your rectum, receptors that are responsive to stretching get activated, and this sends signals to your brain that are ultimately interpreted as discomfort, an urge to defecate, or a need to let one rip. Nerve endings in your rectum and anus allow you to distinguish between solids, liquids, and gases, ensuring that you don't soil your trousers when you simply intend to pass a little flatus. When you finally decide that it's time to break wind (hopefully not in a crowded elevator) or do your duty, the opening of your anus allows stool and flatus to exit your body. The opening and closing of your anus is controlled by your anal sphincters, which, as a reminder, are rings of muscle that constrict and relax to control the flow substances (boluses, chyme, stool) between sections of your gut.[31] You have internal anal sphincters that are controlled involuntarily by your autonomic nervous system, as well as external anal sphincters that are, to a large extent, under conscious control. Damage to the nerves that connect and communicate with these sphincters can lead to an inability to control one's bowels.

25

THE ENTERIC NERVOUS SYSTEM

Your gut has a seemingly impossible job. Each day you consume several pounds of food containing an almost incalculable assortment of nutrients, nonnutrient molecules, and microorganisms—and if you trust a recent report, also thousands of bug bits from mealworms, maggots, roaches, and the like.[32] Not only is your gut responsible for identifying, digesting, and absorbing the nutrients you need to survive, but it's also tasked with protecting your body from toxins and from being infected by the trillions of microorganisms that live in and pass through it day after day. The mucosal lining of your gut is the largest surface of your body exposed to the outside world, with an area that's many times greater than your skin.[33] The job of your gut is analogous to defending the Great Wall of China from hostile invaders while also allowing the flow of goods required to sustain an immense dynasty. This is no easy task.

Given the complex interface between your gut and the outside world, it shouldn't be overly surprising to learn that your gut is home to one of the largest networks of nerve cells in your body. Although estimates vary, your gut houses somewhere between 100 million and 600 million neurons,[33, 34] roughly equivalent to what you'd find in the brain of your pet dog or cat.[35] Practically the entire length of your gut's walls—from mouth to anus—is embedded with neurons, and this network of neurons is so vast that it's often referred to as the body's second brain (it's also commonly called the enteric nervous system). This second brain is officially part of your autonomic nervous system, the branch of your peripheral nervous system that acts primarily on an unconscious level.

There are a couple of important things to know about how your second brain works. First, many of the actions your gut takes are controlled reflexively without instruction from your central nervous system (i.e., your brain and spinal cord).[36] Other bodily reflexes—such as the muscle stretch reflex that your doctor tests by tapping below your kneecap—require signals to be sent to your spinal cord or brain before an appropriate action is taken. In contrast, sensory neurons within your gut are able to detect mechanical or chemical stimuli and reflexively cause an action—smooth muscle contraction, changes in blood flow, secretion of a substance—without ever communicating with your spinal cord or brain.

One prominent example of this type of intrinsic reflex is the control of peristalsis, the wavelike motion that propels boluses through your gut. Peristalsis begins with the stimulation of sensory neurons embedded in your gut, and this stimulation can occur through physical distension or through changes in the chemical environment of the lumen. These sensory neurons then communicate with motor (action) neurons housed entirely within your gut's walls, causing smooth muscle to contract above and relax below a food bolus. This reflex was documented well over a century ago in experiments conducted by British physiologists William Bayliss and Ernest Starling, who showed that elevating pressure within the lumen of a dog's intestine caused reproducible peristaltic contractions even when connections to nerves outside of the gut were severed.[37] This isn't to say that peristaltic movements are free of influence from extrinsic nerve activity (e.g., from the vagal nerve), as research has shown dual regulation through intrinsic and extrinsic nervous system control. Regardless, it's clear that many of your gut's actions aren't wholly dependent on input from your central nervous system.[22] So while your gut can't learn a language or write poetry, it does seem to have a mind—albeit a primitive one—of its own.

Another interesting fact about your second brain is that it sends more signals to your central nervous system than it receives. Your brain and spinal cord are usually thought of as the command centers that run your entire nervous system, hence most of us assume that the flow of information tends to move in a downstream manner from the brain and spinal cord to the gut. On the contrary, much of this communication occurs in a bottom-up fashion, with up to 90 percent of the fibers in your vagal nerve sending information from your gut to your central nervous system.[38] These messages include information about the overall activity of the gut and the presence of certain microbes, immune components, and chemicals, which may help the body respond to changes in the environment.

Intriguingly, studies in animals and humans show that these upstream messages impact mood and emotions.[39, 40] In one innovative study, volunteers underwent several brain scans while being given either fatty acids or a placebo made of saline.[40] Instead of having participants consume the treatments orally, the investigators shrewdly chose to infuse them directly into the participants' stomachs so that they were unaware of what they were being given. This ensured that participants' responses were due to gut-to-brain signaling and not from the taste, smell, or visual properties of the treatments. A few minutes after the investigators began infusing the treatments, they attempted to induce a sense of melancholy in the participants by showing them sad facial expressions and playing sad classical music. (If I had designed this study, I would have made them stare at photos of Kit Harington from *Game of Thrones*, who seems to always have resting sad face.) The study ultimately revealed that reductions in mood were less pronounced with fatty acid infusion, and these effects also showed up as blood flow changes in regions of the brain involved in mood regulation.

The take-home message of this research is that the composition of what a person eats can impact their mood and emotions, and these changes may be mediated by upstream messages traveling from the gut to the brain. While much is still to be learned about the interconnections between the gut, brain, and mood, it's obvious that these links are bidirectional (both upstream and downstream) and that they are likely to have implications for our health and physical function.

27

SUMMARY

GUT ANATOMY AND PHYSIOLOGY

From start to finish, your **alimentary canal** consists of your mouth, esophagus, stomach, small intestine (duodenum, jejunum, ileum), and large intestine (colon, rectum, anus).

Other important digestive organs include your salivary glands, pancreas, gallbladder, and liver.

Sphincters act as your gut's security gates, regulating the flow of boluses, chyme, and stool from one section to another.

Your **esophagus** serves primarily as a transport tube between your mouth and stomach.

Your **stomach** relies on mechanical (churning and peristalsis) and chemical (release of hydrochloric acid and enzymes) processes to digest macronutrients, particularly protein.

Your **pyloric sphincter** regulates the flow of nutrients into your small intestine by opening and closing, a process that's influenced by the specific nutrients coming into contact with sensory tissue in your duodenum.

Your **small intestine** is the main site of absorption in your gut, thanks to circular folds, small fingerlike projections called villi, and tiny hairlike structures known as microvilli, which create a massive surface area.

Your **large intestine** is responsible for absorbing water and electrolytes that escape your small intestine, resulting in the formation of stool.

Your large intestine is home to trillions of **microorganisms** that affect your gut's function and your health, in part via the metabolism of fiber and other poorly absorbed carbohydrates.

Your gut is home to your **second brain**, a network of 100 million to 600 million neurons that is integral to your gut's functions and which plays a role in regulating your mood.

02

THE ORIGINS OF GUT SYMPTOMS

Several years ago I was interviewed for an ultrarunning podcast, aptly titled *Science of Ultra*, and was asked a straightforward but astute question about the origins of gut symptoms. The host, Shawn Bearden, a professor of physiology at Idaho State University, queried, "Do we know, and if so, where GI [gastrointestinal] distress is coming from?" While this may seem like a softball question, the diverse collection of peptic problems experienced by athletes makes it remarkably challenging to answer. As a parallel example, try imagining how an oncologist might explain the cause of cancer, which isn't a single disease but a collection of more than a hundred diseases. Although all cancers are characterized by out-of-control cellular growth, they can be quite different in terms of their underlying causes and pathophysiologies. Similarly, although all forms of gut distress cause discomfort from physiological changes in the digestive tract (or in the brain), each has a unique mechanism (or mechanisms) responsible for its manifestation.

In this chapter, I describe the gut symptoms that routinely afflict athletes before, during, and after exercise; explain the mechanisms behind their appearance; and discuss strategies to prevent and manage each symptom. Finally, I also address other factors known to modify the risk or severity of these symptoms.

NAUSEA AND VOMITING

It was 1996, and medical student Bob Kempainen was running the marathon at the Olympic Trials in Charlotte, North Carolina. Kempainen was already a well-respected runner, having represented the United States at the 1992 Olympic Games in Barcelona, where he finished 17th. On this cool February day, Kempainen was leading the race by a few seconds with about 2 miles to go, when all of a sudden he projectile vomited midstride. Most TV viewers probably expected Kempainen to stop running, but he only briefly slowed and swayed before righting himself and accelerating back to full speed. Perhaps it was the $100,000 paycheck and a ticket to the Olympic Games in Atlanta that pushed Kempainen to continue in spite of his stomach troubles. Amazingly, he managed to win the race in 2:12:45 despite spewing several more times over the final miles. Footage of Kempainen's tenacious effort even showed up in a Nike Air commercial set (very effectively, I might add) to Johnny Cash's cover of the song "Hurt."

Like Kempainen, at some point we've all experienced the irrepressible urge to spew up a food and return it ingloriously to the world. Maybe it was from drinking too much cheap beer (Natty Light, anyone?), from catching a stomach bug, or from taking a boat ride in turbulent waters. (The word *nausea* comes from *nausia* or *nautia*, which in Greek originally meant "seasickness."[1]) Regardless of the causes, all people experience nausea the same way—a feeling of sickness in the stomach marked by an urge to barf.

It's difficult to generalize about how often athletes experience nausea, largely because it varies with the intensity, duration, and mode of exercise, but it definitely isn't the most prevalent digestive trouble. Nevertheless, it's one of the most significant in terms of its capacity to mar an athlete's performance. In a survey of 500 competitors from the Western States Endurance Run and the Vermont 100 ultramarathon, nausea and/or vomiting was experienced by almost 4 of every 10 runners and was the leading reason for quitting the races prematurely (23 percent), far outpacing other causes such as inadequate heat acclimatization (7.2 percent), muscle cramping (5 percent), and exhaustion (3.6 percent).[2]

While 100-mile races are on the extreme end of the spectrum of endurance events, other studies document that nausea also occurs during shorter competitions. In a small survey of runners, 11 percent reported at least some nausea during a marathon, and an identical prevalence was found among 25-kilometer racers.[3] A similar estimate was obtained from a survey of 707 runners, with 12 percent saying they felt nauseated during or after hard training runs and races, which was approximately six times more frequent than with easy runs.[4] In my own research, 21 percent of athletes participating in a 70.3-mile triathlon reported nausea during the bicycle leg, which increased to 30 percent during the run.[5] Broadly speaking, roughly 10–40 percent of endurance athletes suffer from nausea during hard training sessions and competition, though the prevalence is probably higher among athletes exercising for extreme durations or in hot and humid weather.

31

Of all the gut symptoms you can be stricken with, nausea is the most complex in terms of its sources. Blood-borne substances (toxins, drugs, hormones), motion disturbances, stomach distension, and foul odors are just a handful of the triggers of nausea and—if you're unlucky enough—vomiting. When you do vomit, it's thought to be your body's way of ridding itself of potentially harmful substances—at least when we're talking about vomiting associated with eating or drinking. The functional purpose of vomiting in other situations (e.g., seasickness or motion sickness) is less clear, and perhaps an unfortunate by-product of how our vestibular system and brain are wired together.

Regardless of what underlies it, the sensation of nausea originates in the medulla oblongata, a part of your brain that sits just above your spinal cord. If activation of a specific region in your medulla—referred to unimaginatively as the vomiting center—is strong enough, retching is initiated via signals sent through your nervous system to your digestive tract and abdominal muscles. As former president George W. Bush might say, your vomiting center is the Decider because although it receives input from several sources (Cabinet members and the like), these signals are insufficient to initiate yacking without the actions of the Decider.[6]

One of the most important advisors to the Decider is the chemoreceptor trigger zone, also located in your medulla. Unlike most of your brain, this zone isn't fully protected by your blood-brain barrier, the semipermeable membrane that separates circulating blood from your brain. Your blood-brain barrier is critical to defending your brain against substances that could be injurious to your nervous system, and although your brain needs protection from these substances, it also needs to be capable of quickly detecting them so they can be promptly ejected from your gut via vomiting. The chemoreceptor trigger zone is just one of several advisors that helps the Decider figure out whether barfing is the best course of action; others include sensory neurons

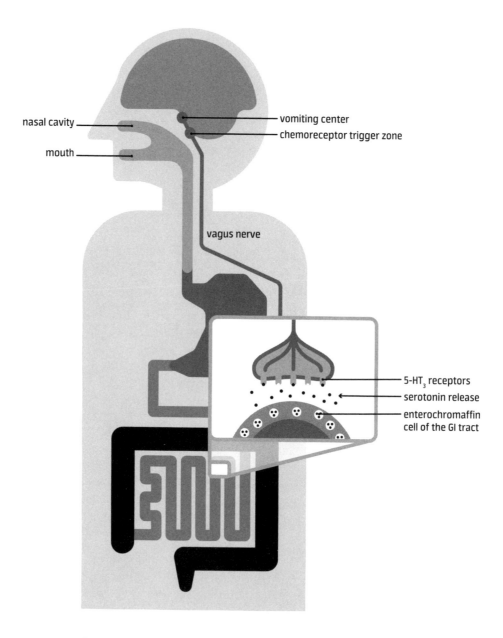

figure 2.1. **PHYSIOLOGY OF NAUSEA AND VOMITING**
···
Activation of the vomiting center in the brain (via the chemoreceptor trigger zone and peripheral sensory nerves) induces feelings of nausea and can trigger vomiting.

distributed within and outside the digestive system.[6] See Figure 2.1 for a simplified overview of the roles that these structures play in triggering nausea and vomiting.

Specific to exercise, the mechanisms responsible for activation of the vomiting center are varied. One presumable source is an abrupt surge in epinephrine and norepinephrine— otherwise known as adrenaline and noradrenaline—which are hormones that help you respond to all kinds of stressors, exercise being no exception. These stress hormones are considered catecholamines and are produced by your adrenal glands as well as by neurons in your central and peripheral nervous systems, and it's been known since the first half of the 20th century that they're released into the bloodstream during exercise.[7]

33

A key piece of evidence supporting the hypothesis that catecholamines can set off exercise-associated nausea is that both surge as exercise intensifies. Decades-old research shows that the more intense exercise is, the larger the secretion of epinephrine and norepinephrine into the blood.[8] Similarly, nausea heightens as exercise gets more intense and is particularly prevalent after sprinting or anaerobic efforts. For example, ratings of queasiness after a Wingate—a test consisting of cycling as hard as possible for 30 seconds—average about 3 on a 0-to-10 scale, though it's not unheard of for people to rate their nausea as 5 or higher.[9] Similar to high-intensity exercise, psychological stressors—going on a first date, bungee jumping, giving a big speech—give rise to catecholamine secretion and can sometimes trigger nausea. (As Garth from *Wayne's World* says when he's nervous, "I think I'm gonna hurl.")

Beyond the scientific literature, there are also numerous anecdotes of athletes puking their guts out after high-intensity exercise, especially in high-pressure settings. The combination of pre-competition anxiety, along with an abrupt surge in adrenaline at the onset of exercise, is a perfect recipe for eliciting nausea and vomiting, and the following examples remind us that, although they may have superhuman speed or supreme endurance, even the world's best athletes are susceptible to the puke-inducing effects of intense exercise:

⊙ Wayde van Niekerk, current world-record holder in the 400-meter sprint, has said that he throws up after nearly every 400-meter race, which is the main reason he has a surprising love-hate relationship with the event.[10]

⊙ British runner and four-time Olympic gold medalist Mo Farah tossed his cookies after setting the 2-mile indoor world record (8:03:04 minutes).[11]

⊙ Early in his career, American miler and running legend Jim Ryun violently vomited after many of his races.[12]

⊙ During the 2016 Olympics in Rio de Janeiro, American swimmer Katie Ledecky squeaked out a victory in the 200-meter freestyle but revealed after the race that she nearly vomited in the pool, saying, "That was a really tough race. . . . the closest I've come to throwing up."[13]

⊙ Though not during a race, the world's fastest human, Usain Bolt, posted a video of himself yacking after a grueling workout in 2014.[14]

The catecholamine-nausea hypothesis is further bolstered by studies of altitude sickness, a cluster of symptoms that develops at high elevations, particularly over 10,000 feet. Nausea and vomiting—among other symptoms such as shortness of breath, headaches, and fatigue—often plague people at high altitude. The thin air causes hypoxia (a deficiency of oxygen), and to compensate, your body dials up sympathetic nervous system activity and catecholamine secretion, increasing your heart rate and the total amount of blood that's pumped from your heart. Some data suggest this surge in sympathetic activity is partly responsible for altitude sickness,[15] though it's hard to rule out other causes of nausea in these situations, including cerebral edema, cerebral blood flow changes, and headache-induced nausea.[16, 17]

One of the earliest written accounts of nausea and vomiting stemming from altitude sickness comes from José de Acosta, a Jesuit theologian and missionary who traveled to the New World in the 16th century. In 1572, Acosta and his fellow travelers crossed several mountain passes in the Andes, including one near the 18,865-foot mountain Pariacaca. In the third volume of his *Natural and Moral History of the Indies* (translated into English by Edward Grimston), Acosta provides one of the most vivid accounts of nausea and vomiting I've come across:

> ❝ *When I came to mount the stairs, as they call them, which is the top of the mountaine, I was suddenly surprised with so mortall and strange a pang that I was ready to fall from my beast to the ground; and although we were many in company, yet every one made haste (without tarrying for his companion) to free himselfe speedily from this ill passage. Being then alone with one Indian, whom I intreated to keep me on my beast, I was surprised with such pangs of straining and casting as I thought to cast up my soul too; for having cast up meate, fleugme, and choler, both yellow and greene, in the end I cast up blood with the straining of my stomacke.*[18]

Straining and *casting* are old-timey ways of saying that Acosta did the technicolor yawn; his case of vomiting was so severe that he spewed up bile and blood and for a brief time even believed he might perish on the mountain.

Clearly, the links between catecholamine secretion, intense exercise, altitude exposure, and nausea provide indirect evidence that catecholamines can induce queasiness. To truly verify the role of these hormones in provoking nausea, it would be ideal to directly administer them to people. Because epinephrine is the first-line treatment for anaphylactic reactions and is also sometimes used to enhance pain relief in medical situations, this type of data actually exists. Trials administering epinephrine for these and other reasons, although not 100 percent consistent, often report nausea as a side effect.[19-21] In a similar way, individuals with tumors (known as pheochromocytomas and paragangliomas) that cause hypersecretion of catecholamines are often racked by nausea, and, amazingly, one study found that removing these growths led to the disappearance of exercise-associated nausea and vomiting in a small group of patients.[22]

Outside of catecholamine secretion, another source of nausea that many athletes have firsthand experience with is ingesting too much food before or during exercise. In these situations, nausea is the product of stomach distension and mechanical jostling, which tends to be most prominent during running. Beyond sheer volume, the types of victuals you ingest also modify this effect, as any foodstuff that delays stomach emptying can trigger nausea during exercise (e.g., hypertonic carbohydrate beverages, solid protein-rich foods, foods loaded with fiber, or fatty foods).

In my own experience, I once had a cheeseburger and large soda an hour or so before a high school cross-country race, and as I came to discover shortly thereafter, gobbling a fatty slab of meat and washing it down with a hypertonic carbohydrate beverage is a fantastic way of inducing nausea during a 5-kilometer race. This is the same lesson that 14-time Grand Slam winner Pete Sampras learned when he drank a can of soda during the fourth set of his quarterfinals match at the 1996 US Open. And it's also the lesson that Steve Carrell's bumbling but loveable character from *The Office*, Michael Scott, learned when he ate an entire plate of fettuccini alfredo just before Michael Scott's Dunder Mifflin Scranton Meredith Palmer Memorial Celebrity Rabies Awareness Pro-Am Fun Run Race for the Cure. (If you have no idea what I'm talking about, it's time for you to binge-watch *The Office*.) If you prefer science to anecdotes, consider that one study found that consuming a 12 percent carbohydrate beverage caused more queasiness than a 6 percent carbohydrate beverage during prolonged cycling in the heat.[23]

While excessive intake of any of the macronutrients can provoke nausea, fat is perhaps the most culpable of the three. This is because the products of fat digestion (i.e., free fatty acids) strongly activate receptors in your small intestine that induce sensations of fullness.[24] On a mechanistic level, activating these receptors releases cholecystokinin into your blood, a hormone that works on your brain to elicit feelings of fullness and sometimes even nausea.[25] Further proof of these effects comes from experiments showing that both cholecystokinin release and perceptions of nausea are largely prevented if the normal splitting of fat molecules in your gut is blocked.[26]

Although other nutrients can initiate the release of cholecystokinin (especially amino acids from protein digestion), the king of this effect is the free fatty acid,[27] and these effects have implications for you as an athlete. When cholecystokinin is released after a fatty meal, it slows emptying of chyme from your stomach, which is usually an undesirable response just before or during exercise. This is a particularly unwelcome response when you're planning to ingest substantial amounts of food and fluid during exercise. Clearly, you want that sports beverage—or any other nutrient you ingest during exercise—to rapidly empty from your stomach so it can be absorbed and utilized to sustain physical work. This effect of fat on stomach emptying is a major reason most sports dietitians recommend curbing fat consumption immediately before and during exercise.

THE ORIGINS OF GUT SYMPTOMS

While avoiding copious quantities of dietary fat before exercise is a simple way to prevent nausea, other insidious forms of this troubling symptom can be more challenging to thwart. One of these insidious versions of nausea is the variety that befalls athletes during extremely prolonged exercise. Indeed, nearly every serious marathoner and ultrarunner has a story of ralphing during or after a race. If you don't believe me, plant yourself at the finish line of a popular marathon and you'll likely witness this happening to several racers, and perhaps even to the winner. In 2011, Emmanuel Mutai set a course record (2:04:40) at the London Marathon and puked seconds after finishing. More recently, Galen Rupp ran a 2:06:07 at the 2018 Prague Marathon and immediately hurled after crossing the finish line.

It's especially challenging to study the origins of nausea at these lengthy distances because, as you might expect, it can be hard to find sufficient numbers of people willing to exercise in a lab at race pace for hours on end. Still, we do have a few ideas about what causes nausea during prolonged exercise, the first of which is that blood flow to the gut progressively declines as exercise duration increases. In one investigation that had cyclists ride at 70 percent of their maximal aerobic capacity for 60 minutes, blood flow in the portal vein, which carries blood from the intestinal tract to the liver, was reduced by about 20 percent after 10 minutes, continued to decline by about 50 percent after 20 minutes, and finished 80 percent below baseline levels by the end of the 60-minute ride.[28] Less blood flow means less oxygen delivery, which can impair the internal machinery of your gut's cells. Dehydration from heavy sweating exacerbates this problem simply because there's less blood to go around; indeed, several experiments have documented a higher incidence and/or severity of nausea when individuals exercise in a dehydrated state.[29-31] Similarly, exercising in the heat makes nausea more likely because heavier sweating accelerates losses of body water and blood volume.[32]

I've had my own encounter with severe nausea during prolonged activity that was likely exacerbated by dehydration and impairments in gut blood flow. When I was in high school, our father took my brother and me on a camping trip to the Beartooth Mountains in Montana. Although the first part of the trip went off without a hitch, our father started displaying signs of altitude sickness after a few days on the trail, which prompted us to terminate our excursion prematurely. Because of his symptoms, he wasn't up to carrying his 30-pound pack back to the trailhead. Being the strapping young lad that I was (or thought I was, anyway), I volunteered to make the trip twice, first carrying my pack down, then going back up for his pack. I hiked more than 20 miles that day, most of which were on anything but flat terrain. If that wasn't dehydration-inducing enough, I ran out of fluids with several miles to go. By the time I reached the trailhead for the final time, my thirst was off the charts, and I was undoubtedly in a state of major dehydration. My teenage brain's remedy for this was to chug a 16-ounce bottle of Gatorade, and much like their advertising would have you believe, it did a marvelous job of quenching my thirst. Within 30 minutes, though, a strong sensation of nausea washed over me, and just as we pulled our Chevy Suburban into the parking lot of another trailhead, I stuck my head out the window and vomited *Exorcist*-style. Obviously, my nausea could have been due to a mixture of factors (including a minor case of altitude sickness), but it seems probable that my water deficit bore some of the blame.

The exact reasons dehydration and a waning flow of blood to the gut bring about nausea are somewhat unclear, but there's one hormone that's almost certainly involved: arginine vasopressin (AVP). Like California's state regulators, this hydration-related hormone's chief job is to conserve water, which it accomplishes by telling your kidneys to reabsorb more water. AVP is secreted from your pea-sized pituitary gland (located at the base of your brain) when your blood volume declines and plasma osmolality rises. Blood levels of AVP increase during moderate-to-intense exercise, and this increase is typically larger when people exercise in a dehydrated state.[33] Consequently, we know that dehydration, AVP release, and nausea are interconnected.

As any researcher worth their salt will remind you, correlation does not equal causation. In other words, it's possible that AVP has no direct role in causing nausea and that other factors are responsible for the simultaneous surges in AVP and nausea during prolonged exercise. However, experiments directly administering AVP to humans confirm that it can make them feel nauseated, at least when it's given in large doses.[34, 35] In one of these studies, administering the drug atropine effectively prevented the nausea-inducing effects of AVP, and because atropine is thought to act on receptors within the brain stem, the researchers concluded that AVP works through the central nervous system to provoke nausea.[35]

Beyond AVP, there are other reasons dehydration and gut blood-flow impairments might make you vomit during prolonged exercise. When your intestinal cells are deprived of life-sustaining blood and oxygen, the bonds that normally keep these cells held tightly together start to loosen, allowing larger than normal molecules to seep through into your blood. While some of these molecules are harmless, they're not all benign. For example, the passage of endotoxins (fat-sugar compounds from the cell walls of bacteria) through your gut barrier can cause an inflammatory reaction in your body that may exacerbate nausea. Indeed, some studies have found correlations between blood levels of endotoxins and the development of nausea during prolonged exercise.[36, 37]

Much like the links between AVP and nausea, we can't definitively conclude that endotoxins directly cause nausea based on correlations alone. Fortunately for us, hundreds of volunteers have agreed to be injected with endotoxins over the years so that scientists can understand how the human body responds to these trespasser molecules. Enough studies have compiled data that we can say with confidence that endotoxin invasion leads to nausea in some people.[38-41] The inflammatory molecules your body produces in response to endotoxin entry may be the real underlying instigator of nausea, as opposed to the endotoxins themselves. These inflammatory molecules help you fight foreign invaders (like viruses and bacteria), but they also act on your brain and other components of your nervous system to cause symptoms like fever, fatigue, and malaise.[42] Interestingly, directly administering inflammatory molecules is sufficient to induce nausea even in the absence of infection,[43] which supports the notion that the inflammatory response to an infection—and not the infection itself—drives the development of nausea.

The final two causes of nausea worth addressing in the context of exercise both start with the prefix *hypo-* (meaning "low" or "below"). The first is hyponatremia, a disorder of low blood sodium that, in exercisers, usually stems from being overzealous with fluid intake. Given that dehydration is a known contributor to nausea, it might come as a surprise that overhydrating can produce the same symptom. To explain this conundrum, it's important to keep in mind that when an athlete's blood sodium rapidly declines due to overdrinking, their body will attempt to reestablish an equilibrium in osmolality between intracellular (inside cells) and extracellular (outside cells) compartments. The eventual result of this equilibration process is swelling in the brain, which

39

contributes to nausea as well as other symptoms like lethargy, headache, dizziness, and mental confusion.[44]

Not all cases of hyponatremia are symptomatic, but when an athlete does develop symptoms of the condition, it can be serious and even deadly in rare instances. The easiest way to ward off hyponatremia is to make sure you don't go overboard with drinking during exercise. How much is too much? Well, one simple rule is that you shouldn't gain weight over the course of an exercise session. If you weigh yourself before and after a 15-mile run, for example, your post-exercise weight should be no greater than your pre-exercise weight. And in actuality, you should expect to lose at least 1–2 pounds if you're running at a pretty good clip. In one highly cited study of Boston Marathon participants, hyponatremia was strongly associated with weight gain over the course of the race; the prevalence of hyponatremia was under 10 percent among runners who lost 1–2 kilograms, while roughly half of the runners who gained more than 2 kilograms developed it.[45]

The other *hypo-* cause of nausea is hypoglycemia (low blood sugar), often defined as a blood glucose of less than 50–70 milligrams per deciliter. Because glucose serves as the most important fuel for brain cells, your body works extra hard to stabilize blood glucose levels within a narrow range. While several organs work as a team to ensure relatively consistent blood glucose levels, your liver is critical to this process for two reasons: (1) it serves as a storage depot for glucose, and (2) it's capable of making its own glucose through a process called gluconeogenesis. During prolonged exercise, stores of carbohydrate in your liver gradually fall due to the demand created by your muscles, and while your body can compensate by ramping up gluconeogenesis, your liver's glucose-producing capacity isn't without limits. If you work out long enough at moderate-to-high intensity, glucose release from your liver won't be able to keep pace with the rest of your body's demand for it, and if this mismatch between supply and demand persists, hypoglycemia will develop. The occurrence of hypoglycemia during exercise varies based on several factors, but it's clearly more common as exercise duration increases, especially when you train in a fasted state or without consuming carbohydrate.[46, 47]

What exactly, you might be wondering, do hypoglycemia and blood glucose regulation have to do with nausea? To that end, it's long been known that people experiencing

hypoglycemia can feel nauseated. The reason nausea sometimes accompanies hypoglycemia has to do with the body's efforts to bring blood glucose levels back to a normal
range. Because of glucose's role in brain function, your body responds aggressively to
hypoglycemia by modifying the release of several hormones. In addition to dampening
the release of insulin (which lowers blood glucose), your body dials up the release of
hormones (epinephrine and glucagon) that stimulate gluconeogenesis and the release
of glucose from your liver. Discharge of these blood glucose–raising hormones is likely
behind the nausea that accompanies hypoglycemic episodes, as well as several other
hypoglycemia symptoms (e.g., shakiness, nervousness, a pounding heart).

41

While I previously covered the evidence linking epinephrine and nausea, it should
be noted that administering glucagon to people also produces nausea,[48] so we shouldn't
assume that epinephrine is solely responsible for the queasiness that accompanies
hypoglycemia. It's exceptionally challenging to parse the mechanisms of hypoglycemia-
associated nausea during exercise, especially because levels of these hormones usually
change simultaneously. **Regardless, athletes partaking in prolonged, intense exercise
should implement strategies that delay or prevent hypoglycemia, the most important being
to start off well-fed and to consume carbohydrate during intense workouts that surpass
60–90 minutes.**

At this point, you've probably figured out that explaining the origins of exercise-
associated nausea is a complex endeavor. The truth is that we don't have all the answers
as to its causes, nor do we know how to prevent it in every situation. That being said, if
you're experiencing nausea regularly during training and competition, there are several
suspects to consider, including hormones, endotoxins, inflammatory molecules, and
poor nutritional choices prior to and during exercise. The hormones at play are released
in response to intense exercise (epinephrine), dehydration/heat stress (AVP), and hypoglycemia (epinephrine and glucagon). The latter two problems—dehydration/heat stress
and hypoglycemia—can be prevented, or at least mitigated, with appropriate nutrition,
training, and cooling interventions.

In contrast, thwarting nausea that stems from sprinting and other types of high-
intensity exercise isn't so simple. Lowering how hard you work is an obvious losing
strategy (during competition, anyway), so in reality, some amount of nausea may be

inevitable in these situations. Even so, there are a couple of strategies worth trying to minimize feelings of nausea with intense exercise, namely avoiding prolonged fasting and high-dose caffeine consumption beforehand. Both fasting and caffeine (especially at high doses) stoke the flames of catecholamine secretion,[49, 50] which we know can contribute to nausea. In fact, nausea is a well-documented side effect of high-dose caffeine ingestion,[51] and this nausea-provoking effect is more pronounced when caffeine is combined with other stimulants like ephedrine.[52, 53] Thus, taking a stimulant-laden pre-workout supplement before hitting the gym could be a formula for feeling nauseated during a tough workout, especially if you do it on an empty tank.

REFLUX, REGURGITATION, AND HEARTBURN

A fundamental function of your gut is to keep food and fecal matter moving in one general direction. Just like when nasty stuff comes up through the sink drain in your house, it's usually an ominous sign when foodstuffs reverse course in your gut. To keep things moving in a top-to-bottom fashion, your gut relies on peristalsis and the opening and closing of its sphincters. The job of your lower esophageal sphincter, for instance, is to prevent chyme as well as chemicals and enzymes in your stomach from flowing into your esophagus. In a fairly large number of people, including athletes and nonathletes, chronic dysfunction of the lower esophageal sphincter leads to repeated reflux of food and gastric secretions into the esophagus. If this reflux is accompanied by a burning sensation in the chest, the term *heartburn* is used to describe the symptomology. Regurgitation, on the other hand, describes a situation in which swallowed food makes its way back to your throat or mouth, giving you one last (unsolicited) opportunity to taste what you had for lunch.

All of us have undoubtedly dealt with reflux-related symptoms at some point, whether it was from eating too much food (think Thanksgiving dinner) or from going horizontal too soon after feasting (think eating a tub of ice cream just before bed). For a significant number of people, however, these episodes transpire all too frequently, and said unlucky individuals have what's known as gastroesophageal reflux disease (GERD). In North America, approximately 18–28 percent of people have GERD, with similar rates found in most other places around the globe.[54]

When it comes to experiencing reflux during exercise, studies show considerable variability in its prevalence, in large part because the terms *reflux*, *heartburn*, and *regurgitation* are often used interchangeably. The survey of 707 marathoners discussed earlier in the section on nausea found that 9 percent of runners felt heartburn during training runs.[4] A similar result emerged from a survey of marathoners recruited from the 1986 Belfast City Marathon, with 13 percent reporting occasional or frequent heartburn while running.[55] These estimates are oftentimes higher, though, when surveys use the terms *reflux* or *regurgitation*,[56-58] which makes sense given that not every episode of reflux is accompanied by burning.

In terms of how it does its job, your lower esophageal sphincter controls the passage of foodstuffs by opening and closing via the manipulation of muscle tone. When your lower esophageal sphincter is functioning normally, it blocks foodstuffs from entering or leaving your stomach by increasing muscle tone. Obviously, it needs to relax and open when you swallow, otherwise food would be indefinitely trapped in your esophagus. To achieve this, sensory receptors in your throat communicate with a region in your brain stem that controls swallowing reflexes, and this signal is then passed to your lower esophageal sphincter, which responds by relaxing.[59] After you swallow, your lower esophageal sphincter ceases its relaxation phase and reestablishes a level of tone that prohibits the movement of foods and fluids.

So what goes wrong with this process when you experience reflux-type symptoms? Well, it depends on the situation, but in many cases your lower esophageal sphincter spontaneously relaxes in the absence of swallowing; the technical term for this event is transient lower esophageal sphincter relaxation (TLESR). It's thought that TLESR is a venting of excess gas from your stomach when it's distended with too much food and air.[60] This distension reflexively initiates TLESR, which some scientists suggest is a way of preventing gas from accumulating in your stomach or from entering your small intestine.[61] This is also why you might have noticed that belching frequently accompanies reflux episodes.

Now that we've established some of the underlying physiology behind esophageal function (as well as dysfunction), let's turn our attention to the effects of exercise. Studies unequivocally show that reflux events are more common during heavy exercise. In one study, cyclists had contractions and pH changes in their esophagi measured while

43

they exercised under three conditions: 1 hour at 60 percent of VO₂max, 45 minutes at 75 percent of VO₂max, and 10 minutes at 90 percent of VO₂max.[62] (VO₂max is the maximal rate of oxygen consumption that one can achieve during exercise.) Upping exercise intensity, particularly to 90 percent of VO₂max, unmistakably reduced the frequency and duration of esophageal contractions and was associated with more regular acid reflux episodes as measured by an electrode. A second study published a year later by the same research group replicated these results in nonathletes.[63] It's still unclear how upping exercise intensity provokes reflux episodes, although there are several possible explanations. Reductions in gut blood flow may impair esophageal function and reduce normal peristaltic contractions. Likewise, relaxation of the lower esophageal sphincter or a heightened pressure gradient between the stomach and esophagus are plausible explanations.[64]

Mode of exercise is another important factor influencing the risk of reflux. In a study published in the *Journal of the American Medical Association,* healthy volunteers experienced more reflux episodes while running in comparison to cycling and weight lifting,[65] and the authors suggested that the jostling of running was the most likely reason for this observation. (It should also be noted that cycling in a hunched position could theoretically increase pressure inside the thoracic cavity and exacerbate reflux in some athletes.) In contrast, a different study of seasoned weight lifters, runners, and cyclists found the most reflux episodes during activity in weight lifters.[66] The discrepant findings could be because the latter study used weight lifters capable of manhandling heavier loads, whereas the former study used people with variable exercise backgrounds. Lifting a heftier load raises pressure within the thoracic cavity, which can push food back into the esophagus against the force of gravity. Increases in pressure are especially pronounced when a person performs the Valsalva maneuver (attempting to exhale against a closed airway) while lifting.[67]

Strategies for avoiding reflux during training and competition can be both nutritional and nonnutritional in nature. Regardless of the particular form, reflux episodes are common when exercise is performed within an hour or so of eating.[62, 63] So the simplest nutritional advice for preventing reflux is to steer clear of eating a full meal within one to two hours of exercising. Moreover, meals rich in fat are particularly effective at causing reflux,[68] so instead of downing a bag of potato chips and a glass of whole milk one to two hours before exercise, perhaps you should opt for modest servings of carbohydrate-rich foods.

During competition, it may be helpful to choose foods and beverages that empty rapidly from the stomach given that any clogs in the system can exacerbate reflux or heartburn.[69] Fatty and solid protein-rich foods are two obvious choices to limit, but you should also pay attention to the carbohydrate concentration of the drinks you consume. Beverages with more than a 10 percent carbohydrate concentration retard stomach emptying and cause more reflux.[70] There are several other foods and beverages (some quite tasty) that can induce or exacerbate reflux-type symptoms and may be worth avoiding prior to and during exercise:[71, 72]

45

- ⊙ Citrus fruits
- ⊙ Acidic foods like vinegar and tomatoes
- ⊙ Chocolate
- ⊙ Alcohol
- ⊙ Coffee
- ⊙ Spicy foods
- ⊙ Carbonated beverages

It's important to keep in mind that every athlete is different in terms of what foods they can tolerate, so trial and error is a critical part of any plan for managing reflux symptoms. Nonnutritional approaches to avoid or control reflux during exercise include lowering the intensity of exercise and trying medication. Much like with nausea, reducing exercise intensity isn't a winning strategy during competition, although it might be feasible during training. Drugs that suppress gastric acid secretion (ranitidine and omeprazole) reduce reflux during exercise as measured objectively through esophageal probes.[73, 74] Somewhat surprisingly, these reductions in acid reflux don't clearly translate to less subjective heartburn while exercising, which is a bit puzzling to say the least. Despite a lack of high-quality evidence in athletes, some sportspersons do obtain relief by using these acid-suppressing medications. Even though versions of these drugs are sold over the counter in the US, be sure to consult with a healthcare provider before using them. (Note: some ranitidine products have recently been recalled because they were found to contain a known carcinogen.)

One intriguing (yet unproven) strategy for reducing reflux during exercise is "zenning out," known more formally as relaxation training. People with boatloads of anxiety are prone to chronic reflux symptoms,[75] and a handful of experiments have even shown that temporarily inducing psychological stress in people with reflux disease aggravates their symptoms.[76, 77] Interestingly, the subjective reports of reflux in these experiments often occur in the absence of any actual pH changes in the esophagus, suggesting that the symptoms arise, in part, from activation of brain regions involved in the perception of gut discomfort. With that in mind, it may be possible for people with stress-induced reflux to improve their symptoms through stress-reduction interventions that aim to shift the mind's focus.

In one study from The University of Alabama, subjects experienced fewer reflux symptoms when a stressful task was followed by a 45-minute relaxation intervention, which involved diaphragmatic breathing, alternating between relaxing and tensing 16 muscle groups, and saying the word *relax* with each exhalation.[77] Notably, relaxation training decreased symptoms by about 50 percent in comparison to a control intervention that focused on educating subjects about GERD. Another study, albeit with only 19 people, showed that four weeks of training designed to change breathing from the chest to the abdomen reduced acid reflux and improved quality of life as compared to a control intervention.[78] Overall, there's considerable reason to think that pre-exercise interventions focusing on relaxation could prevent—or at least mitigate—reflux symptoms during exercise, especially in the context of stressful competition. This hypothesis is yet to be tested in athletes, though there is probably little risk to trying these interventions if you're suffering from stress-induced reflux during competition.

FULLNESS AND BLOATING

Feeling uncomfortably full during training and competition would appear to be a straightforward problem to avoid: don't overeat! As simple as it seems, you might be surprised to learn how many athletes report feeling overstuffed or bloated during exercise. In my study of 70.3-mile triathlon competitors, fullness was the most common symptom affecting the upper half of the gut, with 33 percent and 50 percent of the triathletes reporting at least some of this feeling on the bike and run legs, respectively.[5] While most of the triathletes felt only mild sensations of fullness, a small but meaningful fraction rated it as 5 or more on a 0-to-10-point scale.

Unsurprisingly, the sheer volume of what you eat has an immense impact on perceptions of fullness. As you stuff more and more food down your piehole, stretch

and tension receptors located in your stomach's walls get activated, and these receptors communicate with the brain regions—the hypothalamus, amygdala, hippocampus,
midbrain—involved in the regulation of eating behaviors.[79] In one simple study, on
separate occasions men were given different volumes (300, 450, and 600 milliliters) of
milk that contained the same amount of energy and macronutrients, and 30 minutes
after drinking said milk, they were given access to a buffet-style lunch.[80] After downing
the milk, the men rated their fullness on a 0-to-100 scale, and as you'd expect, ratings
went up with each increase in volume, from 12 to 23 to 40 out of 100. Further, in
comparison to when they consumed only 300 milliliters of milk, energy intake at the
all-you-can-eat lunch was less after the men consumed 600 milliliters.

47

Although stretch and tension receptors help explain why you feel full after gorging
on your favorite foods, a recent fascinating experiment shows that the sensory properties
(taste, smell, etc.) of a food also influence the sensation of fullness. For the trial, men
completed three sessions while their brains were probed noninvasively using functional
magnetic resonance imaging (functional MRI), a high-tech device used to assess activation in different brain regions.[79] For one session, the men had 17 ounces of water infused
through a nasal tube into their stomachs, which was meant to cause stomach distention without sensory exposure in their mouths. In another session, the same volume of
chocolate milk was used instead (which tested the effects of the nutrients in the milk
without sensory exposure in the mouth). In a third session, they drank the chocolate
milk (which tested the nutrient content and sensory effects of the milk). Remarkably,
sensations of fullness went up only when the men drank the chocolate milk, even though
each treatment used the same 17-ounce volume. And while infusing chocolate milk and
water amplified activity in several brain regions over baseline, drinking the milk induced
greater brain activation in several regions involved in sensory perception and taste processing. Ultimately, this study suggests that the sensory properties of foods, as well as
the act of eating itself, are contributors to the sensation of fullness.

Beyond the sheer volume and sensory properties of a meal, the nutrient composition of what you feed on also influences how full you feel. Dietary fat potently
stimulates cholecystokinin release into your blood, which, as a reminder, is a hormone
that provokes feelings of fullness. This is one reason to avoid loads of dietary fat during

exercise. Likewise, drinking large volumes of concentrated carbohydrate beverages also increases fullness perceptions.[23, 70] Really, though, any food or beverage that slows gastric emptying can induce a sense of fullness. **Avoiding sizeable quantities of fat, fiber, solid-protein foods, and concentrated carbohydrate beverages may prevent excessive feelings of fullness during competition and training.** (Outside of these nutrient-specific causes, dehydration and heavy exercise decrease gut blood flow, delay stomach emptying, and possibly contribute to feeling full during exercise.)

One final issue to delve into related to fullness involves a similar term: *bloating*. While the words *fullness* and *bloating* are sometimes used interchangeably, in many situations they don't represent the same phenomenon. Though it has no universally agreed-upon meaning, one common way to define *bloating* is as a feeling of distension from a buildup of gas in the gut. In other cases, though, people who say they feel bloated are trying to convey other sensations: a full belly, abdominal pressure, nausea, needing to pass a BM, or cramping.[81]

For the sake of simplicity, let's assume that bloating is a feeling of distension resulting from a buildup of gas. Based on that definition, there are a number of foods that you may want to avoid in proximity to exercise. Gas-forming foodstuffs tend to be rich in fiber and other carbohydrates that are fermented by bacteria inhabiting your bowels. End-products of this fermentation include gases, which, if produced in excess, can leave you feeling like a float in Macy's Thanksgiving Day Parade. A review of studies on the effectiveness of fiber for hemorrhoid relief, for example, found that bloating was one of the most frequent side effects.[82] So, if you often suffer from uncomfortable bloating during competition, you might consider reducing your fiber intake for a day or two beforehand. Interestingly, the likelihood that fiber and other carbohydrates will elicit bloating may depend on a person's sex. Food residues generally take longer to transit the colon in women,[83] which in theory could leave them more prone to bloating. Indeed, women are more likely to report bloating than men, even after accounting for symptoms related to menstruation.[84]

Aside from fiber, another dietary source of gas is carbonated beverages, which contain dissolved carbon dioxide. There's a longstanding debate as to whether carbonated beverages should be shunned during exercise. While intuitively it makes sense that carbonated beverages would cause bloating during exercise, most studies that have tested this hypothesis have found little to no support for it.[85-87] And while some non-exercise studies show carbonated drinks worsen perceptions of fullness and bloating, a minimum of about 10 ounces of fluid is needed to elicit these effects, and symptoms tend to only appear when beverages are consumed with meals.[88] This means that an athlete who is consuming a few ounces of a bubbly beverage every 15–20 minutes is unlikely to suffer from more bloating than an athlete consuming a noncarbonated beverage. That being said, belching is definitely more prevalent with carbonated beverages,[88] a fact that most of us are aware of without having to consult scientific studies.

49

Paying careful attention to foods and beverages that are associated with gas production is an obvious way to minimize the incidence or severity of bloating. On the other hand, reducing stress and anxiety is perhaps a less intuitive strategy to address bloating symptoms, but research does show that perceived levels of stress and anxiety are tied to bloating.[89] Exactly how one's psychological state can impact bloating is still up for debate, though it may be because stress and anxiety can make people hypersensitive to all sorts of discomforts and pains.

INTESTINAL CRAMPS

Among the smorgasbord of gut symptoms athletes can be hit with during competition, intestinal cramping is near the top of the list, along with the likes of nausea and diarrhea, in terms of its ability to disrupt performance. During the inaugural Tour de France in 1903, Hippolyte Aucouturier—one of the race's favorites—threw in the towel during the 467-kilometer opening stage after developing excruciating stomach cramps. Although Aucouturier recovered to win the second and third stages, he was ineligible to win the race since failing to finish any single stage would warrant a disqualification.[90] One persistent story is that Aucouturier's penchant for indulging in wine was to blame for his cramping ordeal, though his ether-sniffing habit shouldn't be ignored as a possible culprit.

In more contemporary times, elite marathoners have had important races ruined because of painful intestinal cramps. In 1988, American Joan Benoit Samuelson—the winner of the inaugural women's Olympic Marathon in 1984—began suffering from intestinal cramps at mile 14 of the New York City Marathon. The cramps, plus a collision with a boy near an aid station, wrecked Samuelson's chance at taking home the title that day.[91] In 1993, three-time former champion Ibrahim Hussein dropped out of the Boston Marathon after mile 18 because of stomach cramps, which may have been aggravated by the unusually warm April weather.[92] And just a year after setting the Boston Marathon course record of 2:03:02, Geoffrey Mutai failed to finish the 2012 edition because of cramps.[93]

The observation that intestinal cramps can kill an otherwise winning performance isn't just anecdotal. Take for example a study out of New Zealand led by professor of exercise metabolism David Rowlands.[94] The main objective of Rowlands and his colleagues was to test the performance effects of a specific glucose-fructose carbohydrate mixture (a topic discussed in Chapter 4), but they also happened to use some fancy statistics to figure out how their special mixture influenced performance. In comparison to a beverage made up entirely of glucose, the glucose-fructose mixture improved cycling performance by about 1–2 percent, and based on their statistical analysis, an abatement in abdominal cramps was one of the likely factors responsible for the improvements.

Exactly how common is it for athletes to experience intestinal cramping during training and competition? That same survey of 707 runners discussed in relation to nausea and reflux reported that 10–20 percent of runners occasionally or frequently get hit with abdominal cramping during easy runs, which nearly doubles during hard runs.[4] Almost identical findings were produced from a study of runners in the 1986 Belfast City Marathon.[55] My research on triathletes found that roughly 13 percent had occasionally experienced abdominal cramping during the previous three months of training.[58]

The list of potential causes of intestinal cramping is lengthy but includes some of the same suspects from our discussions on nausea, reflux, and fullness. Exercise-induced gut ischemia is a definite culprit, and, ultimately, anything that impedes gut blood flow has the potential to fan the flames of intestinal cramping, including intense exercise, psychological stress, and dehydration. Other than dehydration, two common nutrition-related causes of intestinal cramps are ingesting concentrated sports drinks and overconsuming carbohydrate. When concentrated sports drinks enter your duodenum, water shifts from your blood into your lumen to lower the osmolality (number of particles in a fluid) there. This shift in fluid induces sensations that your brain perceives as cramping, discomfort, or pain. Consequently, quickly slamming an entire bottle of soda or juice—which are about 10–12 percent carbohydrate by weight—isn't the shrewdest strategy during a sporting contest.

Instead, opting for a beverage that has a more modest carbohydrate concentration (4–8 percent) could prevent stomach cramps. Be cognizant, though, that even beverages containing modest concentrations of carbohydrate can induce intestinal cramping if you consume too much of them. This is similar to what happens in people with medical conditions that cause poor carbohydrate absorption. For example, someone who is lactose intolerant—meaning they have low or inadequate amounts of the enzyme lactase—is prone to intestinal cramps and other forms of abdominal discomfort when they consume more than 10 grams of lactose.[95] Similarly, a person who has trouble absorbing fructose will experience intestinal cramping when challenged with a hefty dose (25–50 grams) of this sweet sugar.[96]

All of this tells us that you should keep an eye on the amount and type of carbohydrate that you eat during exercise. For athletes exercising for one to two hours at a time, 30–45 grams of carbohydrate per hour is sufficient to avoid fatigue without overloading the gut. If you decide to push the envelope (i.e., more than 50 grams per hour), it would be wise to consume multiple sugar types (specifically, glucose and fructose) instead of a single source. That's because glucose and fructose are absorbed by different transporters in your intestine, and like a bridge or tunnel, these transporters can only handle so much traffic at one time. If you ingest either glucose or fructose too quickly, these transporters become overwhelmed, resulting in incomplete carbohydrate absorption. Using a mixture of glucose and fructose is equivalent to opening another bridge to increase the maximal flow of vehicles that can cross a river. (Further details of these transporters are covered in Chapter 4.) A simple rule of thumb is to choose a food or beverage that has a 50-50 split of glucose and fructose when you plan to consume 50 grams or more of carbohydrate per hour.

Beyond dietary choices, another source of cramping is nonsteroidal anti-inflammatory drugs (NSAIDs), a group of medications that includes aspirin, ibuprofen, and naproxen. The vast majority of Americans take these pain relievers at some point or another, and athletes are no exception. It's well documented that gut discomfort is a

51

common and expected side effect of frequent NSAID use, of which abdominal cramping is a component.[97] Both NSAID ingestion and exercise (particularly the intense variety) lead to a state of temporary gut leakiness, which means the normal barrier of your intestine performs at less than optimal levels. The combination of intense exercise and NSAID ingestion before and during competition is, for many athletes, a recipe for being stricken with intestinal cramps.

The best example of this from the scientific literature comes from a study of 3,913 participants of the 2010 marathon and half-marathon in Bonn, Germany.[98] Runners were queried as to whether they ingested pain relievers before the races as well as whether they experienced any adverse events during and afterward. While a multitude of pain-relieving medications were taken by the runners, that vast majority were NSAIDs. Strikingly, the incidence of intestinal cramps was roughly *tenfold higher* among participants taking pain relievers before the race than among those not taking them, and while these results are correlational, the effect is so large that it's improbable other factors are to blame. Taking this into account, athletes should carefully consider the pros and cons of popping NSAIDs, especially in high dosages; if evading intestinal cramping is a goal, finding an alternative to NSAIDs is a sensible approach.

SIDE STITCH

One of the most dreaded gut symptoms an athlete can experience during competition is the side stitch, or, as it's referred to in abstruse journal articles, "exercise-related transient abdominal pain (ETAP)." A side stitch, despite what its moniker suggests, can affect any part of the abdomen, though the left and right sides of the midabdominal region tend to be hot spots. Although it can be challenging to delineate a side stitch from other gut symptoms (particularly cramps), localized pain, which becomes sharp or stabbing as the discomfort increases, is what makes ETAP distinct. In fact, the pain can become so unbearable that some athletes cease exercise. In one study, 12 percent of 965 athletes from six different sports (running, cycling, swimming, aerobics, basketball, horseback riding) claimed that at some point over the past year they had been stricken with side stitching severe enough that it forced them to halt exercise.[99] If 12 percent doesn't seem remarkable, consider that an additional 72 percent reported easing up on the throttle during exercise because of side stiches, and at its most severe, the pain was rated as roughly a 5 out of 10.

Side stitching occurs in athletes of all sizes, ages, and abilities, but it tends to rear its ugly head most frequently in runners, swimmers, and horseback riders. The continuous up-and-down displacement and contorting of the torso that occurs with these activities is one putative explanation for the greater incidence of ETAP, although there are numerous others, many of which are discussed in a 2015 paper by Darren Morton, an expert on ETAP.[100] Morton outlined many of the theories on the causes of ETAP, but there is one in particular that's been gaining traction more than any other in recent years, which is that irritation of the parietal peritoneum (a membrane lining the abdominal cavity) is responsible for most cases of side stitch. This theory is supported by the following observations: (1) aggravating a section of the parietal peritoneum that adheres to the abdominal wall causes localized pain characteristic of side stitch, and (2) pain originating from the parietal peritoneum is heightened by physical movement. Perhaps most important, the parietal peritoneum lines the entire abdominal wall, which could explain why, despite being dubbed "side stitch," ETAP affects other areas of the abdomen.

The most effective means of halting ETAP—to the disappointment of most athletes— is curtailing how hard you train or by ceasing exercise until the pain remits. In 2018, two-time Olympian Des Linden was almost a minute ahead of her nearest competitor in the Rock 'n' Roll Philadelphia Half-Marathon when she abruptly stopped running for more than half a minute. Video of the incident shows Linden doing a side stretch in an attempt to alleviate the ETAP that was bothering her. In a testament to her toughness, Linden started running again as the second-place runner approached and, astonishingly, she went on to win despite dealing with persistent pain. In another example, American marathon record holder Deena Kastor has reportedly suffered from side stitches at various points throughout her career. And at the 1926 Boston Marathon, Finnish runner and defending Olympic champion Albin Stenroos surrendered the race lead to an unknown deliveryman from Canada named John C. Miles after developing a debilitating case of side stitch.[101]

Morton's review paper on ETAP listed several other strategies for preventing and mollifying ETAP, but most of these interventions remain untested in rigorous studies:[100]

53

- Avoid large volumes of food and fluid one to four hours before exercise.
- Limit the intake of hypertonic beverages.
- Improve core body strength, posture, and spinal alignment.
- Wear a supportive belt around the waist.
- Practice deep breathing.

FLATULENCE

Of all digestive symptoms, flatulence is the one that society may view most negatively, and this has been the case for millennia. To be sure, most kids learn from an early age that passing gas in public is a no-no. Children's book authors have been nobly fighting back in recent years with norm-busting reads like *Toot*, *Almost Everybody Farts*, and *The Gas We Pass*, but still, breaking wind remains a persistent social faux pas. This is despite the fact that the average person passes flatus every one to four hours[102] and that many esteemed persons throughout history, from Hippocrates to Sir Thomas More to Benjamin Franklin, have extolled the benefits of passing gas.[103] To me, the quote that best sums up the pure essence of flatulence comes by way of physician Charles David Spivak, who in 1905 poetically wrote, "Occasional puffs, buccal or rectal, audible or not, are physiological and therefore useful; though neither ornamental nor always agreeable."[104]

Flatulence is considered by most athletes to be a nuisance, and in stark contrast to nausea, cramping, and side stitches, there's little reason to think that passing gas during competition impairs performance. All the same, most of us would prefer not to leave a gaseous cloud in our wake as we dart across the track, field, or court. Despite our wishes, flatulence is one of the most prevalent bowel complaints reported by athletes. In my study of triathletes, more than 50 percent said they bottom burped occasionally, frequently, or almost always during training over the preceding three months, which was higher than any other symptom.[58] Experiments also show that mild exercise stimulates the clearance of gas from the gut, which may help explain the high prevalence of this symptom in athletes.[105, 106]

Unlike most other gut symptoms, the causes of flatulence are usually straightforward. By definition, flatulence is the expulsion of gas, or flatus (meaning "blowing" or "wind" in Latin), from the anus. As such, anything that forms or traps gas in your bowel is a possible source of flatulence. I covered a number of gas-forming foodstuffs in previous sections, so I'll spare you the rehashing of the granular details here. In brief, gas in your gut comes principally from one of three sources: (1) swallowed air, (2) carbon dioxide produced from the neutralization of stomach acid by bicarbonate, and (3) breakdown of foodstuffs by intestinal bacteria.[107] The bulk of flatus—roughly three-quarters—is made of carbon dioxide, methane, and hydrogen and is produced via bacterial fermentation. Some of these trapped gases get absorbed through your intestinal wall into your blood (particularly carbon dioxide), but the bulk exits your bottom as flatulence.

How the heck, you might be asking yourself, do we know what human flatulence is made of? It's easy enough to collect stool samples from volunteers, but alas, flatus is of a more ephemeral nature. Luckily, flatulence scientists are a clever lot, as they have had to come up with ways of collecting flatus before it escapes the gut and is on the lam forever. One way to do this is to stick rubber tubes up people's rear ends and connect said tubes to collection bags, which is precisely what one study did.[108] (If, like me, you're skeptical that this method could trap all flatus, the researchers made a point of saying they validated the technique by having two volunteers submerge their lower parts in water for an hour and watching for signs of leaking, of which there were none.) Total flatus emissions on a normal diet varied from a low of about 500 milliliters to a high of 1,500 milliliters, with the average around 700 milliliters (or about one-third of a 2-liter soda bottle's worth), and for a majority of this study's volunteers, hydrogen made up at least half of their gas.

Given that trapped gas is the root cause of flatulence, strategies for avoiding or alleviating this pesky symptom obviously involve targeting gas production. Eschewing certain fibers found in plant foods is one option, as studies have shown that ramping up fiber intake to treat constipation moderately increases flatus production.[109] In addition, the flatus collection study mentioned above found that consuming a fiber-free liquid diet caused daily flatus emissions to plummet from about 700 milliliters to 200 milliliters.[108] Dramatically cutting your fiber intake, though, could negatively impact your health in the long run, so it's a tactic you might want to implement only on a temporary basis. Likewise, limiting the intake of lactose, fructose, and short-chain carbohydrates can reduce flatulence in people who have trouble digesting and absorbing large quantities

55

of those carbohydrates, but again, this strategy may not be optimal for gut health over months and years (see the "FODMAPs" section in Chapter 4).

Even well-digested carbohydrates can increase flatus emissions if you consume loads of them. When you ingest too much carbohydrate, a small but significant fraction of the sugar molecules goes unabsorbed in your small intestine and passes into your colon, where the dense population of bacteria residing there ferments it. As it relates to exercise, the amount of carbohydrate consumed was positively correlated—albeit modestly—with flatulence severity in a study of competitors in half- and full Ironman® triathlons,[110] which supports the idea that too much carbohydrate can turn you into a flatus factory. How much carbohydrate is too much? Well, that depends on a host of factors discussed in Chapter 4, but in a nutshell, trial and error during training is critical for determining your individual response to carbohydrate ingestion. If you decide to consume carbohydrate at a high rate (greater than 50 grams per hour), try choosing foods, beverages, and supplements that contain a mixture of glucose and fructose.

Other than altering the substrate (a.k.a. food) that bacteria feed on, another logical way of altering gas production is to directly manipulate the populations of microorganisms that occupy your colon. Consuming probiotics (live microorganisms) in supplement form has been shown to influence bowel habits and gut symptoms, but specific to flatulence, there is contradictory evidence as to whether probiotics are a good idea. Unfortunately, experiments supplementing probiotics in athletes have typically neglected to report on changes in flatulence severity, so we have to rely primarily on studies of nonathletes and people with irritable bowel syndrome (IBS)—a somewhat nebulous condition marked by, among other signs and symptoms, pain, gas, and irregular bowel habits. And although some trials in IBS patients have found modest reductions in flatulence after probiotic supplementation, most have not,[111, 112] and other studies have shown that probiotics can actually make these symptoms worse in some cases.[113, 114]

These null and sometimes contradictory findings on probiotics and flatulence likely stem from the fact that dozens of different species and strains have been used in these trials. To make matters more complicated, the dosage of probiotic and background characteristics of a population (athletes versus IBS versus healthy but inactive) can also influence whether these supplements have a positive, negative, or neutral effect on symptoms like flatulence. Considering all of this, no simple message about probiotics and flatulence is currently possible, but it seems doubtful that supplementing with probiotics is going to be a highly effective strategy for reducing flatulence.

Along the same lines as with probiotics, avoiding carbonated beverages is unlikely to be a highly fruitful approach to mitigating the flow of flatus during exercise. Ultimately, most of the carbon dioxide in these beverages is belched out or absorbed through your intestinal wall.[88] Swallowed air is an unlikely cause of flatulence for the same reasons, though people with a condition called aerophagia may be an interesting (albeit rare) exception. *Aerophagia* is medical jargon for excessive air swallowing, which can cause abdominal distension, belching, and extra flatulence. Though it most frequently appears in people who have mental disabilities and in children, occasionally aerophagia ends up explaining otherwise unexplainable cases of severe flatulence. In a case study published in the *American Journal of Gastroenterology*, a 32-year-old male computer programmer was reported to cut the cheese up to 129 times per day.[115] (To give you some perspective, most people report passing gas 10 to 20 times per day.) Ultimately, he was diagnosed with excessive air swallowing after it was discovered that an unusually high percentage of the gas coming out of his rear end was nitrogen, the main constituent of atmospheric air.

On a final note about flatus, the aforementioned fermentation gases—carbon dioxide, methane, and hydrogen—are all odorless and aren't responsible for the awful smell of some people's flatus. Instead, sulfur-containing gases like hydrogen sulfide (rotten egg smell) and methanethiol (rotting vegetable smell) are the real troublemakers, and foods such as cabbage, broccoli, and garlic are especially effective at producing these odorous gases. Amazingly (or disturbingly, depending on your perspective), a study that played a major role in determining that hydrogen sulfide and methanethiol cause smelly farts somehow convinced two research assistants to judge the unpleasantness of human flatus.[116] To be precise, these fart judges held a syringe filled with flatus up to their noses and "slowly ejected the gas, taking several sniffs."

If you're personally concerned about the smell of your flatus (or are concerned with the well-being of those around you), you could avoid sulfur-gas producing foodstuffs. If you just can't pass on the broccoli, activated charcoal pills have been used for years to tone down the offensiveness of flatus, albeit with little scientific evidence.[117]

57

DEFECATION AND DIARRHEA

Even though a hip injury prevents me from putting in much mileage these days, I can still vividly remember a winter morning in 2009 when my long, slow run of the week morphed into a speed workout consisting of sprinting back to my house to soothe an angry bowel. Thankfully, I was doing loops around my neighborhood and wasn't far from home. I made it back just in time to scurry to the bathroom and reenact Harry Dunne's infamous scene from *Dumb and Dumber*. My experience is by no means an aberration, and it's reasonable to assume that almost every seasoned distance runner has been seized by an irrepressible urge to void their bowels midrun. In the best-case scenario, a runner can find their way to a nearby lavatory, or at least a close bush, but in the worst circumstance, they may actually soil their britches.

While many people struggle to understand how athletes can soil themselves while exercising, a quick search of the internet reveals numerous tales of in-race bowel disasters, some of which involve top-level athletes. In truth, elite endurance athletes may be more predisposed to this sort of mishap simply because of their supernatural ability to push through discomfort. The loss of precious time from stopping to use the toilet may incentivize them to push the limits, poohaps too far. (Hey, if you can't make poop witticisms in a book about gut distress, when can you?)

In other situations, athletes may stop to go number two but decide that making it to the Porta-John isn't viable, either because it would take too much time or because there isn't one nearby. Instead, they might opt to duck behind a shrub or a crowd barrier. One of the most notorious of these cases comes from former women's marathon world-record holder Paula Radcliffe, who, during the 2005 London Marathon, briefly stopped four miles before the finish to go number two in front of the world. Despite sounding like an unpleasant spectacle to watch, it's hard to tell from video of the incident that Radcliffe actually had a poo, as she only briefly pulls over to the course barricade, quickly squats, yanks her shorts slightly aside, relieves herself, and thereafter hastily resumes running. The whole sequence takes about 10 seconds, and if you watched the video without any prior knowledge of the incident, you'd probably assume she merely stopped to pee. Amazingly, despite her bowel troubles, Radcliffe went on to not only win the London Marathon but also set a world record for a women-only marathon. She later reportedly said, "I didn't really want to resort to that in front of hundreds of thousands of people. But when I'm racing, I'm totally focused on winning the race and running as fast as possible. I thought, I just need to go and I'll be fine."[118]

Another high-profile case of dumping during competition comes from the Giro d'Italia, one of the three major European professional cycling stage races. During stage 16 of the 2017 race, overall leader Tom Dumoulin pulled to the side of the road and proceeded to strip off his clothes as he scampered down a grassy embankment. The TV camera remained fixated on Dumoulin before producers realized he had stopped to go poo, at which point the feed cut to other cyclists. Months after the race, which he went on to win, Dumoulin revealed that excessive fructose and lactose in his diet was probably responsible for his gut issues.

As with other symptoms, most studies that have investigated the prevalence of defecation-related issues (urges to poo, diarrhea, watery stool, etc.) come from the world of endurance sports. Running tends to bring on these symptoms the most; that study of marathoners from the Belfast City Marathon found that urges to take a dump were occasionally or frequently experienced by just over 40 percent of runners during difficult runs, which was roughly twice as high as during easy runs.[55] What's more, diarrhea occurs so often during and after running that a unique term exists for it: *runner's trots*. Estimates from other sports are few and far between, but given the pervasiveness of bowel issues in the general population, odds are that almost every athlete has had a run-in with these sorts of issues during training or competition.

Defecation-related symptoms can be either short-lived or long-lasting. Symptoms that last more than a few days or that are particularly severe are a sign that you should speak to your healthcare provider ASAP. Crohn's disease, IBS, and celiac disease are just a few of the disorders that can produce chronic diarrhea. Likewise, use of certain medications is another source of sustained diarrhea. Laxatives are meant to trigger urges to defecate and even diarrhea in some instances, but there are many other drugs for which diarrhea is a side effect, such as antibiotics, metformin (used to treat type 2 diabetes), and selective serotonin reuptake inhibitors (used to treat mood disorders).[119]

Sources of transient diarrhea—much like with more chronic sources like IBS and Crohn's—are varied. Probably the most common cause of short-lived diarrhea is

59

catching a gut bug like *E. coli* or norovirus. By one estimate, just under 50 million cases of foodborne illness occur in the US each year.[120] That adds up to a lot of hours spent toiling away on the porcelain throne. Notably, athletes are probably at heightened risk of acquiring these infections because they frequently have contact with other athletes, are exposed to common food sources in training facilities, and sometimes live in close quarters. This is particularly true when an athlete or team travels to a region where pathogenic microorganisms are endemic in the local food and water supplies. Acquiring a gut infection during international travel is known colloquially as traveler's diarrhea, or more colorfully as Montezuma's revenge or Delhi belly.

Simple strategies for avoiding traveler's diarrhea when making a trip abroad include avoiding tap water, only eating food that's served piping hot, and shunning raw foods and unpasteurized dairy products. (As tasty as it sounds, just say no to the ceviche.) Supplementing with probiotics is an appealing approach to prevent traveler's diarrhea because of its simplicity and safety, but, unfortunately, there isn't strong evidence that it's particularly effective for that purpose.[121] People who suffer from repeated bouts of traveler's diarrhea or who cannot tolerate even the slightest chance of getting sick (competing in the Olympics, for example) should consider speaking with their physician about prophylactic treatment with antibiotics or other drugs.

Another possible cause of defecation-related symptoms in athletes is anxiety. Anecdotally, pre-competition jitters are notorious for triggering urges to release the Kraken. (As you can tell, I'm running out of novel ways to describe pooping.) In terms of research supporting this idea, a study of over 60,000 Norwegians confirmed there's a relationship between general anxiety and the occurrence of diarrhea.[122] This research— along with the overwhelming volume of anecdotes I've heard—led me to carry out my own study on anxiety and gut symptoms in runners. In late 2015, I began recruiting seasoned runners and asking them to journal about their running-related gut symptoms over a month. Each runner rated six symptoms (nausea, reflux, fullness, cramps, flatulence, urge to defecate) on a 0-to-10 scale after every run, and at the end of the month, they completed questionnaires on how stressed and anxious they felt over the previous month. Long story short, ratings on the stress and anxiety questionnaires were positively correlated with the occurrence of gut distress (defined as 3 or higher on the scale). This meant that runners who reported more stress and anxiety were more likely to experience gut symptoms during their runs.[123] That being said, the correlations were modest in size, and the study was purely observational, meaning that we can't draw too many conclusions about cause and effect (i.e., anxiety causes gut distress versus gut distress causes anxiety). However, if you consider these findings along with other sources of evidence, it's hard to imagine how anxiety and stress wouldn't play some sort of role in the defecation-related symptoms that many athletes experience in and around the time of competition. (These links are explored in Part 3.)

61

As with all gut symptoms, competition-day nutrition can play an outsized role in whether you stop midcompetition for the sake of saving your shorts. On the most basic level, eating provokes bowel urges because it initiates what's called the gastro-colic reflex. Stretching of your stomach's walls and the presence of digestive products in your small intestine cause signals to be sent, via your nervous system, to your colon, and these messages notify your colon that it needs to make room for an invading horde of partially digested foodstuffs. Your colon heeds this order by initiating giant migrating contractions, which are intense and sustained contractions that propel colonic contents forward. A study published in the journal *Gastroenterology*, for instance, showed that colonic activity surged immediately after eating a 1,000-kilocalorie meal and peaked at nearly fivefold of baseline levels within about 30 minutes.[124] To be clear, I'm not telling you to avoid eating before or during exercise; instead, this information should reassure you that having to poo is a natural response to eating.

The nutritional choices you make during exercise can affect defecation-related symptoms for reasons other than the gastrocolic reflex. Just as with intestinal cramps and flatulence, overconsuming carbohydrate-rich foods and drinks during exercise can lead to diarrhea. If they fail to be absorbed in your small intestine, carbohydrate molecules enter your large intestine, where they subsequently draw water from your blood into the luminal space, leading to loose stools or diarrhea. As a parallel example, this phenomenon also occurs when a person ingests lactulose, a synthetic, nondigestible sugar that's used as a laxative drug. Undigested lactulose travels through the small intestine and ends up in the large intestine, leading to a highly reproducible and dose-dependent increase in watery stool output.[125] Similarly, anyone who is lactose intolerant is all too familiar with the diarrhea that ensues after downing sizable portions of dairy foods.[126, 127]

Poor absorption of the other two macronutrients, fat and protein, are possible but less probable culprits of defecation-related symptoms. Fat malabsorption is common in some medical conditions like pancreatitis and cystic fibrosis, and administration of pancreatic enzymes relieves symptoms in these situations. Fat malabsorption is characterized by passing foul-smelling stools that have a pale, oily appearance.

Finally, dietary supplements can also bring about unwelcome bowel urges. In the world of sports, two of the most scientifically supported supplements are caffeine and sodium bicarbonate. Caffeine improves performance in practically every competitive context, while sodium bicarbonate (otherwise known as baking soda) enhances high-intensity anaerobic exercise performance.[128] However, both substances (but particularly sodium bicarbonate) can cause gut woes that, if severe enough, compromise performance. A cautionary tale of how sodium bicarbonate's side effects can harm performance comes from an article written by sports science journalist and former competitive runner Alex Hutchinson. In a piece published in *Runner's World*, Hutchinson recounts what happened to one of his teammates who used baking soda before a race at the team's conference championships:

> ❝ *He had explosive diarrhea and had to scratch from the 4 × 800-meter relay. I was the alternate, so I got my big chance to run on the relay team. I set a three-second PR and earned a spot on the team for nationals.*[129]

Even though things worked out exceedingly well for Hutchinson (he set a PR and made it to nationals as a member of the relay team), his teammate's baking soda experiment shows that even supposedly beneficial supplements can crush your chances of winning if applied inappropriately. Specific guidelines on how to avoid or minimize the ill effects of sodium bicarbonate supplements are provided in Chapter 10. Creatine and ketones are two other sports supplements that can cause diarrhea (at least when taken in large single doses),[130, 131] but this can largely be avoided by spreading your intake over an entire day.

CONSTIPATION

On the opposite end of the spectrum from a bad case of the runs is constipation, which involves infrequent bowel movements and/or difficulty emptying one's bowels. Over the course of a year, it's projected that roughly up to one in six Americans will end up being fecally challenged in this way,[132] and rather astonishingly, over half a million emergency room visits each year are attributable to this troublesome symptom.[133] In contrast to the frequent occurrence of diarrhea in athletes, constipation during exercise isn't a widespread problem. Although the science is somewhat equivocal, there's some evidence that exercise increases colon motor activity and reduces transit time through the colon,[64] both of which typically decrease constipation. In fact, a lack of exercise is often blamed for the constipation that arises when people are forced into immobility (e.g., after surgery).

The causes of constipation vary and can be multifactorial. In some people, colonic transit is slowed (perhaps due to a disease or medication), which increases water absorption into the body, resulting in hard, pebble-like stools that are difficult to pass. In other people, continuously suppressing their urges to go number two may be to blame. In an article subtitled with one of the great questions of our time ("Can constipation be learned?"), researchers asked 12 brave men to suppress their urges to poo over a week.[134] In comparison to a normal week when they promptly answered nature's calls, the number of stools fell from 8.9 to 3.7 during a week when the men did their best to hold back the brown. What's more, three of the men were able to go a full three days without dropping a deuce. In the words of the authors, the "volunteers succeeded in suppressing the urge to defecate to an amazing extent." The most surprising finding from this and other studies is that postponing your toilet obligations may slow transit through other parts of your gut and even delay stomach emptying,[134-136] which is generally not what you want to happen. Basically, holding stool in your rectum may trigger a reflexive response in the rest of your gut so as not to overload your colon with digestive material. Poor fluid intake has also been linked to constipation, but increasing water intake isn't helpful unless adequate fiber is supplied in the diet.[137] Numerous medications can make you constipated, including tricyclic antidepressants, opioids, certain antacids (aluminum hydroxide and calcium carbonate), and some antihypertensive drugs.

Likewise, diseases such as diabetes, multiple sclerosis, and Parkinson's as well as spinal cord injuries can lead to persistent constipation. Beyond making sure not to suppress your natural urges, management strategies for constipation include fiber supplementation, laxatives, prosecretory medications, biofeedback training, and avoidance of constipation-inducing drugs.[138]

BLOODY STOOL

One of the most alarming gut symptoms an athlete can experience is the appearance of blood in their stool. Hemorrhoids, ulcerative colitis, and colon cancer are just a few of the medical concerns that can cause this, and these conditions usually cause blood to show up in the stool on a chronic basis, either continuously or intermittently. Intense or prolonged exercise is also capable of producing bloody stools, albeit this is more temporary. In most cases, a small amount of blood in the stool after exercise is benign, although severe gastrointestinal hemorrhaging, even necessitating emergency surgery, has been observed on rare occasions.[139] That said, repeatedly losing blood in the stool can be deleterious to your health and fitness, as it can give rise to iron deficiency or outright anemia in severe cases.

One of the larger surveys examining the frequency of gut symptoms among marathoners found that a small percentage—maybe 1-2 percent—reported occasional bloody bowel movements during or after runs.[4] These self-report surveys would seem to indicate that bloody stools are fairly uncommon during and after exercise. However, failing to see blood in your stool with your naked eye doesn't necessarily mean it isn't there. For one thing, the amount of blood is usually small. In addition, blood in the gut, like most other substances, is susceptible to digestive processes, and if it gets partially digested, blood ends up as melena, which is the technical term for stool that appears dark and tarry looking. These were the sort of symptoms that Derek Clayton came down with in 1969 after setting the world record in the marathon and being the first person to break the 2:09 barrier, saying, "I was vomiting black mucus and had black diarrhea."[140]

One way to detect blood that's imperceptible to the naked eye is to conduct a fecal occult blood test. These tests look for the presence of specific blood components through chemical or immunologic reactions. When used in endurance athletes, these tests usually show that occult (hidden) blood is present in the stools of more athletes than what's found in studies that rely on self-reports. As an example, 29 of 125 runners who volunteered for a study at the eighth annual Marine Corps Marathon ended up with a positive fecal occult blood test after the race when they initially had negative results beforehand.[141] Another study of marathoners found that 13 percent were positive for fecal occult blood loss after a race.[142] The occurrence of fecal occult blood loss in this pair of studies (13–23 percent) is considerably higher than the 1–2 percent that typically report visible blood in the stool after running.

Exercise duration is an important factor dictating the prevalence of fecal blood loss. A study of 35 participants from a 100-mile running race revealed that 85 percent had a positive post-race test,[143] which is undoubtedly more common in comparison to shorter races.[144] Similar to the effect of increasing exercise duration, the repetitive impact of running leads to more occult bleeding in comparison to low-impact activities. In stark contrast to the 85 percent of ultrarunners who tested positive for occult bleeding, a study of 100-mile bike race competitors found a positive test rate of only 8 percent.[145]

What exactly is behind this large discrepancy between running and nonimpact physical activities? One possibility is that the jostling of running causes transient trauma or damage to the intestinal lining that, over increasing distances, worsens blood loss in the stool.[146] A physician named Alan Porter proposed over 35 years ago that repetitive slapping of the cecum (a pouch that makes up the first part of your colon) against the abdominal wall is a cause of this trauma and bleeding. Porter's description of what he called the "caecal [cecal] slap syndrome" in a 53-year-old first-time marathoner was published in the *British Journal of Sports Medicine*:

> ❝ *A jog around the garden demonstrates that as the right foot moves forward, the abdominal muscles in the right iliac fossa relax. As the foot hits the ground, the muscles tighten and there is a brief check in momentum. The posterior wall of the caecum would now slap against the fixed anterior wall. . . . it might do this up to 20,000 times during the course of the race.*[147]

Porter's hypothesis seems logical, but to this day there remains no concrete evidence that repetitive slapping of the cecum is responsible for running-associated fecal blood loss. And given the anatomical location of the cecum (i.e., beginning of the colon), bleeding that originates from the upper portion of the gut (stomach and small intestine) obviously wouldn't fit nicely with this hypothesis. In all probability, the origins of bloody stools likely vary in importance depending on the situation and other predisposing factors (such as NSAID use) known to cause gut damage and bleeding.

As mentioned earlier, a small amount of blood in the stool after a run is often benign, but recurrently losing blood in the stool can give rise to iron deficiency. Your body relies on red blood cells to transport oxygen to your organs and muscles, and the molecule that facilitates this is hemoglobin, an iron-containing protein that loves to bind oxygen. People with low hemoglobin levels (less than 13.5 g/dL for men and 12 g/dL for women) are anemic and often suffer from fatigue, shortness of breath, and pallor. However, a person can be iron deficient without being anemic, which is the case for many endurance athletes. While anemia causes symptoms that are often readily noticed, iron deficiency without anemia is more insidious, frequently going unrecognized until an athlete's blood is tested for iron markers like ferritin, an iron storage protein. Anywhere from 20 percent to 60 percent of female athletes are iron deficient depending on the population studied and the ferritin threshold used.[148] The prevalence in males is usually lower, in part because they don't have monthly menstrual blood losses. Although it's not the main cause of iron deficiency in most athletes, blood losses in the stool may be a contributor to poor iron status in some runners.

It goes without saying that anyone who is regularly seeing blood in their stool should promptly see a medical provider. Unfortunately, there's limited research on how to stop gastrointestinal bleeding that appears with exercise. A few case reports have had athletes stop running, avoid NSAIDs, manage exercise-induced gut ischemia through proper hydration, employ gradual increases in training volume, or a combination of these interventions.[149, 150] While these strategies might help resolve fecal bleeding, it's hard to conclude which, if any of them, are actually effective given the anecdotal nature of case study investigations. A couple of larger experiments have shown that taking acid-reducing medications (cimetidine and pantoprazole) before competition reduces the risk of fecal bleeding, although these studies still had only a few dozen participants and were mostly limited to ultraendurance exercise.[143, 151]

FACTORS INFLUENCING THE OCCURRENCE OR SEVERITY OF GUT SYMPTOMS

A host of factors can amplify or ease peptic problems during exercise. The final part of this chapter is devoted to some of the established demographic and training factors that exacerbate or temper your risk of gut symptoms. Other possible causes of gut problems, including nutritional and psychological, deserve more extensive attention and are reserved for Parts 2 and 3 of *The Athlete's Gut.*

67

Form of exercise. All other things being equal, running has a tendency to elicit more severe gut symptoms than other forms of exercise, and most attempts to explain this phenomenon rely on the simple fact that running is a jarring activity. In one study, researchers attached small sensors to the bellies of six participants during bouts of running and cycling.[152] Participants ran and cycled on the same stretch of asphalt at 60–70 percent of max effort, and overall output from the device, which can be thought of as a measure of abdominal displacement, was over twice as high during running.

Exercise intensity and duration. Most athletes know that ramping up exercise intensity can trigger gut woes. Likewise, exercising for an hour or longer puts you more at risk of troublesome symptoms than brief bouts of exercise done at the same intensity. While the underlying causes are undoubtedly multidimensional, one shared pathway by which these factors heighten gut problems is through reductions in gut blood flow.[139] Fortunately, exercise training dampens these gut blood flow decrements over time,[153] which may help explain why older and more seasoned athletes suffer from fewer gut issues than their younger and less experienced comrades (see the "Age" and "Training experience" sections that follow). With that said, the volume of training undertaken doesn't seem to correlate with the incidence or severity of gut problems during exercise.[58, 123, 154] In a nutshell, most athletes can expect their gut issues to decline in severity over time as they become fitter and more experienced, but they shouldn't necessarily presume that a larger training volume (in terms of mileage) will accelerate this adaptation process.

Age. The physical aging process—from the greying of our hair to the sagging of our skin— isn't something most of us look forward to with anticipation. For athletes, the cosmetic aspects of aging are usually accompanied by lagging race times, slowed reaction speeds, and diminished coordination. In many respects, it's hard to see any advantages, at least physically, to adding another candle to your birthday cake. A curtailment in several gut symptoms is one such consolation prize of getting older, however, and this decline in symptoms occurs in athletes and nonathletes alike.[4, 155-157] One simple explanation for this is that as athletes age, they don't train as hard as they used to. Heavy exercise is a strong stimulus for impairing gut blood flow, so it's possible that older athletes are experiencing less profound blood flow alterations as they spend more time training at lower exercise intensities. In addition, the vascular system of aged athletes seems to be less responsive to catecholamines (stress hormones that impact blood flow distribution), and as a result, older athletes may experience smaller declines in gut blood flow during exercise.[158]

Training experience. As you probably know from your own life experiences, the more time you spend doing an activity, the better your body adapts to that stressor. Case in point, training in the heat boosts your tolerance to heat stress. Similarly, long-term exercise training improves the way your gut responds to the physiological stresses of acute exercise. Experiments in animals and humans reveal that exercise training helps prevent some of the blood flow declines to the digestive tract during acute exercise, at least when you test them at the same absolute workload before and after a training intervention.[153] These findings are also supported by observational studies that show seasoned athletes have fewer gut symptoms than their novice counterparts.[57, 123, 155] It's important to keep in mind that experience and age correlate with one another, making it difficult to tease out precisely how much of these improvements are due to cumulative training history versus the aging process.

Sex. Women have the upper hand in several aspects of the battle of the sexes. Take, for example, that they tend to live longer and are, on average, more socially and emotionally intelligent than men. When it comes to gut ailments, though, women often find themselves getting the short end of the stick. While not true for all symptoms (heartburn is an exception), many of them (abdominal pain, constipation, nausea) are reported more frequently in women.[156, 159, 160] Exactly what's behind this sex gap remains somewhat of a mystery, but one possible explanation is that women are more in tune with their internal state, which may be the result of living through events (menstruation, pregnancy, menopause) that regularly call attention to their bodies.[161] Also, the socialization process for children, at least in most societies, encourages females to more openly acknowledge all kinds of distress and discomfort. And finally, women sometimes experience changes in gut symptoms across their menstrual cycles, which suggests that female sex hormones play a role in some situations.[162] Although most women will probably be disappointed to hear these facts, a sliver of good news is that differences in symptoms between men and women diminish with age.[156]

69

A history of gut symptoms. A powerful predictor of the future is the past. Simply put, the past is prologue. And when it comes to gut grievances, this age-old turn of phrase holds true. In one of my own studies, the frequency of gut symptoms experienced by athletes over three months of training was modestly correlated with symptoms during a 70.3-mile triathlon,[58] and these results are in line with earlier investigations.[110, 163] It remains unclear to what extent these correlations are driven by modifiable versus nonmodifiable factors. As an example of a largely nonmodifiable factor, a person born with a stenosis of the celiac artery—a vessel supplying oxygen-rich blood to the upper gut—might have greater impairments in flow during exercise, leading to more distressful symptoms.[164] On the modifiable side of things, it's plausible that some of the athletes in these studies were guilty of choosing poor dietary strategies or using symptom-provoking medications like NSAIDs during both training and competition. In essence, athletes who have made poor choices in the past may be making these same mistakes over and over again.

Sleep. It may not be the most obvious upside of sleep, but consistently getting seven-plus hours of shut-eye per night has a positive impact on gut function. Like most other organ systems, your gastrointestinal tract runs on a 24-hour rhythmic biological clock, enabling it to anticipate and prepare for future events such as meals, activity, and sleep. Inputs from the environment such as light, eating, and sleep influence this internal clock and can impact your gut's function.[165] However, there's a chicken-or-egg dilemma with this observation: do sleep disturbances cause gut symptoms, or do gut symptoms cause sleep disturbances? While the latter explanation is certainly true in some cases (e.g., a person waking up at night because of severe heartburn), there's evidence that the former explanation is also true. Indeed, shift workers report more digestive symptoms than their non-shift-work counterparts and have higher odds of being diagnosed with disorders like IBS and GERD.[166, 167] Although other lifestyle factors differ between shift workers and non-shift workers, sleep disruption is probably the most reasonable explanation for the uptick in gut problems among those working nocturnally. Even more convincing, one experiment showed that inducing sleep deprivation (less than three hours of sleep) for one night intensified heartburn among individuals with GERD,[168] and these findings are in agreement with research demonstrating that inducing sleep deprivation worsens perceptions of pain, possibly by amplifying inflammation in the body.[169] Given all the other health and performance upsides of sleep, athletes should make getting sufficient slumber a top priority.

REVIEW OF COMMON GUT SYMPTOMS AND THEIR POSSIBLE CAUSES

Table 2.1 offers an abbreviated overview of the symptoms covered in this chapter. It's worth noting that not every possible cause is listed for each symptom, and you should refer to the text in this and other chapters for deeper insights. In addition, this table doesn't include chronic diseases that contribute to these symptoms. For descriptions of various conditions that can cause gut woes, refer to Appendix A.

table 2.1. **PREVALENCE OF GUT SYMPTOMS AND UNDERLYING FACTORS THAT CONTRIBUTE TO THEIR DEVELOPMENT**

SYMPTOM	PREVALENCE	POSSIBLE CAUSES
Nausea and vomiting	• Prevalence is roughly 10% during marathons or hard training runs. • Prevalence increases during ultraendurance events. • It's a common reason for athletes to drop out of ultraendurance races.	• Catecholamine release with intense exercise • AVP release • Dehydration • Reduced gut blood flow • Ingesting fatty foods just before or during exercise • Ingesting hypertonic fluids during exercise • Ingesting large volumes of food or fluid during exercise • Hyponatremia • Hypoglycemia • High-dose caffeine or stimulant use • Psychological stress/anxiety
Reflux, heartburn, and regurgitation	• Prevalence is 10% or higher during endurance running, depending on the terminology used in the survey. • These symptoms are possibly more common during running or weight lifting.	• A diagnosis of GERD • Reduced gut blood flow • Intense exercise • Ingesting foodstuffs within 1 hour of exercise • Ingesting fatty foods before or during exercise • Ingesting hypertonic fluids during exercise • Aggressive carbohydrate intake during exercise • Ingesting large volumes of food or fluid during exercise • Consuming chocolate, citrus fruits, spicy foods, acidic foods, coffee, alcohol, or carbonated fluids • Psychological stress/anxiety
Fullness and bloating	• Prevalence is variable depending on the type and duration of exercise as well as nutritional choices.	• Dehydration • Reduced gut blood flow • Ingesting fatty, solid-protein, or fiber-rich foods immediately before or during exercise • Ingesting hypertonic fluids during exercise • Aggressive carbohydrate intake during exercise • Ingesting large volumes of food or fluid during exercise • A high-fiber diet • Psychological stress/anxiety
Intestinal cramps	• Prevalence is 10% to 20% during endurance running. • Prevalence goes up as exercise duration and intensity increase.	• Reduced gut blood flow • Ingesting hypertonic fluids during exercise • Aggressive carbohydrate intake during exercise • Carbohydrate malabsorption • NSAIDs • Psychological stress/anxiety

71

continues

table 2.1. **CONTINUED**

SYMPTOM	PREVALENCE	POSSIBLE CAUSES
Side stitch	• Over one year, roughly 70% of athletes may experience a side stitch severe enough to necessitate a reduction in exercise intensity. • This symptom is common in swimmers, runners, and horseback riders.	• Reduced gut blood flow • Movement causing up-and-down jostling or twisting of the abdomen • Ingesting hypertonic fluids during exercise • Irritation of the parietal peritoneum
Flatulence	• This is possibly the most common symptom experienced by athletes. • Half of endurance athletes experience flatulence at least occasionally during training.	• Aggressive carbohydrate intake during exercise • Carbohydrate malabsorption • High fiber intake
Defecation and diarrhea	• Urges to have a bowel movement are reported by about 40% of runners during hard runs. • Having to stop for a bowel movement is less common.	• Reduced gut blood flow • Ingesting hypertonic fluids during exercise • Movement causing up-and-down jostling • Aggressive carbohydrate intake during exercise • Carbohydrate malabsorption • Gastrointestinal infections • Medications (antibiotics, metformin, selective serotonin reuptake inhibitors, etc.) • Various supplements (caffeine, sodium bicarbonate, etc.) • Psychological stress/anxiety
Constipation	• Roughly one in six Americans suffers from chronic constipation. • Because of the possible impact of exercise on colonic transit and motility, constipation is not common during exercise.	• Slowed colonic transit • Inadequate fluid intake • Low-carbohydrate or low-fiber diet • Overall low dietary energy intake • Consciously suppressing urges to defecate • Medications such as antihypertensive drugs, tricyclic antidepressants, opioids, and antacids • Psychological stress/anxiety
Bloody stool	• 13% to 23% of marathoners test positive for fecal occult blood, although only 1% to 2% report visible blood loss.	• Reduced gut blood flow • Movement causing abdominal jostling • Cecal slap syndrome • NSAIDs

SUMMARY

THE ORIGINS OF GUT SYMPTOMS

The prevalence of gut symptoms varies quite a bit between studies, but it's fair to say that **most athletes occasionally experience gut problems** during training or competition.

73

There are many potential causes of gut symptoms, and each symptom often has its own unique contributing factors. That said, **reductions in gut blood flow** are likely to contribute to most of these gut symptoms.

Gut problems experienced during exercise are often **multifactorial** in nature, meaning **several management strategies** may be needed to obtain substantial relief.

Gut symptoms may be inevitable for some athletes in certain situations (e.g., extremely intense or prolonged exercise), but there are usually strategies that can be implemented to lessen the severity of such problems.

Nausea/vomiting, abdominal cramping, side stitching, and diarrhea can quickly **kill a solid performance**. Other symptoms (e.g., belching, fullness, gas) can be bothersome but are perhaps less likely to impact an athlete's performance.

Younger age, less training experience, female sex, and a history of gut symptoms are all associated with **more frequent** and/or more severe gut symptoms during exercise.

NUTRITION
AND THE ATHLETE'S GUT

03

ENERGY

Every human on this planet needs energy: energy for chemical work, energy to produce body heat, and, especially for athletes, energy to perform physical work. Food is where we get this life-sustaining energy. More specifically, plants harness energy from the sun's rays to convert a gas, carbon dioxide, and water into carbohydrate. Animals— cows, chickens, bison, ostriches—consume these plants and carbohydrates and convert some of them into fat. Ultimately, the carbohydrates and fats found in the plants and animals that we feed on are used to make a high-energy molecule—known as adenosine triphosphate (ATP)—that powers everything our bodies do. Although we can use protein to make ATP, our bodies prefer to save it for building muscle and other vital tissues and substances. Consequently, dietary carbohydrate and fat make up the largest sources of energy in humans' diets and are the two fuels that our bodies prefer for manufacturing ATP.

The amount of daily energy you consume—relative to your body's needs—has important implications when it comes to your gut's function. Over the long run, consuming less energy than your body needs increases your chances of experiencing several gut symptoms; conversely, gut discomfort and problems can also arise if you are the type of athlete who needs to consume huge quantities of energy (e.g., more than 4,000–5,000 kilocalories per day) in order to meet training demands or to put on body mass. In this chapter, we explore what energy is, how to determine how much energy athletes need, and the consequences that can arise from under- and overconsuming energy in the diet.

MEASURING ENERGY

It may not be plainly obvious, but both underconsuming and overconsuming dietary energy can give rise to gut problems. Both scenarios are covered later in this chapter, but let's take a minute to get on the same page when it comes to defining and measuring energy in foods. Even though ATP powers all your bodily processes, you likely already know that nutrition labels don't list quantities of ATP but instead report energy in the form of calories (at least in the United States). Still, you might be wondering what in the world a calorie actually represents. The short answer is that a calorie is the amount of energy needed to raise the temperature of 1 gram of water by 1 degree Celsius.

Sounds fairly straightforward, but how do we apply this concept to quantify the calories in food? How many calories, for example, are in a Twinkie? A head of lettuce? A double cheeseburger? A pound of milk chocolate? To figure this out, a device called a bomb calorimeter can be used to measure the energy content of these and other foods. Scientists place a sample of food inside the bomb calorimeter, which consists of a sealed container surrounded by water. Then the sample is ignited, and the resulting combustion releases heat, which can be measured by the degree of temperature change of the surrounding water. Although this is a precise way of determining the energy content of foods, most manufacturers don't go to these lengths. Instead, they calculate the calories in foods based on the amounts of carbohydrate, protein, and fat they contain, as the energy content per gram of each macronutrient is fairly consistent.

Before moving on to talk about the energy needs of athletes, there's a brief point I need to make in regard to how energy is listed on the Nutrition Facts label in the United States. This may be a tad confusing, but the word *calorie* that's used on the Nutrition Facts label doesn't mean exactly the same thing as the definition I just gave you. Instead, 1 calorie on the Nutrition Facts label actually represents 1,000 calories, or 1 kilocalorie. As an example, 1 cup of cereal that lists 200 calories on its label actually contains 200,000 calories, or 200 kilocalories. I'll use the term *kilocalorie*, or *kcal* for short, to describe energy concepts, and this will identify the same amount you're used to thinking of as calories or seeing on Nutrition Facts labels.

ENERGY NEEDS AND ENERGY BALANCE

It's a given that you need energy to survive, but exactly how many kilocalories should you consume each day to maintain your health and physical function? Even if you were to lie in bed all day and binge-watch your favorite TV show (I'd probably choose *The Office*), your body would still expend anywhere from 1,000 to more than 2,000 kcal over 24 hours. This is the energy required to keep your lungs breathing, heart pumping, kidneys cleansing, liver detoxifying, appendix appendicizing, and brain cogitating—it's the energy needed to simply keep the lights in the building turned on. The technical term for this minimal energy requirement is *resting metabolic rate*, or RMR for short. (It's also sometimes called resting energy expenditure or basal metabolic rate.) After adding in energy expended through physical activities (which, for nonathletes, is usually several hundred kilocalories), most people living in modern societies end up burning 2,000–3,000 kcal per day, or if you prefer to measure energy in candy bar form, about 8 to 12 Snickers' worth.

Ultimately, if you eat fewer kilocalories than you burn, you'll lose weight. Alternatively, if you eat more kilocalories than you burn, you'll gain weight. If the number of kilocalories you ingest equals the kilocalories you burn, you'll maintain your weight. The physics are simple, and meticulous feeding studies show us that this energy balance principle works.[1] Outside the confines of a controlled lab, however, numerous factors complicate the application of this simple energy-balance equation by affecting your energy intake, energy expenditure, or both. For example, eating a 2,000 kcal diet that contains an abundance of protein, water, and fiber would blunt your hunger much more than eating a 2,000 kcal diet consisting entirely of sugar or oil. If you started eating a 2,000 kcal diet of pure sugar or oil, soon thereafter your ravenous brain would propel you to up your energy intake (perhaps to something like 2,500 kcal) due to persistent hunger. I recognize that all-sugar and all-oil diets are extreme, unsustainable examples, but they illustrate the point that the type and quality of food you eat impacts the dynamic processes that regulate energy intake.

Similarly, there are factors that subtly influence the expenditure side of the energy-balance equation. If you were to lose a considerable amount of weight over a few months (say, 30 pounds), your RMR and total energy expenditure would also decline (assuming you didn't compensate by doing more physical activity). In fact, each pound you

79

lose equates to about a 5 kcal drop in RMR. So, if your daily energy expenditure is 2,500 kcal and you follow a weight-loss diet of 2,000 kcal (equating to an initial negative balance of 500 kcal), your weight loss progress would slow to a crawl after several months because your RMR (and total energy expenditure) would decline over time. In order to continue to shed pounds, you'd need to either decrease your energy intake even further (maybe to 1,500 kcal) or boost your energy expenditure by doing more physical activity.

CONSEQUENCES OF HIGH ENERGY INTAKES

For the public, a failure to remain in a neutral energy balance has contributed to the explosive growth of obesity over the past half century, and today, almost 4 out of 10 American adults are obese. While most athletes don't have to worry about suffering from the untoward effects of obesity in the midst of their playing careers, they do need to be conscious of how much energy they consume because consuming either too much or too little can have undesirable performance consequences. Excess intake can lead to body fat gain, while chronically underconsuming energy is a path toward metabolic and hormonal dysfunction.

Eating the appropriate amount of energy for weight maintenance can be challenging for athletes because, in comparison to couch potatoes, their total energy expenditures often vary much more from day to day. Amazingly, athletes training or competing for multiple hours each day routinely expend twice as much energy as their lazybones counterparts. A cyclist participating in one of the Grand Tours, as an example, can burn through 24 to 32 Snickers' worth of energy (6,000–8,000 kcal) every day.[2, 3] During the most extreme athletic endeavors—such as participating in a 24-hour adventure race—daily expenditures can swell to 15,000–20,000 kcal, or between 60 and 80 Snickers bars[4] (see Figure 3.1).

It goes without saying, then, that many athletes have to eat almost nonstop during heavy training and competition periods in order to maintain energy balance, or at least prevent severe deficits. The sheer volume of food required to sustain this demand can undoubtedly be a source of gut discomfort. As a result, these athletes often choose foods and beverages that are energy dense, meaning they have more kilocalories crammed into each gram. Examples of energy-dense foods include butter, oils, nuts, sugar, sweets/desserts, and high-fat cheeses.[5] Conversely, foods on the other end of the energy-density spectrum contain more energy-free or low-energy nutrients (such as water and fiber), with examples being vegetables, fruits, lean meats, and low-fat dairy products.

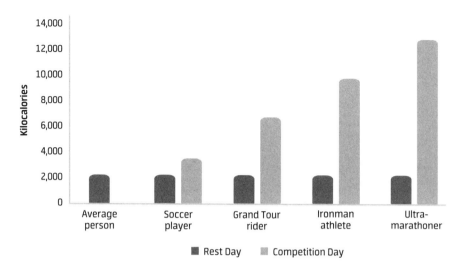

figure 3.1. **DAILY ENERGY NEEDS OF VARIOUS ATHLETES**

The day-to-day energy needs of athletes can fluctuate drastically depending on their training volume and competition loads, with some athletes even burning 10,000+ kilocalories in a single day.

Cyclists competing in the Tour de France are prime examples of athletes favoring energy-dense foods. Case in point, a 1989 study of five cyclists competing in the Tour de France found that sweet cakes and a concentrated carbohydrate drink were the foremost contributors to the athletes' energy intakes.[2] Another study published about a decade later reported that biscuits and confectionery were the leading sources of dietary energy among 10 cyclists competing in the Vuelta a España (Tour of Spain).[6] Returning to our Snickers bar system of measurement, a cyclist would need to consume 24 bars to achieve a daily intake of 6,000 kcal, and at a weight of 53 grams per bar, that adds up to 1.27 kilograms (or 2.8 pounds) of Snickers. As a point of comparison, 1 cup of cubed cantaloupe, coming in at 160 grams, contains only about 50 kcal, and that same cyclist would have to eat 120 cups' worth of cantaloupe, or over 19 kilograms, to get those same 6,000 kilocalories! This is an outrageous example, but it demonstrates how energy density influences the amount of food that's needed to meet an athlete's energy demands.

A more realistic comparison is shown in Table 3.1. Although each menu provides roughly 2,500 kcal, the low-energy density version contains larger amounts of food. And remember that many athletes will need to eat much more than 2,500 kcal per day.

table 3.1. **ENERGY DENSITY COMPARISON**

	LOWER ENERGY DENSITY	HIGHER ENERGY DENSITY
Breakfast	• 16 ounces fat-free milk • 1 cup cooked steel-cut oatmeal • 1 cup blueberries • 1 large banana • 3 ounces Swiss cheese	• 10 ounces 2% fat milk • 1 cup cooked steel-cut oatmeal • 1 ½ Tbsp. honey • Small omelet with cheese
Snack 1	• 1 large apple • 3 ounces baby carrots • 3 Tbsp. hummus	• 16 ounces orange juice
Lunch	• 3 ounces low-fat turkey • 2 slices whole-grain bread • 2 Tbsp. low-fat mayo • 1 medium orange • 16 ounces fat-free milk • 1 cup cucumber salad with vinegar dressing	• 1 chicken salad sandwich • 10 ounces 2% fat milk • ½ cup mixed roasted nuts
Snack 2	• ½ cup pretzels	• 15 ounces Naked Green Machine smoothie drink
Dinner	• 4 ounces grilled chicken breast • 1 cup cooked whole-grain rice • 3 ounces steamed broccoli • 1 cup raspberries • 12 ounces fat-free milk	• 3 ounces cooked salmon • 1 cup mashed potatoes • ½ cup onions and tomatoes sautéed in extra virgin olive oil

For athletes who have very large daily energy needs, including more energy-dense foods reduces the overall volume of food they need to consume.

In sum, athletes with high energy needs who attempt to get all of their energy from nutrient-dense, lower-energy foodstuffs can sometimes find themselves suffering from symptoms like excessive fullness, bloating, flatulence, and frequent urges to poo.

CONSEQUENCES OF UNDERCONSUMING ENERGY

While the massive volume of food that some athletes eat can sometimes lead to gut problems, eating too little energy over extended periods of time (days to weeks) can also be a source of digestive difficulties. As an example, individuals living with anorexia nervosa are often afflicted with symptoms affecting the upper portion of their digestive tracts (i.e., bloating, premature or excessive fullness, nausea, and stomach pain). The heightened prevalence of upper gut symptoms in anorexia stems, in part, from a delay in the release of chyme from the stomach; indeed, even a few days of severely undereating curtails gastric emptying.[7] In a way, it's as if the stomach forgets what it's supposed to do after being off the job for a few days.

Obviously, not all athletes with small builds or very low body fat levels have anorexia. Yet, athletes are generally at greater risk of developing eating disorders like anorexia as well as disordered eating patterns (i.e., problematic but not necessarily diagnosable eating abnormalities). This is particularly true for those competing in sports where performance depends on having a low body weight or being lean. Despite evidence that upper gut symptoms are common in anorexia nervosa, there's scarce data directly supporting the notion that athletes who subtly but chronically restrict energy intake are more prone to experiencing these problems. However, it's logical that this would be the case, and while these symptoms may not directly impact the performance of every athlete, situations exist where slowed stomach emptying from chronic undereating would be problematic. An example is a marathoner competing in a hot and humid environment, who, as a result of heavy sweating, needs to drink large quantities of fluid to stave off the effects of dehydration. If this athlete suffers from impaired stomach emptying because of disordered eating, they would be more likely to experience fullness and nausea if they try to maintain an appropriate level of hydration.

Just as with the upper half of the gut, long-term restriction of dietary energy can induce symptoms that affect the lower half of the digestive tract, most notably constipation. Interestingly, constipation may be an adaptive slowing of the digestive process that the body makes in response to a dwindling supply of incoming food, allowing it to squeeze out as many nutrients as possible.[8] Again, anorexia nervosa serves as an extreme but illustrative example of this sort of functional change. In a study from Johns Hopkins Hospital, the time it took substances to transit the gut was nearly twice as long in individuals with anorexia (67 hours) than in controls (38 hours).[9] Furthermore, this plodding transit is reversed when adequate nutrition is returned to an anorexic patient's diet.[10] Similar to the situation with upper gut symptoms, there's not much research directly tying energy restriction to constipation in athletes, but the evidence linking disordered eating to constipation in nonathletes is robust.[7]

In the end, you need energy to run all your body's systems, including your digestive tract. Cutting your caloric intake to slightly below your needs (a deficit of a couple hundred kilocalories) for a few days is unlikely to produce much in the way of gut problems, but more severe or prolonged restrictions could reduce gut motility and put you on a path to experiencing bloating, premature fullness, nausea, and constipation. The more severe the caloric deficit is and the more time that deficit is sustained, the more likely it is you'll encounter these problems. Any athlete experiencing these symptoms—especially in the presence of other signs of disordered eating—should consult with a healthcare provider. Some signs and symptoms of disordered eating in athletes are listed below.[11] On their own, none of these are 100 percent accurate for identifying disordered eating, but the presence of multiple signs and symptoms at the same time is cause for concern:

⊙ Dramatic/sudden weight loss
⊙ An irregular or absent menstrual cycle in females
⊙ Loss of sexual drive
⊙ Stress fractures
⊙ Memory loss or poor concentration
⊙ Low blood pressure or heart rate
⊙ Heart palpitations
⊙ Fatigue

⊙ Inability to tolerate cold
⊙ Insomnia
⊙ Depression and/or anxiety
⊙ Poor healing
⊙ Reoccurring or frequent respiratory infections
⊙ Signs of frequent vomiting (e.g., swollen salivary glands, severe tooth erosion)

DETERMINING YOUR ENERGY NEEDS

In order to prevent the sequela of chronic low energy intake (especially if you expend more energy than the average person), it's important to have an idea of how much energy you burn from day to day. How exactly would you go about figuring that out? Unfortunately, the most accurate methods of measuring energy expenditure are impractical, expensive, and mainly used in meticulous research studies. In reality, there are no exceptionally accurate, practical ways of measuring energy outputs in the real world. That being said, you could try a few different approaches to get a ballpark approximation of your energy needs.

The first approach is to purchase a wearable monitor that provides estimates of energy expenditure. Companies like Fitbit, Apple, Garmin, and Tanita make these devices, which are typically worn on the wrist, at the hip, or around the chest. The estimates generated by these monitors correlate pretty well with research-grade methods, but they still often end up being off by a few hundred kilocalories or more.[12] As a rule of thumb, they are more likely to underestimate than overestimate energy expenditure. Also, the estimates are more inaccurate when you do a lot of physical activities other than straight walking or running. Examples include weight lifting, climbing stairs, yardwork (digging holes, raking, etc.), and swimming.

The second approach is to track all your activities using a website or smartphone app such as MyFitnessPal, Lose It!, or Cronometer. The key to getting a semiaccurate estimate from these sources is making sure to log every activity you do for 24 hours, whether it is watching TV, snoozing, or chopping wood like a lumberjack. At the same time, it's also critical that you don't overreport the time you spend exercising and doing other physical activities. For example, if you went to the gym for an hour but only spent 20 minutes of that hour actually lifting weights, you should log that as 20 minutes of weight lifting, not 60 minutes. Not surprisingly, most people overestimate the time they spend doing all sorts of activities, including housework, childcare, and walking; consequently, estimates derived from this method are often higher (sometimes grossly so) than the real values.

The final (and most crude) approach to estimating energy expenditure involves determining your resting metabolic rate (RMR) and multiplying it by a standard activity factor. You could contact your local university's exercise science or nutrition department or a dietitian to see if they offer RMR testing, or you could use a published equation to estimate it. There are many equations available, but one that tends to be fairly accurate is the Mifflin-St. Jeor equation, shown here for each gender:

MALES
(10 × weight in kilograms) + (6.25 × height in centimeters) – (5 × age in years) + 5

FEMALES
(10 × weight in kilograms) + (6.25 × height in centimeters) – (5 × age in years) – 161

Once you determine your RMR, multiply that number by the most appropriate activity factor in Table 3.2 to obtain your projected daily energy expenditure.

One obvious shortcoming of this method is that the activity descriptions have relative meanings. Very high physical activity might be an hour of exercise for the average person, whereas it might be several hours for an athlete. For example, if an ultrarunner took his estimated RMR (say 1,800 kcal) and multiplied it by the factor for very high physical activity (2.0), he would get an estimated expenditure of 3,600 kcal. While that seems like a lot of energy to burn through, on a day that he trains 3–4 hours, his real energy expenditure is probably 4,000–5,000 kcal.

The fact that these methods have some inaccuracies doesn't mean they're completely useless. What it does mean is that it isn't feasible to measure your energy needs with 100 percent certainty. Instead, figuring out if you're chronically underconsuming energy is best achieved through a multipronged approach that includes an assessment of your energy intake and expenditure over several days, tracking your weight over weeks and months, and monitoring for the signs and symptoms of disordered eating.

table 3.2. **TOTAL DAILY ENERGY NEEDS**

ACTIVITY FACTOR	DESCRIPTION	EXAMPLE
1.2	Little to no physical activity	Sitting all day
1.4	Light physical activity	30 to 60 minutes of walking plus some housework
1.6	Moderate physical activity	60 to 90 minutes of walking plus some housework
1.8	High physical activity	60 minutes of jogging or playing soccer
2.0	Very high physical activity	90 minutes of jogging or playing soccer

A rough estimate of your total daily energy needs can be estimated by multiplying your RMR by the physical activity factors in the left column.

SUMMARY

ENERGY

Your **total energy requirements** depend primarily on your resting metabolic rate (RMR) and how much energy your burn during physical activities.

Most people expend 2,000–3,000 kcal daily, whereas athletes can burn **two to five times as much** in a single day.

Although difficult to assess accurately, estimates of your energy needs can help ensure that you're not **chronically underconsuming** energy.

Over the long run, **consuming energy below your body's needs** increases your chances of experiencing several gut symptoms (bloating, premature or excessive fullness, nausea, stomach pain, and constipation).

Severe energy restriction may induce these symptoms by impairing stomach emptying, reducing gut motility, and prolonging gut transit time.

Athletes who require large energy intakes (more than 4,000 kcal per day) can **sometimes experience gut discomfor**t if they try to meet 100 percent of their needs by eating foods that have low-energy densities; they may benefit from periodically eating more energy-dense foods like oils, nuts, seeds, sports recovery beverages, and higher-fat dairy products.

CARBOHYDRATE

Most athletes know ingesting carbohydrate can improve performance under the right circumstances. It's no coincidence that carbohydrate-containing drinks and supplements are a ubiquitous presence on the sidelines of sporting events and at endurance-race aid stations. Decades' worth of well-controlled studies support the notion that consuming carbohydrate during intense, prolonged exercise—whether it's from a "scientifically formulated" sports beverage or a handful of candy—can help delay the onset of fatigue.[1]

At the same time, ingesting food during intense exercise (even in the form of easily digested carbohydrates) represents a challenge to your gut. Many a seasoned athlete has had an important race or contest ruined by an aggressive or poorly planned nutrition strategy. In some of these cases, overingestion of carbohydrate—or eating the wrong type of carbohydrate—is the root cause. Clearly, there's a delicate balance when it comes to selecting the optimal amount of carbohydrate to ingest during exercise, a happy medium that exists somewhere between the extremes of consuming too little, leading to a bonk, and consuming too much, sending you straight to the roadside privy. Before we discuss finding this delicate balance, it's worth briefly reviewing the reasons carbohydrate is often touted as the champion of fuels during exercise.

FUELS BURNED DURING EXERCISE

When it comes to supplying the ATP needed to sustain exercise, two fuels reign supreme: carbohydrate and fat. During a mile race, an Ironman, a soccer match, or any other event that lasts more than a minute, you're continuously breathing in oxygen and transporting it throughout your body to convert that avocado, fancy sports beverage, or plate of pasta into ATP. It's this conversion of foodstuffs into mechanically useful energy that allows you to power your limbs, so you can run, bike, paddle, or swim, not to mention keep your vital organs functioning. Carbohydrate and fat burning are by far the most important sources of ATP production for the majority of athletic endeavors lasting longer than a couple of minutes.

Of these two fuels, the amount of carbohydrate stored in your body—known as glycogen—is much more limited. To put it into perspective, even super-lean athletes usually have a few days' worth of fat stores to burn through before they risk running dry during exercise. Think of your capacity to store carbohydrate as a gas tank on a small car that holds 10–15 gallons of fuel and your capacity to store fat as gas tanks on a big rig that hold 150–300 gallons of fuel. The actual amount of glycogen a person stores varies with body size and diet, but an average person (150 to 175 pounds) might store 400–500 grams (1,600–2,000 kcal) of glycogen, mostly in their muscles and liver. In contrast, an athlete weighing 150 pounds (68 kilograms) with 10 percent body fat stores roughly 6,800 grams of fat (about 61,000 kcal). I'll say it again. That's 400 grams of carbohydrate versus 6,800 grams of fat. To take this illustration even further, a person weighing 300 pounds (136 kilograms) with a body fat of 50 percent has 68,000 grams of fat (over 600,000 kcal) stored away!

Given the body's capacity to store massive quantities of fat, why don't we exclusively rely on it to power all forms of exercise? The short answer is that fat burning is limited by one or more steps in the chain of events responsible for converting a fatty acid molecule into mechanical energy. This relative inability to burn fat becomes more pronounced as exercise intensity increases. Research by many independent scientists has shown that, on average, fat burning supplies half of the energy needed to power exercise at about 60 percent of VO_2max (see Figure 4.1). As exercise intensity hits 80–90 percent of VO_2max, fat burning typically contributes to 10 percent or less of energy production.[2, 3] Eating a high-fat diet would allow an athlete to burn more fat at these higher intensities, but it would by no means completely abolish the need for carbohydrate burning during intense exercise.

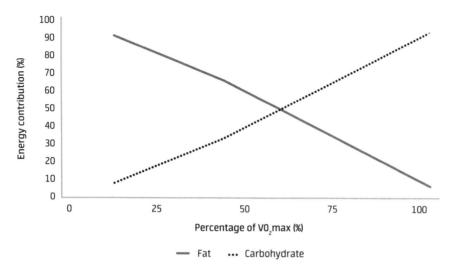

figure 4.1. **FUEL USE DURING EXERCISE**

As exercise intensity increases, the relative contribution of fat to energy production declines and carbohydrate utilization ramps up.

Although scientists continue to debate what's behind this fat-burning limit, the balance of evidence points to the transport of fatty acids into the power plants of our cells: the mitochondria. These incredible organelles are where fatty acids are oxidized for energy. But before this can happen, they must first be transported deep inside the mitochondria, which happens with the help of the molecule carnitine and several enzymes. High-intensity exercise (e.g., 200-meter dash, 60-second hockey shift) is believed to directly slow the mitochondrial transport of fatty acids, possibly through a reduction in free carnitine availability.[4] Regardless of the true cause, it's clear that burning fat alone cannot provide ATP fast enough to supply all the energy needed for high-intensity exercise.

Given the limits to carbohydrate storage—and its well-documented importance for fueling high-intensity exercise—it's no surprise that most dietitians tell serious athletes to pay close attention to the amount of carbohydrate they eat. **Athletes training at high volumes require somewhere between 2 grams and 5 grams of carbohydrate per pound of body weight for the whole day to maintain muscle glycogen stores.**[1] (This carbohydrate range roughly corresponds to one to four hours of moderate-to-intense exercise in

table 4.1. **EXAMPLE OF DAILY CARBOHYDRATE NEEDS**

	FOODS	CARBOHYDRATE CONTENT (g)
Breakfast	1 large bagel	50
	16 ounces orange juice	45
	1 large banana	30
Snack 1	12 ounces sweetened yogurt	60
	1 cup pineapple chunks	30
Lunch	1½ cups cooked white rice	65
	16 ounces lemonade	70
Snack 2	2 sports gels	50
	12 ounces fat-free milk	15
Dinner	1 cup pasta	45
	½ cup tomato sauce	15
	1 apple	25
	¼ cup raisins	30
	12 ounces beer	15
Snack 3	2 slices white toast	30
	2 Tbsp. jam	25

This sample menu shows the amounts and sources of carbohydrate that a 150-pound athlete would need to consume in order to replenish glycogen stores on a day when they train for two to three hours at a moderate to high intensity.

a day.) Table 4.1 provides an example of the amounts and sources of carbohydrate that a 150-pound athlete would need to eat to achieve an intake of 4 grams of carbohydrate per pound of body weight, which is an appropriate amount to fuel a training day that involves two to three hours of moderate-to-high-intensity training.

Even though this menu represents a hefty amount of carbohydrate in comparison to what the average person eats daily, athletes competing in extreme events are known to consume even more. As an example, four-time Tour de France champion Chris Froome reportedly consumed 1.3 kilograms of carbohydrate on the day of stage 19 of the 2018 Giro d'Italia,[5] and based on a reported weight of roughly 152 pounds, that calculates out to about 8.6 grams of carbohydrate for every pound of Chris Froome.

RECOMMENDATIONS FOR CARBOHYDRATE DURING EXERCISE

I've tried to make it clear that athletes engaging in intense training for an hour or more each day benefit from additional carbohydrate in their diets. This allows them to maintain muscle glycogen stores and sustain periods of vigorous training without fatiguing mentally and physically. Beyond ensuring they consume enough carbohydrate each day, how much carbohydrate should athletes be consuming during exercise itself? Unfortunately, there's not a straightforward recommendation that will fit every situation, as an athlete's needs depend on a range of factors.

Perhaps the two most important factors dictating during-exercise carbohydrate intake recommendations are exercise intensity and duration. As covered in Part 1, exercise intensity has a profound effect on the physiology of your gut. As intensity amps up, blood is shunted away from your gut to meet the oxygen demand imposed by your muscles. A simple way to think about this phenomenon is that your body only has so much blood to go around, and during intense exercise the priority isn't digesting what you ate for breakfast. This makes sense from an evolutionary perspective, given that, you know, outrunning a predator or fighting a serious threat was important for survival. Simply put, it's difficult for your gut to tolerate much of any ingesta during very intense exercise (e.g., greater than 90 percent of VO_2max).

The fatigue that develops while exercising continuously at these very high intensities results less from carbohydrate depletion and more from reductions in central nervous system firing, disturbances in acid-base balance, and impairments in calcium release in the muscle.[6] Long story short, carbohydrate consumption is unlikely to boost performance or delay fatigue when exercise lasts less than one hour. During exercise lasting more than 60–90 minutes, stores of glycogen begin to run out, or at least run low, and it's in these situations that eating carbohydrate becomes advantageous.

Although ingesting carbohydrate during a 30-to-60-minute game or race is unlikely to enhance your endurance, there's one carbohydrate-based strategy that has the potential to improve your performance in these situations. Emerging science over the past decade has shown that simply rinsing a carbohydrate beverage in your mouth for 5–10 seconds, followed by spitting it out, can improve power output or running speed during exercise tasks lasting roughly 30–60 minutes.[7] It's believed that swishing a carbohydrate drink tricks your body into thinking that additional fuel is on its way, thereby

activating brain regions that are involved in motor control and the regulation of fatigue.[8, 9] An athlete interested in this strategy can try swishing a carbohydrate drink for 5–10 seconds immediately before and every 10–15 minutes during exercise. Most popular sports drinks will do, but even a homemade concoction consisting of 6–10 grams of table sugar for every 100 milliliters of water should work. One final note about carbohydrate mouth rinsing is that it seems to be most effective if you haven't eaten for 8–12 hours.

In contrast to brief bouts of exercise, glycogen depletion and low blood glucose become likely causes of fatigue as exercise duration extends beyond an hour. With that in mind, how should you go about planning your carbohydrate intake for prolonged competition? First, it's important to recognize that because the average intensity for these events is somewhat lower, most competitors can comfortably stomach larger amounts of carbohydrate. Organizations like the American College of Sports Medicine recommend that individuals consume between 30 and 90 grams of carbohydrate per hour during exercise that lasts longer than one hour,[1] and the variation in feeding rates—from a low of 30 grams to a high of 90 grams—is due to the fact that feeding tolerance increases in parallel with exercise duration. Specifically, most athletes can tolerate 30–60 grams of carbohydrate per hour during exercise that lasts from one to two and a half hours, while some can handle up to 90 grams per hour when exercise lasts longer than two and a half hours.

A quick calculation tells us that 90 grams of carbohydrate equates to about three large bananas or four sports gels, clearly not a protocol meant for those with temperamental stomachs. If you tried to meet that 90-gram target with just a standard sports beverage (Gatorade, Powerade, etc.), you'd have to drink 1.5 liters every hour. Since the majority of athletes' fluid intakes during endurance contests and intermittent sports are between 0.3 and 0.6 liters per hour, most athletes who attempt to consume a lot of carbohydrate end up ingesting carbohydrate-rich foods along with smaller volumes of fluid. This mixing of carbohydrate foods with smaller volumes of fluid allows them to avoid the disastrous stomach discomfort that would come with consuming 1.5 liters of a sports drink every hour.

Chad Haga, an American cyclist who has competed in all three Grand Tours, told me in an interview that he targets 90 grams of carbohydrate per hour from a combination of fluids, bars, and gels. He also said, "That's adaptable, though. If I'm hungry, I'll eat more, or if it's super-hot and solids aren't appetizing, I'll do more bottles and gels." Haga recognizes that fueling during competition is, to some extent, situation and environment specific. Regardless of whether you lean more on solid foods or sports drinks to meet your needs, you should repeatedly practice your plan before attempting to deploy it during an actual race or competition, particularly if you're planning to consume carbohydrate on the higher end of the range.

One important caveat to these recommendations is that they're really meant for athletes pushing the boundaries of what their bodies can do. If you're running a marathon and are simply trying to finish the race by walking and jogging, by no means do you need to consume 60–90 grams of carbohydrate every hour. If you're more of a middle-of-the-pack runner, you can experiment with consuming more modest amounts of carbohydrate (e.g., 30–45 grams per hour) to see how your body responds.

SUGAR TYPE

Sugar is a term used to describe simple carbohydrates—those made of only one or two carbohydrate molecules. In chemical-speak, these simple sugars are referred to as monosaccharides and disaccharides. Monosaccharides include glucose, fructose, and galactose, and these sugars join with one another to form disaccharides, which include sucrose (table sugar), lactose (milk sugar), and maltose (found in beer, among other foods). Long-chain carbohydrates are made of strands of glucoses bound together, forming polysaccharides, such as starch and maltodextrin.

While the basic process of digestion for all carbohydrates is similar, subtle nuances in how they're absorbed and metabolized have important implications for certain athletes. Differences in the absorption and metabolism of two sugars, glucose and fructose, are the most consequential. Glucose is the carbohydrate that circulates at the highest concentrations in your blood and serves as a fuel for your nervous system and brain. Much of the glucose in your diet starts as starch or is bound to another monosaccharide, like fructose or galactose. As I covered in Chapter 1, the process of digesting starch and other long-chain forms of glucose begins in your mouth with salivary amylase. Once you swallow, carbohydrate digestion comes to a screeching halt in the acidic environment of your stomach. Later, amylase from your pancreas reinitiates the digestion of long-chain carbohydrates in your small intestine. Eventually, short-chain carbohydrates consisting of two or slightly more glucose units remain, which are eventually split into individual glucose molecules at the brush border.

Before glucose molecules can circulate in your blood, they need to first pass through the metaphorical castle wall that is the outer layer of cells lining your intestines. The cells that make up this layer are double-sided, consisting of an outer part known as the apical membrane (a.k.a. brush border) and an inner part known as the basolateral membrane. Much like a castle with two walls, an important function of your intestinal cells is to keep foreign invaders (i.e., pathogens) out while simultaneously providing a way to let in much-needed supplies. Transporters that function like doors are responsible for allowing the passage of sugars through the apical membrane (the outer castle wall) and into your intestinal cells.

In scientific jargon, the door used for shuttling glucose through the apical membrane is the sodium-glucose linked transporter 1 (SGLT1).[10] Dietary fructose—which is found primarily in fruit, as a part of sucrose, or in high-fructose corn syrup—also relies on a transport system for absorption. Fructose uses a door known as GLUT5. While these differences in absorption might seem trivial, they can impact not only gut tolerance during endurance exercise but also race performance. Ultimately, both SGLT1 (the glucose door) and GLUT5 (the fructose door) have limits in terms of how much carbohydrate they let into your intestinal cells.

A simple analogy to understand this concept is an off-ramp for the interstate. As you've undoubtedly experienced, the speed at which cars can exit the interstate using an off-ramp is inherently limited, and just as traffic backs up when too many cars try to get off the interstate during rush hour, ingesting too much carbohydrate causes a backup of sugar in your lumen. This accumulation of carbohydrate in the lumen can manifest

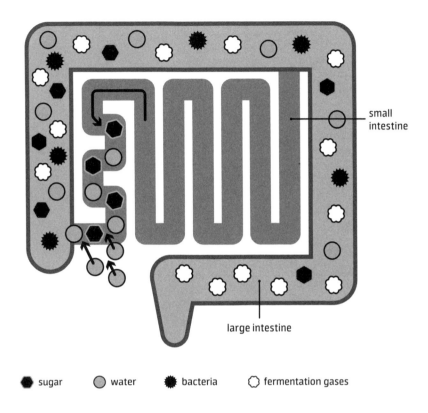

figure 4.2. **CARBOHYDRATE MALABSORPTION**

When carbohydrate molecules go unabsorbed in the small intestine, they drag water into the intestinal lumen and end up in the colon, where they get fermented by bacteria. Bloating, flatulence, and loose stools can ensue.

as bloating, abdominal cramps, flatulence, and diarrhea.[11] As shown in Figure 4.2, these symptoms arise because unabsorbed carbohydrate molecules cause fluid to shift from your blood into your lumen, leading to abdominal cramping and diarrhea. Some of this unabsorbed carbohydrate is fermented by bacteria, leading to gas production, bloating, and flatulence.

Fortunately, you can combat this problem of limited capacity for absorption by ingesting a mixture of fructose and glucose. To return to our interstate analogy, ingesting glucose and fructose together is like opening additional off-ramps. SGLT1 has an absorptive capacity of about 50–60 grams of glucose per hour, while GLUT5 can handle somewhere around 30–40 grams of fructose per hour.[11] If we add those capacities together, a total of about 90 grams per hour emerges, which, if you recall from our discussion of the guidelines from the American College of Sports Medicine, is the maximum amount of carbohydrate recommended for exercise lasting two and a half hours or longer.

Based on an abundance of research, we can say with confidence that consuming glucose-fructose mixtures during prolonged exercise lessens gut symptoms in comparison to consuming an equal amount of either glucose or fructose alone.[11] However, there are several important caveats to this statement. The first—and most important—is that this strategy only influences gut tolerance if someone is aggressively consuming carbohydrate. If you only consume 30–40 grams per hour (which is likely during one-to-two-hour events), then your absorptive limits for SGLT1 and GLUT5 won't be reached. This is why ingestion of glucose-fructose mixtures is most relevant for relatively intense exercise that lasts two to three hours or longer.

A final qualifying comment about this strategy is that the majority of studies have been conducted using cyclists. Studying this strategy separately in runners (and in other athletes) is important because it's naturally easier to consume more carbohydrate while cycling. During running, the mechanical jostling created with each foot strike puts extra stress on your gut, making food and fluid intake a delicate dance, and this is part of the reason runners usually eat less during races. Consequently, it's more difficult for runners to achieve the carbohydrate intake levels necessary to see benefits of glucose-fructose co-ingestion. Even so, research I conducted while earning my PhD seemed to confirm the benefits of glucose-fructose co-ingestion when runners consume more than 60 grams of carbohydrate per hour.[12] After running for two hours at roughly 65 percent of their VO_2max, runners were able to finish a 4-mile time trial roughly 2 percent faster when they ingested a glucose-fructose beverage in comparison to when they ingested a 100 percent glucose beverage. In addition, gut symptoms tended to be less severe when they consumed the beverage that contained both glucose and fructose.

Any runner thinking of using this strategy would be wise to practice it during training runs. You would have to eat almost 3.5 medium-sized bananas every hour in order to achieve a carbohydrate intake of 90 grams per hour, and that's obviously not something you want to try for the first time during an important race. That said, one of the world's best marathoners serves as a firsthand example that it's possible to consume upward of 90–100 grams of carbohydrate per hour if you use glucose-fructose sources. During his 2:01:39 world record–setting 2018 Berlin Marathon, Eliud Kipchoge reportedly consumed in the neighborhood of 100 grams of carbohydrate per hour, mostly from a combination of maltodextrin-fructose-containing products made by Swedish company Maurten.[13] (Note: Maltodextrin is a long-chain form of glucose.)

SIMPLE SUGARS VERSUS LONG-CHAIN CARBOHYDRATES

Another issue to discuss related to carbohydrate source is the impact that molecule size has on digestion. When mixed into fluids, large carbohydrate molecules like maltodextrin result in a lower beverage osmolality in comparison to using monosaccharides and disaccharides. Recall from Chapter 1 that osmolality is just jargon for the concentration of dissolved particles in a solution, and when it comes to fluid absorption, beverages that have an osmolality just at or slightly below that of blood usually get absorbed fastest. This is partly because osmolality influences how fast beverages empty from your stomach, particularly when you consume concentrated carbohydrate drinks (greater than 10 percent carbohydrate by weight). When hypertonic beverages (beverages with osmolalities higher than your blood plasma) empty into your duodenum, they stimulate sensory tissue there, which slows emptying from your stomach. Because maltodextrin contains glucose molecules linked together instead of individual molecules, it results in a lower osmolality when it's mixed into a solution. Practically speaking, you may be less likely to experience gastrointestinal issues if you choose a product with maltodextrin as the main carbohydrate when you're planning to consume a beverage with a 10 percent or higher concentration of carbohydrate. However, if you're consuming a solution with a more typical carbohydrate concentration, say 4–8 percent, then the benefits of maltodextrin are probably negligible.[14]

CARBOHYDRATE FORM: SOLID, GEL, OR LIQUID?

One common question that athletes have about choosing a carbohydrate source is whether they should go with a solid, a liquid, or something in between, like a gel. Studies have attempted to delineate whether there are differences in gut and metabolic responses when ingesting different forms of carbohydrate, and overall, bars and gels seem to elicit worse gastrointestinal symptoms than beverages, with bars being the most consistent offenders.[15-17] The reason bars cause more problems isn't 100 percent clear, but it may have to do with the average particle size of a food. Some studies have shown that blending solid foods, or asking people to chew foods longer, accelerates the gastric emptying of those foods,[18-20] and we've discussed at length that faster stomach emptying generally equates to fewer upper gut issues. **The less severe gut symptoms with carbohydrate drink and gel ingestion may be due to their being relatively homogenized, easlily digestible products.**

Despite some differences in gut tolerance, solid, liquid, and gel carbohydrate foods usually lead to fairly comparable metabolic responses (e.g., blood glucose levels and carbohydrate burning). Like most nutrition strategies, athletes often differ with respect to how they respond to specific carbohydrate-containing products, so if you know through experience that bars don't cause your stomach any trouble, then by all means go with whatever option fits your race plan. Considerations like convenience, portability, and taste all factor into the equation. Just remember that if you choose a sports bars for the first time during a race, it might be worth your while to spend an extra 15 seconds chewing before swallowing.

WHAT ABOUT HYDROGEL TECHNOLOGY?

There has been an interesting development in the sports nutrition industry in the last few years. I mentioned earlier that during his world-record Berlin Marathon, Eliud Kipchoge used products made by Swedish company Maurten (consuming an impressive 100 grams of carbohydrate per hour). Interestingly, Maurten advertises that their products are based on hydrogel technology, which basically means the carbohydrate is encapsulated in a gel-like substance in the stomach after coming into contact with hydrochloric acid. Even the carbohydrate in their drink mixes converts to a hydrogel in the stomach, and supposedly this encapsulated hydrogel allows carbohydrate to pass into the duodenum without activating sensory tissue. Recall that activation of this sensory tissue can retard stomach emptying, and some preliminary data suggest that carbohydrate hydrogel beverages empty faster from the stomach than regular carbohydrate solutions, at least at rest.[21]

While there are certainly anecdotes of athletes tolerating higher rates of carbohydrate ingestion when using these hydrogel products, we're still awaiting results from experiments evaluating their impact on gut symptoms and performance. One of the only studies published to date failed to find any metabolic, gastrointestinal, or performance benefits during three hours of running when runners ingested a hydrogel-based carbohydrate beverage in comparison to a standard carbohydrate beverage.[22]

REVIEW OF RECOMMENDATIONS FOR CARBOHYDRATE DURING EXERCISE

Take a look at Figure 4.3 for a summary of carbohydrate recommendations based on the anticipated duration of exercise. In addition, keep in mind the following points when deciding how much carbohydrate to consume:

- These recommendations apply to situations where you're exercising at a moderate intensity or higher, and when peak performance is important.
- There are often substantial differences in how different athletes respond to the same feeding strategy.
- Trial and error should be used to determine individual tolerance to a particular ingestion protocol.
- If you do plan to consume lots of carbohydrate (more than 50 grams per hour) during competition, it's especially important to practice this strategy during training.
- Although the American College of Sports Medicine states that glucose-fructose mixtures are useful for competitions that last longer than two and a half hours, there are also situations where they could be advantageous for events lasting one and a half to two hours.

101

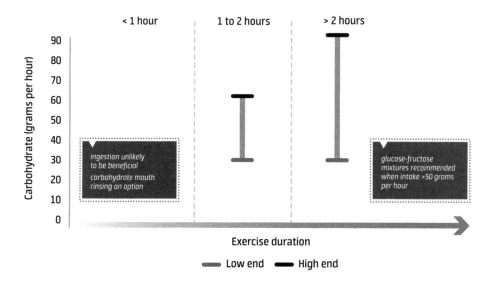

figure 4.3. **CARBOHYDRATE CONSUMPTION DURING EXERCISE**

Recommendations for ingesting carbohydrate during exercise largely depend on exercise duration and intensity, ranging from no intake to up to about 90 grams per hour during prolonged, relatively intense events.

CARBOHYDRATE AND GASTROINTESTINAL INTEGRITY

There's overwhelming evidence that consuming carbohydrate during intense, prolonged exercise delays fatigue. However, that's not the only upside of consuming carbohydrate in these situations. Another potential advantage of downing a sports drink, a sports gel, or some dried fruit—particularly when running in the heat—is the prevention of gastrointestinal cellular injury. Remember, prolonged exercise compromises gut blood flow, leading to reductions in oxygen delivery and other perturbations that impair the internal machinery of gut cells. What's more, heat exposure exacerbates this problem by causing a redirection of blood to the peripheral areas of your body, namely your skin, to cool you off. This response helps you dissipate heat by bringing warm blood closer to the surface of your body and by increasing sweating. While this can keep your body temperature in check, the diminished blood flow to your gut leads to a loosening of the tight junctions that normally keep your intestinal cells together. As a result, large molecules that are usually kept out of your body can seep through these widening cracks (see Figure 4.4); the more consequential of these molecules are the endotoxins discussed in Chapter 2. Once endotoxins invade your body, they're identified and targeted by the immune system, ultimately causing the release of inflammatory molecules that raise core body temperature. Indeed, endotoxemia (high levels of endotoxins in the blood) may partly be responsible for the development of exercise-related heat illnesses.[23]

A little bit of gut leakiness is probably inevitable during prolonged exercise. Still, there are nutritional interventions you can employ to minimize gut leakiness and the likelihood of endotoxemia. Fluid and carbohydrate ingestion during exercise blunt the passage of large molecules through the intestinal barrier,[24, 25] though some evidence indicates that adding carbohydrate to a beverage is superior to plain water alone.[26] Ingesting fluid helps maintain your blood volume, which is critical for sustaining adequate blood flow to your gut as well as to the peripheral parts of your body during heat stress. Carbohydrate ingestion likely prevents gut leakage by stimulating blood flow to your gut and by providing a fuel source for intestinal cells. Notably, protein and fat feedings also stimulate gut blood flow[27] and may prevent gut leakiness during

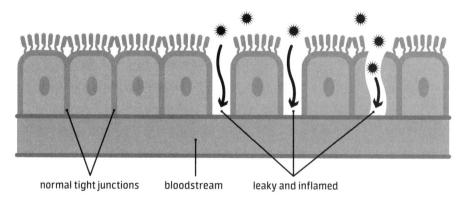

normal tight junctions   bloodstream   leaky and inflamed

✹ endotoxin

figure 4.4. **LEAKY GUT**

Intense and prolonged exercise can loosen the tight junctions that normally characterize the spaces between the gut's epithelial cells, leading to the passage of endotoxins into the body and triggering an inflammatory response.

exercise;[25] however, it makes more sense to go with carbohydrate injestion because, under normal circumstances, protein isn't a primary fuel source for muscles, and fat isn't quickly digested during exercise. In terms of dosage, studies showing reductions in gut permeability have fed subjects 40–60 grams of carbohydrate per hour.

FODMAPs

FODMAPs (short for fermentable oligosaccharides, disaccharides, monosaccharides, and polyols) have received increasing attention from the sports and fitness media in recent years. The headline of a 2017 *Runner's World* story, for example, posed the question, "Can avoiding FODMAPs solve your running-induced GI problems?" Even though the moniker seems somewhat indecipherable, FODMAPs are just short-chain carbohydrates that, if left unabsorbed, are fermented by bacteria in your gut. End products of this fermentation include short-chain fatty acids and gases such as hydrogen and methane. Fermentation of these carbohydrates as well as of fiber is generally thought to be a good thing for microbe diversity in the gut; however, if excess gas is produced from this fermentation of FODMAPs, bloating and flatulence become prevalent and can lead to a feeling of general unpleasantness. And in contrast to fiber, these short-chain carbohydrates are more likely to cause watery or loose stools if they go unabsorbed. Years' worth of research on people living with IBS demonstrates that FODMAPs play a role in the burden of the disease and that low-FODMAP diets can reduce symptoms.[28]

Given the prevalence of bowel issues in athletes and that restricting FODMAP intake can calm gut symptoms in people with IBS, it makes sense that researchers would test the effectiveness of low-FODMAP diets in athletes. Yet surprisingly, scarce research on this topic has been carried out in athletes. One simple reason for this dearth of research is that a low-FODMAP diet can be very challenging to adhere to. If you search the internet for examples of FODMAP-restricted diets, you'll quickly learn that almost every food group (with the exception of meats and oils) includes numerous examples of FODMAP-laden foods. Certain fruits, vegetables, dairy products, grains, legumes, and sweeteners contain FODMAPs, and this lack of intuitive predictability as to what foods are rich in FODMAPs makes restricting them time- and work-intensive. (See Table 4.2 for example foods that are high or low in FODMAPs.)

table 4.2. **FODMAPs**

FOOD GROUP	FOODS HIGH IN FODMAPs	FOODS LOW IN FODMAPs
Fruits	Apples, apricots, blackberries, cherries, dates, pears, plums, peaches, mango, and watermelon	Raspberries, strawberries, grapes, pineapple, and kiwi fruit
Vegetables	Onions, cabbage, asparagus, artichoke, and mushrooms	Cucumber, kale, lettuce, green beans, carrots, and tomatoes
Dairy	Cow's milk, yogurt, kefir, soft cheeses, sour cream, and ice cream	Almond milk, soy milk, and hard cheeses
Grains/starches	Products containing wheat, barley, and rye	Oats, corn flakes, rice, and quinoa
Nuts and legumes	Chickpeas, kidney beans, lentils, soybeans, and pistachios	Peanuts and walnuts
Sweeteners	Agave, honey, mannitol, sorbitol, xylitol, fructose, and high-fructose corn syrup	Table sugar, maple syrup, dextrose, and rice malt syrup

These are examples of selected foods that are high or low in FODMAPs.

So what does the limited research on low-FODMAP diets in athletes say about their effectiveness? On the positive side, a few studies have found that recreational runners obtained some gut symptom relief after following a low-FODMAP diet.[29-31] That said, one of the studies didn't completely equate total carbohydrate and fiber intakes between high- and low-FODMAP diets,[29] while another found a reduction in daily gut symptoms without a reduction in symptoms during exercise.[30] The most promising results come from a trial published in 2019 showing that a 24-hour low-FODMAP diet somewhat lessened the severity of GI symptoms during two hours of moderate-intensity running in the heat.[31] Although it's a promising strategy, the overall scarcity of research means it's too early to say just how useful it is for reducing gut symptoms in athletes across a broad range of competition scenarios. Further, it's not clear that a low-FODMAP diet will help stave off something like the severe nausea or abdominal cramping that runners sometimes experience near the end of a race. That said, athletes who are consuming large amounts of FODMAPs (greater than 20–30 grams per day) could potentially benefit from restricting some of these carbohydrates. While most standard diet-tracking software programs don't provide estimates of FODMAP intakes, researchers from Monash University in Australia have developed an app (Monash University FODMAP Diet) that can be used to determine the FODMAP contents of foods.

If you ever decide to try a low-FODMAP diet, keep in mind that it's unclear what the long-term health implications are. Restricting FODMAPs changes the composition of the gut microbiome,[32] and these alterations could, in theory, affect long-term health because the diversity of gut microorganisms is associated with a range of diseases. One way around this issue is to temporarily follow a low-FODMAP diet just before competition, as opposed to eating that way all the time. Another workaround is to just cut out lactose and/or fructose, as there is some reason to think that both of these sugars (but particularly lactose) are the primary contributors to gut symptoms in athletes.

Notably, restricting fructose and lactose (or even just one of them) in the diet is a heck of a lot simpler to follow than a low-FODMAP diet. This is the type of approach that Dutch cyclist Tom Dumoulin tried after being plagued by gut problems during the 2017 Giro d'Italia. While he was wearing the pink jersey during stage 16, Dumoulin made a pit stop on the side of the road in order to answer the call of nature, costing him minutes of precious time. Months after the race, Dumoulin revealed that excessive fructose and lactose intakes were possible culprits for his gut issues.

FIBER

Different definitions of dietary fiber abound, though most indicate that fiber is an edible component of food that's resistant to digestion by humans. While these definitions don't always explicitly say so, most fibers are considered carbohydrates. You don't have the requisite enzymes needed to break apart the bonds holding carbohydrate fibers together, but bacteria residing in your gut can ferment at least some of this roughage. This fermentation—and its associated production of methane, hydrogen, and carbon dioxide—is responsible for fiber's well-known flatulence-inducing effects. According to the Institute of Medicine, most adults should consume between 25 and 38 grams of fiber every day, with the lower recommendation for women and the higher recommendation for men.[33] Recent representative surveys report that the average adult American falls well short of these recommendations, coming in at about 16 grams per day.[34]

When it comes to managing gut symptoms in athletes, fiber can have both positive and negative effects, depending on the situation, individual athlete, type of fiber, and timing of intake. Let's begin with fiber eaten during and around the time of competition. Consuming fiber—especially viscous fiber—slows emptying of the stomach's contents.[35] This is because viscous fiber interacts with water to form a gel-like substance that drains more slowly from the stomach, sort of what it's like when you pour cold maple syrup out of a bottle. Rich sources of viscous fiber include legumes, oats, apricots, and Brussels sprouts.

107

While pumping the brakes on stomach emptying may be advantageous for maintaining a sense of fullness and preventing a steep rise in blood glucose after a meal,[35] it isn't desirable in close proximity to exercise when the goal is to digest and absorb carbohydrate and fluid as speedily as possible. Hence, sports nutritionists have long advised athletes to avoid hefty doses of fiber in pre-competition meals, and recent guidelines from the American College of Sports Medicine state that, generally, foods with a low-fiber content "are the preferred choice for this pre-event menu because they are less prone to cause gastrointestinal problems and promote gastric emptying."[1]

Overall, eating more than 5–10 grams of fiber right before intense exercise, say, within 30 minutes, probably isn't a wise choice. Is it really necessary, however, to go super-low fiber when your last pre-exercise meal isn't in such proximity to competition? Surprisingly, little to no experimental evidence supports recommendations to avoid fiber in meals eaten two to four hours before competition. Although experiments in nonathletes show that viscous fiber slows stomach emptying at rest, it's highly doubtful that including moderate amounts of fiber in a pre-exercise meal will dramatically impact gut symptoms if said meal is eaten several hours before exercise. In addition, a handful of studies have demonstrated that endurance exercise capacity at moderate intensities is actually improved when some fiber is included in a pre-exercise meal,[36-38] which could be because fiber may prevent spikes in blood glucose and insulin at the onset of exercise.

Even though the picture on pre-exercise fiber ingestion is somewhat muddied, there's little reason to consume much fiber *during* heavy exercise. The potential for delayed stomach emptying, which would have dual effects of slowing nutrient delivery and increasing feelings of fullness, provides sufficient rationale for minimizing one's fiber consumption during a race or game. That being said, the potential downsides of fiber consumption are dependent on exercise duration, as athletes competing in prolonged endurance events (more than two to three hours) can generally tolerate more solid food and fiber. Indeed, surveys of participants from ultramarathons and ultratriathlons find that most competitors consume 1–2 grams of fiber every hour.[39, 40] At these relatively low intakes, no consistent correlations between fiber consumption and gut problems have been found.

Let's now turn our attention to how fiber could affect your health and performance over the long run. As mentioned previously, the Institute of Medicine recommends a daily fiber intake of 25 grams for women and 38 grams for men. These recommendations are based on large epidemiologic studies showing lower rates of cardiovascular disease among people who consume approximately 14 grams of fiber per 1,000 kcal of energy. (Since women generally require less dietary energy, their recommendations for fiber are lower.) There are several potential reasons as to why fiber may cut the risk of heart problems, the primary ones being that adequate fiber intake brings about modest reductions in LDL cholesterol and blood pressure.[33]

Besides potentially lowering the risk of cardiovascular disease, fiber also influences gut health. Experiments feeding individuals varying amounts of roughage clearly show stool weight increases with added fiber in the diet.[41] Whether bulkier stools are good or bad depends on the situation and what your goals are. If you typically have difficulty producing BMs, then yeah, upping your roughage intake may reduce your struggles in the privy. Indeed, trials feeding people additional fiber have shown modest improvements in stool frequency (more poos) and stool consistency (softer poos) among people with chronic constipation,[42] as well as reductions in symptoms among hemorrhoid sufferers.[43]

Some epidemiologic studies have found an inverse relationship between fiber intake and the risk of colon cancer, meaning the more fiber you eat, the lower your risk. Unfortunately, the associations seen in observational studies haven't been replicated in experiments. Several large trials in the early 2000s recruited individuals with colorectal adenomas (precursors to colon cancers) and had them increase fiber intake through whole foods or supplements.[44-46] After several years, reoccurrence rates of adenomas weren't lower among those getting extra fiber in comparison to people in control groups. It could be that looking at cancer precursors (instead of cancer occurrence itself) isn't ideal, that the interventions were too brief, or that the fiber dosages used were too small.

Regardless, the discrepancy between the epidemiological research and controlled experiments is a bit perplexing and suggests that fiber could play less of a role in protecting people from colon cancer than previously thought. Personally, I don't see much of a downside to eating lots of fiber, so the purported benefits on colon cancer risk (even if unconfirmed) are still worth considering.

Although diets rich in fiber likely have some health benefits, little is known about how long-term fiber intake affects gut function during exercise. A critical issue remaining to be addressed is whether athletes would benefit in terms of their performance (irrespective of health) by regularly eating loads of fiber. As much as I'd like to supply an answer to this question, there's no research directly addressing the issue. Diets high in fiber also tend to be rich in other plant compounds that have broad physiological properties, so while fiber per se seems unlikely to directly influence performance and recovery, it's plausible that diets rich in fiber from fruits, vegetables, and whole grains could improve certain aspects of athletic performance and/or recovery.

On the other hand, it's also conceivable that consuming an abundance of dietary fiber would increase the frequency and/or severity of symptoms like flatulence, bloating, and urges to defecate, which, if severe enough, could negatively impact performance. So if you have had trouble with these symptoms during competition in the past, you may want to consider tapering fiber intake prior to important competitions in order to avoid these issues. The time required for fiber to pass through the gut varies, but typically it takes anywhere from one to two days.[47] So athletes wishing to reduce gas and stool frequency might taper fiber in their diet starting three to four days before competition.

SUMMARY

CARBOHYDRATE

Carbohydrate is a **key fuel** you use to make ATP, particularly at exercise intensities above 60 percent of VO_2max.

Your body's **storage capacity** for carbohydrate is much more limited than it is for fat.

Depending on their training volume and intensity, most athletes should consume between **2 and 5 grams of carbohydrate** per pound of body weight each day, although extreme amounts of exercise may further raise carbohydrate need.

Contests and training sessions that last less than **one hour** don't usually benefit from carbohydrate consumption during exercise.

Carbohydrate rinsing may boost performance in competitions lasting 30–60 minutes, especially when you've fasted for several hours prior.

For intense exercise lasting one to two hours, **eating 30–60 grams** of carbohydrate per hour is recommended.

For relatively intense exercise lasting more than two hours, eating up to 90 grams of carbohydrate per hour may be tolerated if **glucose and fructose are consumed simultaneously**.

Restricting dietary FODMAPs might reduce gut symptoms in athletes who have a high FODMAP intake, although doing so for long periods of time may have unfavorable effects on the gut microbiome.

Limiting the intake of **lactose and/or fructose** is probably an easier approach to reducing gut symptoms than following a diet low in all FODMAPs.

Large doses of fiber (greater than 10 grams) should be avoided immediately before and during intense exercise because they slow stomach emptying.

Despite recommendations to choose low-fiber foods for pre-event meals, moderate intakes of fiber are **unlikely to cause major gut problems** if a meal is eaten more than two hours before exercise.

05

FAT

Perhaps nothing in the field of nutrition is more controversial than the recommendations surrounding dietary fat. How much of our diet should be fat? What kind of fat should we eat? From what foods should we get our dietary fat? These and other questions are on the minds of many people interested in improving their health through the foods they eat. And yet, even with the thousands of studies that have been conducted on dietary fat and health, there remains substantial disagreement among scientists and health practitioners about the answers to these questions. I should mention that there are a few points of agreement (e.g., trans fats raise the risk of heart diseases; omega-3 fat is essential; replacing fat with sugar and refined carbs isn't an improvement), but it's clear the scientific uncertainty has made much of the public vulnerable to the huckstering of self-proclaimed health gurus. Indeed, spend five minutes on the internet and you can find someone espousing the virtues of nearly every source of fat on the planet, from coconut oil to olive oil to bacon fat to butter.

This overwhelming array of opinions parallels a controversy in the field of sports nutrition, too. For many years, carbohydrate was considered the most important macronutrient for performance, especially for athletes doing prolonged endurance exercise. Over the past two decades, though, more and more studies have questioned whether this dogma is truly justified for all athletes and situations. Today, the overall evidence indicates that both high-carbohydrate and high-fat diets have their place in sports, but as with many subjects, our hyperpolarized world—partly driven by social media—has created entrenched camps of athletes and coaches who unwaveringly commit to high-fat diets even in situations where they may do more harm than good. Similarly, there are those who dismiss the potential of high-fat diets even though they may offer benefits in certain situations.

Ultimately, my goal with this chapter is to cut through some of this confusion and provide a balanced, scientifically informed perspective on the topic of dietary fat, athletic performance, and gut function. As you'll come to see, the utility of high-fat diets—like many nutrition strategies—is context specific. First, though, I will briefly review what the heck dietary fat is and how much of it the average person eats.

FAT DEFINED

The term *fat* is typically used to describe triglycerides, a type of lipid. A lack of chemical polarity prevents lipids from dissolving in polar substances like water, unless you have a third substance with both polar and nonpolar features (i.e., an emulsifier) to add to the mix. This poor solubility in polar substances such as water is the unifying feature of all lipids (triglycerides, cholesterol, phospholipids, etc.), which can otherwise have rather different functions in your body. Of these lipids, triglycerides are the type found most abundantly in the diet and the human body.

Dietary fat is what makes many of our favorite foods so palatable, and that's one reason food companies started adding sugar to many products during the height of the low-fat diet craze in the 1990s. When you remove fat from a food, it tastes like cardboard, and some extra sugar can go a long way toward keeping the food edible. For survival reasons, we probably evolved as a species to derive a certain pleasure from eating calorically dense foods, and at a whopping 9 kcal per gram, fat packs one heck of an energy punch.

Based on surveys that accurately reflect the American population, the average adult eats about 80 grams of fat each day (700 kcal's worth), an amount that's been fairly stable over the past four decades.[1] To give some context, that's about the amount of fat you'd find in 6 tablespoons of olive oil or almost an entire stick of butter. Bear in mind, though, the dietary fat requirements of athletes can differ greatly from those of the general public. For an ultrarunner who burns over 10,000 kcal on the day of a 100-mile race, eating the average American's 80-gram allotment of fat wouldn't even supply 10 percent of their energy needs. For these types of athletes, extra fat in the diet can be an efficient means of meeting energy demands without having to put away a mountain of food. That said, these athletes need to be cognizant of when fat-rich foods are eaten, because the timing of fat ingestion is key when it comes to preventing several gut symptoms during exercise, particularly those that impact the upper gut (nausea, fullness, reflux, etc.).

FAT CONSUMPTION BEFORE AND DURING EXERCISE

There are several reasons it's usually ill-advised to wolf down fatty foods just before and during exercise. Because we evolved to readily stockpile fat during periods of energy abundance (which is basically 100 percent of the time in today's developed world), there's no real risk of running out of fat stores during exercise. In addition, dietary fat tends to pump the brakes on gastric emptying more than protein and carbohydrate, in large part because fat is such an energy-dense nutrient. As a rule of thumb, the more energy-dense a food is, the longer it takes to leave your stomach. Notably, protein and carbohydrate contain roughly 4 kcal per gram, or about half as much as fat.

In a way, the rationale for limiting fat consumption during exercise is similar to the reason for restricting fiber. Undoubtedly, fatty or fibrous food sitting idly in your stomach is a recipe for gut distress. With that said, tolerance to fat ingestion—much like fiber ingestion—is influenced by exercise intensity, and athletes partaking in relatively low intensity exercise over very long periods (e.g., a 24-hour race or multiday event) don't need to worry as much about fat causing adverse gut symptoms. A study of competitors from a 160-kilometer race supports this idea; runners consumed about 0.5 grams of fat every kilometer, equating to about 80 grams of fat over the entire race, and average fat intakes weren't different between runners who did and did not experience digestive troubles.[2]

Beyond restricting fat during exercise (except possibly during lower intensity activities), avoiding greasy foods immediately before exercise is a prudent decision as well. A study of male triathletes, for example, found that fat intake during the 30 minutes prior to a half-Ironman race was greater in those who vomited or had an urge to vomit than in competitors without such symptoms.[3] The most obvious explanation for this finding is a delay in stomach emptying and the release of cholecystokinin. Furthermore, a study published in the journal *Medicine and Science in Sports and Exercise* found that only about 10 percent of the fat in a meal consumed one hour before cycling eventually got burned during exercise.[4] This is because most of the fat you absorb is transported in your blood as a part of chylomicrons, which don't readily release triglycerides to the muscle during exercise.[5]

While limiting fat consumption within an hour of exercise is sensible, what to do two to four hours beforehand is less clear. Carbohydrate ingestion during this window clearly improves subsequent exercise performance in comparison to fasting or to consuming an energy-free placebo, but studies that have compared feeding carbohydrate- and fat-rich meals containing an equal amount of energy several hours before exercise have often failed to find differences in performance. Several of these studies, conducted from the mid-1990s through the mid-2000s, showed that while the composition of a pre-exercise meal (fat versus carbohydrate) does alter levels of glucose, insulin, and fat in the blood, these metabolic differences don't necessarily translate to changes in performance.[6-8]

Furthermore, the risk of nausea, vomiting, regurgitation, and excessive fullness from eating a high-fat meal is probably pretty low if you eat a few hours before exercise, since most of the fat will have left your stomach by the time you get going with exercise. One study fed men two meals (both 600 kcal) with drastically different fat contents (71 percent versus 7 percent) and tracked how quickly each meal vacated from their stomachs.[9] Despite being equivalent in energy, it took 140 minutes before half of the fat-laden meal had emptied, contrasted against 100 minutes for the low-fat, high-carbohydrate meal. Given that most athletes don't eat meals that are 70 percent fat, we can extrapolate that the bulk of a moderate-fat (35–50 percent of energy), moderate-energy (500–800 kcal) meal would empty from the stomach after a few hours. The theoretical representation of how the timing of moderate-to-high-fat meals impact the risk of gut symptoms is shown in Figure 5.1.

One caveat to keep in mind is that eating a fat-loaded meal that's also an energy bomb (more than 1,000 kcal) would prolong gastric emptying time more than usual and could certainly cause gut issues. In more simplistic terms, eating an entire Chipotle burrito with extra sour cream and guacamole probably is not the savviest pre-event fueling tactic, even if you eat it several hours before hitting the start line. Remember

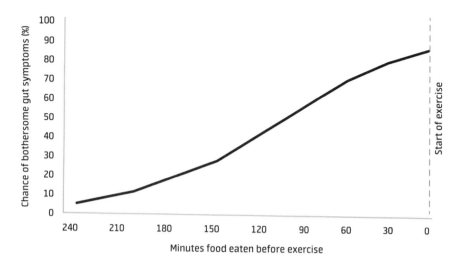

figure 5.1. **PRE-EXERCISE FAT INGESTION**

This theoretical representation shows the likelihood of gut symptoms when consuming meals at least moderately rich in fat at various points in time before exercise.

Michael Scott's Dunder Mifflin Scranton Meredith Palmer Memorial Celebrity Rabies Awareness Pro-Am Fun Run Race for the Cure? (If not, you really, really need to binge-watch *The Office*.)

CHRONIC HIGH-FAT DIETS AND PERFORMANCE

Although high-carbohydrate diets are a mainstay for most high-level athletes engaging in heavy training and intense, prolonged competition, interest in high-fat diets remains robust, particularly among ultraendurance athletes. Unfortunately, the cupboard of science is pretty bare on this topic, which is largely because it's incredibly difficult to recruit participants for controlled experiments that involve multiple exercise trials lasting several hours or more. (Who's up for staring at a lab wall and getting poked and prodded while exercising for five straight hours?) Even so, there's some evidence that high-fat diets can improve (or at least not harm) performance in competitions that last more than a few hours.[10] This is largely due to the fact that competitors in these events exercise at lower percentages (relatively speaking) of their VO_2max and are more reliant on fat burning. Examples of ultra-athletes who have reportedly had success on higher-fat diets include Zach Bitter (current 100-mile world record holder) and Timothy Olson (two-time winner of the 100-mile Western States Endurance Run).

Still, there's little reason to eat a high-fat diet if you're regularly training for and competing in events that involve high-intensity (75 percent-plus of VO$_2$max) exercise. This sort of pedal-to-the-metal activity relies heavily on carbohydrate burning, and while eating loads of butter, Ben & Jerry's, and guacamole would undoubtedly upregulate your capacity to rely on fat for energy, it would also simultaneously impair your ability to utilize carbohydrate.[10] A downtick in carbohydrate burning may not hurt an ultrarunner much during a 100-kilometer race, as the relative exercise intensity over that distance is lower, but it would likely slow an elite runner exercising at 75–90 percent of her VO$_2$max for any substantial length of time. Indeed, a recent experiment led by renowned sports scientist Louise Burke showed that, in comparison to following high-carbohydrate diets, following a very-low-carbohydrate, high-fat diet impaired carbohydrate burning, reduced exercise economy, and hurt 10-kilometer race performance in elite racewalkers during an intensified three-week training period.[11] To give some context for those of you who don't closely follow racewalking, a 10-kilometer race lasts about 37–45 minutes for elite athletes. There's obviously a big difference between a 10-kilometer race and races that last many hours, so perhaps you're wondering at what distance or duration a high-fat diet becomes potentially advantageous. Although I can't give you a precise threshold, races that last more than a few hours are the most likely candidates.

CHRONIC HIGH-FAT DIETS AND THE GUT

If you ever decide to shun carbs in favor of a high-fat lifestyle, what can you expect with respect to gut function and digestive symptoms? By default, most people following high-fat diets (though not all) cut back on nature's stool bulker, fiber, primarily because fruits, starchy vegetables, and whole grains are replaced with low-fiber, high-fat foods. This avoidance of fiber leads to less stool productivity in terms of total output and the frequency with which a person answers the call of nature. In one study, total stool weight dropped by about 27 percent after participants followed a high-fat, low-carbohydrate diet for eight weeks.[12] In addition, participants on the low-carbohydrate diet had reductions in counts of bifidobacteria, microorganisms that are important for the health of the digestive system. On the other hand, the low-carbohydrate dieters reported breaking wind less often, which makes sense given that the products of fiber fermentation include methane, hydrogen, and carbon dioxide.

Whether these changes in gut function ultimately influence exercise performance is uncertain and likely depends on the athlete and the situation. If you're experiencing severe flatulence, bloating, or urges to go number two during training and competition, then a high-fat, low-carbohydrate (and low-fiber) diet could reduce these symptoms. This potential benefit needs to be weighed against the growing—albeit preliminary— evidence that avoiding dietary carbohydrate and fiber alters the gut microbiome in ways that may not be optimal for gut health in the long run. Moreover, diets low in or devoid of fruits and vegetables may increase the risk of cardiovascular disease and some cancers.[13] And while nonstarchy vegetables can certainly be eaten in abundance on low-carbohydrate, high-fat diets, they're sometimes neglected in athletes who aren't vigilant with their nutritional choices.

In the end, the utility of high-fat, low-carbohydrate diets for managing gut issues may be similar to that of low-FODMAP diets. If you're regularly bothered by excessive flatulence and bloating, then temporarily eating a higher-fat diet could, in principle, mitigate the severity of these symptoms during competition. On the other hand, high-fat diets may undermine performance during competition that takes place at or above 70–75 percent of your VO_2max, especially if the event is expected to last more than 30 minutes. Much like with other nutrition strategies, athletes interested in these diets should trial them to determine their individual responses with respect to gut function and exercise performance.

MEDIUM-CHAIN VERSUS LONG-CHAIN TRIGLYCERIDES

Triglycerides are made of a three-carbon molecule called glycerol, which serves as the backbone of the triglyceride molecule, and three fatty acids. These fatty acids are essentially carbon chains that vary in length from a few carbons to several dozen, and their length determines whether they are considered short-chain, medium-chain, or long-chain fatty acids. In the previous section, the discussion of dietary fat's influence on gut function was based on the assumption that people primarily eat fat as *long-chain* triglycerides,[5] which make up 90–95 percent of the triglycerides in the average diet. Foods rich in long-chain triglycerides include fatty fish, nuts, olive oil, and fat-rich animal meats. The remaining small percentage of dietary triglycerides comes mostly in the medium-chain variety, which have different physiological properties than long-chain triglycerides (see Figure 5.2) and are found in coconut oil and palm kernel oil and to a lesser extent in dairy products.

Most of the fat you ingest within hours before exercise isn't burned for energy. Because they're insoluble in water, long-chain triglycerides from food must first be incorporated into chylomicrons before they can be dumped into your blood. Even before chylomicrons enter your blood, however, they first go through your lymphatic system. From there, they ultimately reach the blood circulation at veins located under the collarbone. Medium-chain triglycerides (MCTs), in contrast, are more soluble in water and don't need to be incorporated into chylomicrons before being dumped into blood. Instead, fatty acids from MCTs—which typically range from 6 to 10 carbons long—can enter your blood directly and are usually transported bound to the protein albumin.[5]

Another major difference between long-chain and medium-chain fats is the rate at which they exit your stomach. A seminal study in Great Britain showed that fatty acids equal to or longer than 12 carbons are more potent than shorter fatty acids at hindering stomach emptying.[14] Receptors in your small intestine detect these long-chain fatty acids and tell your body to release hormones such as cholecystokinin that slow the release of chyme from your stomach.[15] This is likely an adaptive response that's intended to prevent too much semidigested food and energy from being dumped into your small intestine all at once.

These differences in the digestion and metabolism of triglycerides led some researchers to speculate that ingesting MCTs would be a good way to boost fat burning during exercise without causing gut problems. A little over a dozen studies conducted between 1980 and the early 2000s—several of which were led by physiologist and Ironman triathlete Asker Jeukendrup—fed athletes variable amounts of MCTs either before or during exercise in an attempt to favorably alter metabolism and performance. While some of these studies showed that ingested MCTs can be burned during exercise,

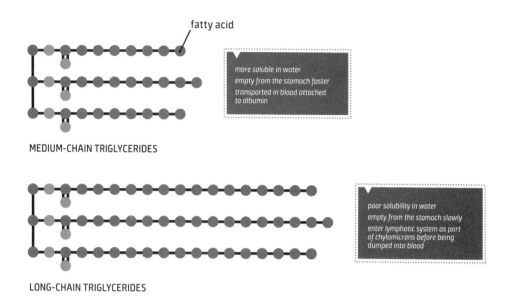

fatty acid

> more soluble in water
> empty from the stomach faster
> transported in blood attached
> to albumin

MEDIUM-CHAIN TRIGLYCERIDES

> poor solubility in water
> empty from the stomach slowly
> enter lymphatic system as part
> of chylomicrons before being
> dumped into blood

LONG-CHAIN TRIGLYCERIDES

figure 5.2. **TRIGLYCERIDE CHAIN LENGTH**

In comparison to long-chain triglycerides, medium-chain triglycerides empty from the stomach more quickly and are absorbed directly into blood circulation.

the majority found no differences in overall fat metabolism, nor did they find improvements in performance.[5] What's more, large single doses of MCT oil (perhaps more than 2 tablespoons), or smaller dosages (about 2 teaspoons) taken every 15 to 20 minutes during exercise, can cause nausea, abdominal cramping, and diarrhea. In one of the earliest studies on the topic, exercise physiologist John Ivy and his colleagues found that 100 percent of their subjects developed abdominal cramping and diarrhea when 50 grams or more of MCTs were fed an hour before exercise.[16]

These digestive side effects can ultimately blow up a performance on race day, as was shown by a later study out of South Africa.[17] Cyclists completed two roughly five-hour trials, one of which involved consuming a 10 percent carbohydrate beverage, while the other involved consuming a 10 percent carbohydrate plus 4.3 percent MCT beverage. After four and a half hours of cycling at a moderate intensity, performance was assessed by having the cyclists complete a set amount of work as fast as possible. While few gut symptoms were reported when the cyclists consumed the carbohydrate-only drink, half of them complained of such symptoms when MCTs were added to the beverage, and these symptoms probably contributed to the additional time that was required for them to complete the performance test when receiving the MCT beverage (14:30 versus 12:36 minutes).

It's not completely clear why MCTs wreak havoc on the gut at high doses, but it may be because they increase osmolality in the lumen. Just like with carbohydrate malabsorption, a surge in osmolality can trigger fluid secretion into the lumen, leading to a bad case of the trots. Intriguingly, a person's ability to handle MCT ingestion may improve over time with repeated exposures over several days or weeks.[18, 19] Starting with small doses (say, 2 teaspoons per day of MCT oil) and increasing by that same amount every couple of days may further improve gut tolerance.[20]

Even if tolerance to MCT ingestion can be improved, there are still no scientific data that strongly justifiy consuming MCTs before or during exercise. As a result, it's probably best if most athletes focus instead on established strategies for augmenting performance—carbohydrate ingestion, caffeine ingestion, and proper hydration, to name a few.

FAT

Fat is the **main fuel you burn** at rest and during exercise at less than 60 percent of VO$_2$max.

Most of the fat you ingest in a **pre-exercise meal** isn't utilized for fuel in muscle during the subsequent exercise, at least during exercise lasting a couple of hours or less.

Eating loads of fat (especially **long-chain triglycerides**) in a single sitting slows stomach emptying in comparison to eating other macronutrients.

Although **chronic high-fat diets** can boost your ability to burn fat during exercise, they also interfere with your ability to burn carbohydrate, especially at high intensities.

High-fat diets may have positive (or at least equivalent) effects on performance for **ultraendurance competitions** that last a few hours or longer.

High-fat diets are more likely to **hinder performance** in competitions that rely heavily on sustained carbohydrate burning (75 percent of VO$_2$max or higher).

In comparison to high-carbohydrate, fiber-rich diets, high-fat diets reduce stool weight, bowel movement frequency, and flatulence and may **unfavorably alter the gut microbiome**.

Ingesting MCTs hasn't been shown to enhance performance and can cause **nausea**, **abdominal cramping**, and **diarrhea** during exercise if they're ingested in large dosages (greater than 20–30 grams).

PROTEIN

Proteins play a myriad of roles in your body. Not only do they serve as building blocks for many of your tissues, but as enzymes, they catalyze the billions upon billions of reactions taking place inside you every second. Proteins consist of hundreds or thousands of smaller units called amino acids, and the order in which these amino acids are strung together dictates a protein's function. Your body uses 20 different amino acids to make thousands of proteins and polypeptides (small strands of amino acids) that do such wondrous things as stimulate growth (somatotropin), metabolize sugars (insulin and glucagon), tell you when you're hungry and sated (ghrelin and cholecystokinin), and help you achieve orgasmic bliss (oxytocin). Nine of the amino acids that we humans use to make proteins must be consumed in the diet because we are incapable of producing them—these nine are referred to as essential amino acids.

While most of the average human's body is actually water, a considerable chunk (15-20 percent) is protein. To get all this protein into you, your gut must first digest intact proteins from food. This process is sort of like taking apart a sectional couch so that it can get through the front door of your house and then reassembling it once it's in your living room. Along the same lines, your gut must first deconstruct proteins until they are small enough to be absorbed through your intestine's epithelial cells. Once inside you, most of these remnants of digestion eventually get repackaged into intact proteins.

You might recall from Chapter 1 that your stomach is a hot spot of protein digestion. Pepsinogen is secreted from specialized cells there, and its discharge is accompanied by

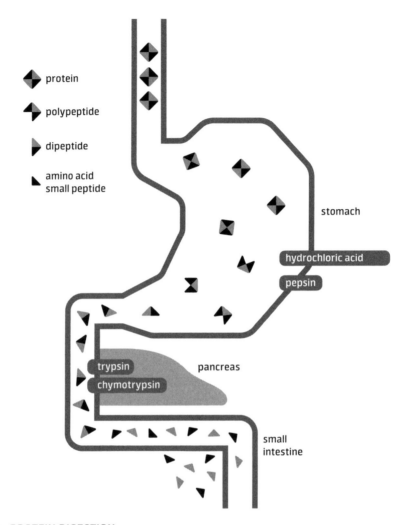

protein

polypeptide

dipeptide

amino acid
small peptide

stomach

hydrochloric acid

pepsin

trypsin

chymotrypsin

pancreas

small
intestine

figure 6.1. **PROTEIN DIGESTION**

*The digestion of protein kicks off in the stomach via hydrochloric acid and the enzyme pepsin and
continues in the small intestine through the actions of several enzymes released from the pancreas.*

the release of hydrochloric acid, which converts pepsinogen to pepsin. Hydrochloric
acid also unravels proteins, which allows pepsin to split apart proteins into smaller molecules. Upon arriving in your small intestine lumen, the pancreatic enzymes trypsin and
chymotrypsin continue working on the intermediates of protein digestion (polypeptides

and peptones) until they are obliterated into individual amino acids or very small peptide chains. (Figure 6.1 provides an overview of protein digestion.)

The aim of this chapter is to identify the ways in which ingesting protein affects your gut. In addition, given the popularity of protein and amino acid supplements, I also detail how these products can impact gut symptoms.

PROTEIN CONSUMPTION BEFORE EXERCISE

When it comes to eating protein before a game or race, the American College of Sports Medicine states that foods high in protein may need to be avoided to prevent gut issues.[1] However, this recommendation is based largely on theoretical grounds. Specifically, researchers and practitioners who recommend avoiding protein before exercise usually claim that it impedes stomach emptying, but, in truth, different types of protein vacate from the stomach at different rates. Intact milk protein and solid forms of animal protein (beef, chicken, etc.), for instance, typically leave from the stomach more slowly than processed sources like whey, and therefore may be more likely to cause upper gut problems if eaten in close proximity to exercise.

There are anecdotal accounts of athletes eating large amounts of protein before competition and experiencing gut distress. In one such case, Scottish-American runner Jock Semple ate a thick, juicy steak an hour or so before the 1934 Boston Marathon; despite being considered a favorite to win, things did not go swimmingly for Semple, thanks in large part to crippling nausea. To be clear, few studies have fed athletes relatively large amounts of protein before exercise and quantified its effects on gut symptoms or rates of gastric emptying. One such study, though, conducted out of the University of Otago in New Zealand, provides some justification for the recommendation to avoid loads of protein.[2] For the study, basketball players were fed meals 90 minutes before completing a high-intensity, 90-minute basketball-specific exercise protocol on two occasions. On one occasion, the players consumed a roughly 600 kcal meal that had a measly 6 grams of protein, while on the other occasion, the 600 kcal meal contained a hefty 69 grams of protein, primarily in the form of whey. Notably, athletes experienced more nausea and burping during exercise after they consumed the high-protein meal, although the symptoms didn't seem to be severe enough to impact sprinting and jumping performance.

Obviously, 69 grams of protein is a whopping dose (it's almost as much as what the average American eats in an entire day), so it would be unfair to extrapolate these findings to situations where athletes consume moderate portions of protein. Take for example an investigation of female cyclists which found that consuming a dairy-based meal with about 35 grams of protein didn't lead to more gut discomfort during 90 minutes of cycling than a nondairy meal that contained about 12 grams of protein.[3] Of note, the meals were consumed approximately two hours before cycling, which should have provided sufficient time for much of the food to exit the participants' stomachs. Undoubtedly, dosage and timing of ingestion are important factors that determine how well your gut will respond to pre-exercise protein consumption. Eating a jumbo-sized serving of protein-rich food 30 to 90 minutes before intense exercise—much like Jock Semple did—is basically asking for nausea and reflux. But consuming more moderate doses (say, 20–40 grams found in 10 ounces of low-fat Greek yogurt or 4 ounces of chicken breast) two to four hours before exercise seems unlikely to induce gut problems in most athletes.

There may also be a potential downside to completely avoiding or heavily restricting protein prior to exercise: increased hunger. On a per-gram basis, protein elicits somewhat greater feelings of fullness and declines in hunger than carbohydrate.[4] As a result, athletes who eat their final meal three to four hours before exercise may end up feeling famished if they choose a high-carbohydrate meal that's also very low in protein. This problem may be further exacerbated if the athlete also curbs fiber intake, which also increases satiety. While limiting fat, fiber, and protein to modest amounts one to two hours before competition is a prudent approach to preventing gut issues, the recommendation to drastically restrict these nutrients for three to four hours beforehand is probably overkill.

Like other nutrients, the likelihood that protein will give you gut troubles depends on a host of factors including the type, quantity, and timing of ingestion, as well as the intensity and duration of exercise you engage in. Accordingly, each athlete should experiment during training to determine how these factors influence their gut symptomology. If eating solid protein like chicken, fish, beef, or tofu one to four hours before exercise causes you considerable gut issues, you might consider switching to faster-digesting sources like whey or soy protein supplements or simply eating those same foods well in advance of exercise. Also, the presence of large food particles in the stomach can modestly slow gastric emptying,[5] so make sure to chew well when you're eating solid protein-rich foods in close proximity to exercise. (It turns out your mom's scolding reminders to chew your food served a purpose after all!)

PROTEIN CONSUMPTION DURING EXERCISE

During the 19th century and even into the early 20th century, many scientists believed that protein breakdown was what primarily fueled physical work, an idea popularized by German chemist Justus von Liebig.[6] This view originated, in part, from his observations that the analysis of animal muscles failed to reveal any trace of fat or carbohydrate. As a result, protein recommendations at the turn of the 20th century were quite high for the average man, ranging from 110 to 150 grams per day depending on activity levels.[7] (That's roughly what you'd get from eating an entire 16-ounce sirloin steak from Texas Roadhouse.) As time went on, work from a variety of physiologists and chemists challenged Liebig's views, and today it's widely acknowledged that protein contributes to only a small fraction (a few percent) of the energy needed for exercise. A poorly fueled athlete who engages in prolonged exercise may see this relative contribution of protein increase to 10–15 percent near the end of exercise,[8] yet even during the most arduous endurance events, fat and carbohydrate supply the lion's share of the ATP needed for muscular contraction.

Because protein isn't a primary source of fuel during exercise, it isn't surprising that most contemporary physiologists focus on carbohydrate ingestion as a strategy for improving endurance. Nevertheless, protein ingestion during exercise has received an increasing amount of scientific attention, and although several experiments have shown improvements in endurance when protein is added to carbohydrate beverages, these benefits were likely due to the extra energy and not the protein itself.[9] In fact, investigations comparing carbohydrate drinks against carbohydrate-protein drinks have consistently found that the addition of protein offers no performance edge when the energy content of the beverages is matched.

On the other hand, these studies haven't shown any detriments from adding a little protein to a sports drink, and even suggest there's a benefit if you're ingesting carbohydrate in smaller amounts (less than 30–45 grams per hour). Furthermore, adding some protein to a sports beverage could speed post-exercise recovery. It's worth noting that the majority of studies adding protein to sports beverages used whey, in large part due to its solubility in water; therefore, athletes looking to use this strategy should probably stick with preformulated beverages or use whey if they plan to make their own concoctions.

CHRONIC HIGH-PROTEIN DIETS

The current minimum recommendation for daily protein intake from the Institute of Medicine is 0.8 grams per kilogram of body mass, or just under 0.4 grams per pound. For a 150-pound runner, that equates to a little over 50 grams of protein per day, or about an 8-ounce chicken breast's worth. For a 250-pound footballer, that equals 90 grams of protein, or roughly the amount in a 12-ounce steak. To put these numbers in perspective, most American adults consume somewhere between 50 and 100 grams of protein per day.[10]

Regrettably, the Institute of Medicine's recommendation for protein is almost certainly suboptimal for a few populations, including athletes. (Note that this isn't because a huge amount of protein is burned during exercise, as Liebig thought, but is instead largely due to an increased demand from tissue remodeling and building.) Based on an array of research since the Institute of Medicine came up with its initial guidelines, it's now recognized that intakes of 1.2–1.6 grams of protein per kilogram of body mass (or roughly 0.5–0.7 grams per pound) are more optimal for serious athletes, individuals losing weight, and perhaps even the elderly.[11] That's not to say that eating an amount closer to the Institute of Medicine's recommendation will cause someone to literally wither away, but it does mean that some people are losing out on important health and performance benefits because of a dietary protein shortfall.

What are these benefits of consuming additional protein above the Institute of Medicine's recommendation? To be sure, there's ample science showing that, at least in the short term, high-protein diets help people shed extra pounds, sometimes even more effectively than other energy-restricted diets.[11] Moreover, elevating protein intake aids in the retention of lean body tissue as one loses weight. As an example, a 2010 study examined the effects of differing protein intakes while athletes followed one of two energy-restricted diets for two weeks.[12] A group consuming 1 gram of protein per pound of body weight lost significantly less lean tissue as compared to a group that ate only 0.45 grams of protein per pound.

Despite some potential advantages of protein-abundant diets, there are concerns that these regimens could be detrimental to your gut over the long term. When people drastically up their intakes of protein, consumption of either carbohydrate or fat is sometimes pared down. Carbohydrate is curtailed more heavily than fat in many of these cases, and as a result, intakes of fiber and other fermentable carbohydrates can drop quite dramatically. When fewer of these fermentable carbohydrates make it to your colon, the populations of microorganisms there begin to shift, leading to changes in the metabolic milieu of the large bowel.

In one study, feeding obese men a high-protein, low-carbohydrate diet for four weeks reduced the amount of butyrate appearing in their stools;[13] remember, butyrate is a by-product of carbohydrate and fiber fermentation in the gut, and, as it so happens, it's an important energy source for your intestinal cells and may even promote the death of colorectal cancer cells. Interestingly, including moderate amounts of carbohydrate in the diets (181 grams) was enough to offset much of this decline in butyrate production. The high-protein diets used in this study also amplified the appearance of so-called N-nitroso compounds in the stool, which are known carcinogens. While these sorts of short-term studies cannot tell us whether these metabolic changes lead to more cases of colon cancer or other gut problems, individuals following high-protein diets should think about including at least modest amounts of carbohydrate and fiber in their nutritional plans.

You might also be wondering what impact loading up on protein has on the incidence and severity of gut symptoms. Regrettably, this is an area bereft of research. This isn't because of a lack of studies on high-protein diets, but is instead due to their failure to collect meaningful information on gut symptoms. Despite the limited data, a handful of studies suggest that several gut symptoms are more prevalent on high-protein diets.

In a study published in the *Journal of the American Medical Association*, bloating and fullness were twice as prevalent (12 percent versus 6 percent) when participants were on a higher-protein diet (about 25 percent of energy) than when they followed either a carbohydrate-rich diet or a diet rich in unsaturated fats.[14] That said, most of the extra protein came from dairy and plant sources (legumes, nuts, seeds, etc.), so it's possible that other components of these foods (lactose and fiber, for example) could have triggered the bloating. Another study, published in the *Annals of Internal Medicine* around the same time, found that in comparison to those following a low-fat diet, overweight adults who were following a very-low carbohydrate, high-protein diet (which contained about 30 more grams of protein on average) experienced more constipation (68 percent versus 35 percent) and diarrhea (23 percent versus 7 percent).[15] It's nearly impossible to tell if these bowel problems were due to the additional protein, additional fat, or because the low-carbohydrate diet was also likely lower in roughage. Perhaps the most likely explanation is that these extra gut symptoms arose from a combination of these factors.

At the end of the day, the effects of a high-protein diet on gut symptoms depend on which foods and supplements are consumed to boost protein intake, as well as which foods are restricted as a consequence of including extra protein in the diet. Dramatically increasing the consumption of protein-rich milk and yogurt, for example, could increase bloating and flatulence in a person who is lactose intolerant. Likewise, even though they're relatively good sources of protein, eating loads of garbanzo and kidney beans could trigger gas and bloating because they're also rich in fermentable fibers. **For these reasons, athletes considering adding extra protein-rich foods to their diets should put some serious thought behind the sources of protein they choose, as well as the gut symptoms they're most concerned with preventing or managing.** If constipation is your main concern, following a meat-laden, low-carbohydrate, low-fiber diet is probably not your best choice. Alternatively, eating an abundance of legumes, nuts, and seeds may not be the best approach if you wish to avoid gas and bloating.

PROTEIN SUPPLEMENTS

Besides vitamins and minerals, protein is one of the most widespread types of supplements used by athletes. Gym bros and bodybuilders are not the only ones crushing protein supplements these days, as one analysis of surveys published in the journal *Sports Medicine* estimated that 25–49 percent of all male athletes and 7–22 percent of female athletes use protein supplements, and an additional 10–15 percent use individual amino acid supplements.[16] Probably the most popular protein supplement is whey. As it relates to gut function, whey empties from the stomach rather rapidly, whereas other supplemental forms like casein tend to leave somewhat more slowly (casein curdles in the acidic environment of the stomach, which delays emptying).[17] Regardless of how quickly they're digested and absorbed, most supplemental forms of protein are well tolerated and have relatively few digestive side effects.

131

One exception to this general rule is if an athlete is lactose intolerant and consumes a large amount of whey protein concentrates. Because whey comes from milk, it typically contains lactose and can trigger symptoms like gas, bloating, and loose stools in those of us who aren't efficient at breaking down lactose. For lactose-sensitive athletes, whey protein isolates are a better choice because they have undergone additional processing that removes almost all lactose.

Beyond whey concentrates, another possible gut-offending category of supplements is that of amino acid products like arginine and branched-chain amino acids. Arginine serves as a precursor for nitric oxide synthesis, and because nitric oxide regulates blood flow in tissues such as the skeletal muscle, arginine is frequently used as a pre-workout supplement in an attempt to, as your typical gym bro would say, "get my muscle pump on." Despite the positive anecdotes you may hear at the gym, much of the research on arginine and athletic performance is lackluster.[18] In addition, clinical trials that have rigorously collected information on the adverse effects of arginine supplements often report diarrhea as a side effect, particularly when 9 grams or more are taken in a single sitting.[18, 19]

Branched-chain amino acids are another popular supplement used by serious athletes and weekend warriors alike, and as with arginine, the hype surrounding them exceeds their true benefits, at least in terms of muscle-building potential.[20] And just as with arginine, side effects like diarrhea and nausea have been reported in some studies of branched-chain amino acids.[21, 22]

PROTEIN

132

Although protein was at one time believed to serve as a major source of energy for physical activity, today it's recognized that only a **small percentage** of total ATP production comes from burning protein.

Ingesting large amounts of protein (more than 40–50 grams) within **90 minutes of exercise** could provoke symptoms that affect your upper gut (nausea, fullness, burping).

Adding protein to carbohydrate beverages offers **no performance advantages** except possibly when your rate of **carbohydrate ingestion** is relatively low (less than 30–45 grams per hour).

Elevated daily protein intakes of about 0.5–0.7 grams per pound of body weight likely benefit a number of populations, including serious athletes, those attempting to lose weight, and even the elderly.

High-protein, low-carbohydrate diets may negatively alter the **microorganism populations** in your gut as well as the **metabolites** that are produced there (butyrate and N-nitroso compounds).

Gut symptoms from following higher-protein diets aren't well documented but likely depend on the main sources of protein you eat as well as the composition of carbohydrates and fat in your diet; plant-based proteins are more likely to **worsen bloating** and **flatulence**, while meat-laden, low-carbohydrate eating plans can be constipation inducing.

Arginine and branched-chain amino acid supplements can cause **diarrhea** and **nausea** when taken in high doses.

07

FLUID AND HYDRATION

Although the human body may look solid, one-half to two-thirds of it is actually water.[1] Of all the nutrients you must obtain in your diet, water requires the most consistent replacement. If water intake is restricted for several days and losses of greater than 7–10 percent of weight occur, the body struggles to maintain adequate blood pressure and blood delivery to vital organs like the brain, liver, and kidneys. Eventually, organ failure and death ensue if severe fluid deficits aren't remedied, and these deficits can set in rapidly in hot and humid environments.

While obviously not as dire as severe dehydration, moderate deficits of body water can still negatively affect you during exercise. In order to meet the swelling energy demands of exercise, your body must deliver more oxygen to your working muscles. This is precisely why your heart rate soars during exercise; every additional squeeze of this four-chambered muscular organ ejects additional blood and increases flow to your working muscles. Water is a critical component in this process because approximately half of your blood volume is water. In fact, one of the earliest adaptations to endurance training the body makes is to increase blood volume, which it mainly accomplishes by retaining extra water.[2] Specifically, an uptick in thirst and a decline in urine output cause your body to store this extra aqua, and these adaptations serve to increase maximal cardiac output (the amount of blood the heart pumps per minute) and aerobic fitness.

During heavy exercise, heat production is a threat to your well-being and performance. Your body must rid itself of this heat, lest your brain be cooked. The human

133

machine utilizes several avenues to cool itself, but sweating becomes an increasingly important method in sweltering conditions. The relevance of this is that heavy sweat losses can translate to less blood volume, and in order to maintain cardiac output, your body adjusts by making your heart pump faster. However, if fluid and blood volume losses are large enough, then your body won't be able to completely compensate by ramping up heart rate. In sum, the following chain of events will ensue:

1. Fluid losses decrease your blood volume.
2. Reductions in blood volume compromise blood flow to your muscles.
3. Compromised blood flow means you can't deliver as much oxygen to your muscles.
4. A reduction in oxygen delivery slows your production of ATP.
5. A reduced rate of ATP production reduces your work output.

Although there are additional reasons you fatigue in the heat, one reason is the inability to deliver the proper amount of blood and oxygen needed to maintain a particular exercise intensity.

Beyond its effects on blood volume and cardiac output, dehydration can also adversely affect body temperature regulation.[3] You only have so much blood to go around, with your skeletal muscles, heart, gut, brain, liver, kidneys, and skin all competing for a piece of the proverbial pie. During exercise, your skeletal muscle—sort of like a Kardashian to the paparazzi—gets much of the attention. Not to be forgotten, however, is your skin; a main mechanism by which your body cools itself is by sending warm blood from your core to your periphery. The extra blood flowing through your skin enhances sweating, and the evaporation of sweat decreases skin temperature and cools your blood before it returns to your core. When you're substantially dehydrated, blood flow to your skin and sweating become compromised, causing a more rapid rise in body temperature.

What exactly does all of this have to do with gut function, you ask? It turns out that this loss of body water and blood volume can hamper stomach emptying and provoke gut symptoms by reducing gut blood flow.[4] This can be a vicious cycle; as you become more and more dehydrated, it becomes progressively more difficult to reverse this dehydration

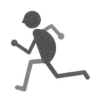

ORGAN	BLOOD FLOW (LITERS/MINUTE)		
	At rest	Intense exercise in heat, hydrated	Intense exercise in heat, dehydrated
Brain	0.75	0.75	0.75
Heart	0.25	1.25	1.25
Kidneys	1.00	0.25	0.20
Skin	1.00	4.00	3.00
Skeletal muscles	1.00	18.00	16.50
Gut	1.25	0.75	0.30
Total	5.25	25.00	22.00

table 7.1. **DEHYDRATION'S IMPACT ON THE GUT**

Moderate-to-severe dehydration can impair blood flow to the gut, especially in hot and humid environments where your skin is competing for blood flow as well.

because the fluid you drink sits idly in your stomach. Table 7.1 shows an example of how blood flow to the skin and gut can change as you go from rest to exercise; in addition, it displays how dehydration can impair blood flow to the skin and gut in the heat. As you can see, total cardiac output surges fivefold from about 5 liters per minute at rest to about 25 liters per minute during intense exercise in the heat. Simultaneously, blood flow to the skin surges, while blood flow to the gut might decline by 40 percent. As shown in the far right panel, when you experience substantial dehydration (4–5 percent body mass loss or more) from heavy sweating, your cardiac output declines and you start to fatigue. Likewise, blood flow to your gut drops even further, leading to delays in gastric emptying and more severe gastrointestinal symptoms.

Because fluid losses can compromise blood flow to muscle and skin as well as impair heat regulation, an indisputable rule in the field of sports nutrition is that dehydration, if severe enough, harms performance. Decades of research—combined with aggressive marketing campaigns from sports beverage producers—has solidified our collective belief that athletes need to be extra vigilant about hydrating during exercise.

136

While it's undeniable that moderate-to-severe dehydration usually impairs exercise performance, recently there's been a growing debate as to whether milder forms of dehydration have the same effects. On top of that, there are concerns that drinking loads of fluid during exercise has its own downsides. Consequently, in the subsequent sections of this chapter, I address the evolution of hydration guidelines over time, as well as the effects of different hydration strategies on gut function and symptomology.

RECOMMENDATIONS FOR FLUID REPLACEMENT DURING EXERCISE

In 1996, the American College of Sports Medicine released a paper detailing their position on hydration and exercise.[5] Along with describing the health and performance consequences of dehydration, the authors recommended that athletes consume enough fluid so that "water losses due to sweating during exercise be replaced at a rate equal to the sweat rate." While the authors acknowledged that, in the real world, athletes rarely achieve those levels of consumption (in large part due to gut intolerance), they nevertheless suggested that athletes "consume the maximal amount of fluids during exercise that can be tolerated without gastrointestinal discomfort up to a rate equal to that lost from sweating." Other sports medicine organizations mirrored these guidelines; for instance, the National Athletic Trainers' Association published a paper in 2000 stating that "athletes should aim to drink quantities equal to sweat and urine losses."[6]

These recommendations may be realistic for an average sweater (one who loses between 15 and 30 ounces of sweat per hour), but how well would they apply to an athlete who sweats like Ted Striker from the movie *Airplane!*? (If you don't get the reference, just google the GIF.) Is it practical for prolific sweaters to replace upward of 50–70 ounces of fluid per hour? (That would be equivalent to downing four to six cans of soda each hour!) The obvious answer is no, especially because the heaviest sweaters are typically exercising the hardest, making their guts less able to tolerate food and fluid intake.

While these sports medicine organizations admitted that athletes rarely met these hydration objectives of their own volition, they probably understated the potential risks of gut distress when athletes consume large volumes of fluid during exercise. After about a decade, the American College of Sports Medicine updated their position on exercise and hydration, in part as recognition that their recommendation to match drinking to sweat rates was unrealistic for many athletes. The updated paper no longer explicitly stated that athletes should consume fluid at a rate equal to sweat losses. Instead, the authors remarked that the general goal of drinking was to prevent greater than a 2 percent body mass loss, though they acknowledged that several factors (exercise duration, opportunities to drink, etc.) will ultimately influence exercise hydration plans.[7]

Around the same time, other organizations and researchers began questioning the wisdom of avoiding anything greater than a 2 percent body mass loss during prolonged exercise. Take for example an article from the International Marathon Medical Directors Association, in which the authors argued that body mass loss isn't a completely accurate marker of fluid loss during prolonged exercise and that the wide spectrum of weather conditions, body sizes, and running speeds that characterize races (and that determine sweat losses) makes formulating a universal hydration recommendation impractical.[8] Furthermore, the research used as the basis for developing the 2 percent threshold often wasn't reflective of real-life conditions. Some studies, for example, had people begin exercise in a fluid deficit (which is clearly different from developing dehydration gradually during exercise), while others implemented problematic methods to induce dehydration before exercise (e.g., exhausting exercise or heat exposure).

In support of these criticisms, a relatively recent scientific review found that if a person starts exercise in a hydrated state, drinking fluid to prevent a 2 percent body mass loss doesn't necessarily lead to superior performance on realistic, racelike tests (i.e., finishing a set distance as fast as possible).[9] In this analysis from researcher Eric Goulet, it was shown that dehydration levels of about 2 percent weren't associated with reduced performance and that drinking to the dictates of thirst likely improved performance in comparison to drinking more or less. Yet, this analysis was based entirely on cycling studies with exercise durations lasting around one to two hours, so whether these findings translate to other sports and longer exercise durations is unclear.

137

To add to the lack of clarity, a second analysis from Goulet published about a year later found that body weight losses of 2 percent or more did in fact reduce exercise capacity on what are referred to as time-to-exhaustion or fixed-power tests.[10] An example of this type of test is asking a person to cycle or run for as long as they possibly can at a fixed intensity (e.g., 75 percent of VO_2max). While this type of test doesn't exactly replicate most endurance races or sporting events, it does imitate some types of training as well as activities that are common in military and occupational settings.

Hydration science is inherently difficult to do rigorously (you can't blind someone to whether they're drinking fluid, right?), but if I were to distill these findings into a basic recommendation, it's this: **Drinking fluid based on the dictates of your thirst is a reasonable hydration strategy for competitions that last one to two hours.** This conclusion was largely reaffirmed by a more recent analysis from Goulet.[11] That said, situations exist where it may be better to use a more aggressive hydration approach; examples include competitions held in extremely hot/humid conditions, when exercising at a constant intensity for as long as possible, and during more protracted exercise (more than two hours).

Given that we know dehydration can reduce blood volume, it seems somewhat counterintuitive that drinking to thirst would optimize performance in many situations even when it can cause 2–4 percent body mass losses in a relatively short amount of time (one to two hours). If drinking more can prevent such significant losses in body mass and blood volume, then why wouldn't it also lead to better performance in these situations? While there are a few answers to this question, the most important one comes back to gut tolerance. In brief, drinking well above thirst makes it more likely you'll be plagued by excessive fullness, stomach discomfort, and nausea. Indeed, a 1991 experiment showed that drinking about 1,600 milliliters (about 54 ounces) of fluid per hour during two hours of cycling doubled stomach fullness ratings as compared to intakes that were about half as much.[12] Another study conducted a few years later found that attempting to fully replace sweat losses during one hour of intense cycling led to more gut distress and caused cyclists to cover less distance than when they ingested no fluid.[13]

These findings were extended to runners in a study that demonstrated that drinking a carbohydrate beverage at a rate of about 30 ounces per hour during a two-hour run was associated with fullness ratings that were nearly twice as severe than from drinking

13 ounces per hour.[14] In another study, 10 runners completed two half-marathons in hot conditions while ingesting water to the dictates of thirst or based on prescribed rates that aimed to prevent 2 percent body mass losses.[15] Fluid consumption was dramatically different between trials (roughly 20 versus 70 ounces), and the prescribed strategy led to gut discomfort ratings that were twice as high by the end of the half-marathon.

While the gut discomfort that accompanies aggressive fluid intakes doesn't automatically hurt performance, it clearly can in some situations. Take for example an experiment that examined how drinking different volumes of a carbohydrate beverage influenced running performance.[16] Nine men completed a 10-mile run on three occasions while drinking (1) no fluid, (2) as much fluid as they pleased, or (3) a prescribed volume to minimize dehydration. The amount drank in the prescribed trial was about three to four times as much as when subjects drank whatever they pleased (10 versus 35 ounces), and although prescribed drinking led to less dehydration (0.6 percent versus 1.4 percent body mass loss), it caused the runners to finish the race about one minute slower! The most plausible explanation for the less-than-stellar performance during the prescribed trial was gut intolerance, as discomfort ratings by the end of the race were twice that of the ratings from when they drank as much as they pleased. The gut discomfort was likely the result of fluid remaining in the participants' stomachs since the max rate of emptying is not much more than 30–35 ounces per hour and is further reduced at intensities above 70 percent of VO_2max.[17] Interestingly, performance with prescribed drinking was essentially the same as when the runners consumed no fluid, substantiating the idea of a Goldilocks zone for fluid intake.

Hydration recommendations during exercise will likely continue to remain ambiguous because of the markedly different environments, modalities, and durations of exercise people engage in. With that said, an optimal hydration zone likely exists for each athlete and each situation (see Figure 7.1). If you drink too little during prolonged exercise, dehydration can ensue and endurance may suffer. Additionally, consuming too little fluid can aggravate gut woes by impairing gut blood flow. On the opposite end of the spectrum, drinking too much can also cause stomach discomfort and performance may suffer. Ultimately, the goal is to consume an optimal volume of fluid that minimizes the risks of dehydration and gut discomfort at the same time.

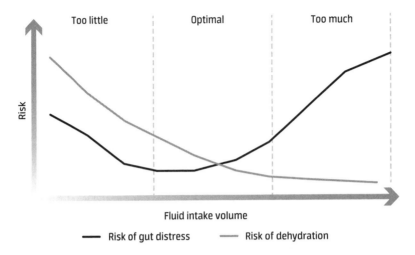

figure 7.1. **OPTIMAL FLUID INTAKE**

Both over- and underconsuming fluid during exercise carry certain risks, including gut distress, and each athlete may need to use trial and error to find their own Goldilocks zone.

Like other nutrition strategies, trialing different drinking plans during training should help you dial in your own optimal hydration zone for competition, whether it be drinking to thirst or to a preplanned schedule. In addition, the following recommendations may be of use when making decisions about hydration:

⊙ For competitions that last between one and two hours, drinking based on thirst may be the easiest and most effective strategy for optimizing gut comfort and performance in the vast majority of cases.

⊙ Heat and humidity increase sweating and the risk of dehydration, and therefore drinking to thirst may be an insufficient strategy for a majority of one-to-two-hour competitions held in hot and humid environments.

⊙ Hydration guidelines for events lasting longer than two hours are murkier because most experimental studies testing different hydration strategies haven't used exercise tests lasting that long; although using thirst is a perfectly acceptable option for some athletes, others may require more regimented approaches to prevent levels of dehydration that impair performance.[18]

- Athletes choosing preplanned hydration strategies should obtain estimates of their sweat rates using body weight changes and fluid intakes (see Table 7.2).
- Environmental conditions and exercise intensity both impact sweating, so athletes will need to estimate their individual sweat rates for the situations they expect to compete in; this obviously makes preplanned hydration strategies more burdensome on the athlete.
- If using a preplanned strategy, replacing 50–75 percent of sweat losses is a reasonable goal when sweat rates are expected to be between 17 and 34 ounces (500–1,000 milliliters) per hour.
- When sweat rates are expected to exceed 34 ounces (1,000 milliliters) per hour, replacing roughly 25–50 percent of sweat losses is a reasonable target.

141

table 7.2. **CALCULATING SWEAT RATES**

	IMPERIAL EXAMPLE (POUNDS AND OUNCES)	METRIC EXAMPLE (KILOGRAMS AND MILLILITERS)
Formulas for sweat rate†	[(Weight loss) × 16 + Fluid intake] / Exercise duration	[(Weight loss) × 1,000 + Fluid intake] / Exercise duration
Pre-exercise weight (after urinating)	150 pounds	75 kilograms
Post-exercise weight	147 pounds	73 kilograms
Weight loss	3 pounds	2 kilograms
Exercise duration	2 hours	1.5 hours
Fluid intake	20 ounces	600 milliliters
Example calculations	[3 × 16 + 20] / 2 [48 + 20] / 2 68 / 2 = 34 ounces per hour	[2 × 1,000 + 600] / 1.5 [2,000 + 600] / 1.5 2,600 / 1.5 = 1,733 milliliters per hour

† For the Imperial system, weight loss needs to be multiplied by 16 to convert pounds to ounces. For the metric system, weight loss needs to be multiplied by 1,000 to convert kilograms to milliliters.

⊙ The higher the sweat rate, the lower the percentage of replacement; for example, an elite marathoner who sweats 80 ounces of fluid per hour is much more likely to tolerate replacing 30 percent of losses (24 ounces) than 50 percent of losses (40 ounces).

⊙ There's some evidence that repeatedly drinking large volumes of fluid over multiple exercise training sessions can reduce gut discomfort over time (discussed in Chapter 9), which reenforces the point that it's important to practice preplanned hydration strategies over the long term.

FLUID LOADING

What we've learned so far is that drinking fluid well above and beyond your perception of thirst may create gut discomfort that, in some cases, negatively impacts performance. This is despite the fact that drinking above thirst can prevent a loss of blood volume and improve thermoregulatory responses to exercise in some situations. What if there were a way to stay hydrated without having to down loads of fluid? A way of sort of bypassing your gut during exercise? At first thought this may seem like an improbable idea, but there are a couple of strategies that might bear some fruit.

One approach would be to hook someone to an IV so they can receive a constant stream of fluid directly into the vascular system, but that's obviously impractical/unethical outside the confines of a lab. An alternative strategy—known simply as fluid loading—may allow you to avoid the problems of dehydration without having to choke down bottles of water and sports drink during exercise. Fluid loading is similar to the more well-known strategy of carbohydrate loading, and just as carbohydrate loading increases reserves of high-octane fuel in your body, fluid loading expands your stores of water. In basic terms, the more fluid there is in you before exercise, the less you may need to drink during exercise, or at least that's how the theory goes.

From a practical perspective, ingesting loads of water by itself isn't a super effective method of increasing water stores. Plain aqua is low in electrolytes like sodium, so when it's absorbed and incorporated into your vascular space, your blood concentrations of sodium decline. The body reacts to this dilution of blood sodium by producing more urine, causing you to pee out, over the next few hours, much of the water you drank.

One way that scientists have tried to enhance the retention of ingested water is by adding glycerol to beverages. Glycerol is a three-carbon molecule that, through osmotic forces, allows your body to hold on to more of the water you drink. Notably, a review of studies, again conducted by hydration researcher Eric Goulet, found that including glycerol in pre-exercise beverages improved performance by an average of 2.6 percent on exercise tests lasting about one to two hours.[19] Of note, most studies used dosages of about 0.5 grams per pound of body weight mixed with 1.5–2.0 liters of water. In addition, a glycerol beverage should be consumed over a period of about one hour, with the goal of finishing the entire beverage 30–60 minutes before exercise commences.

Until recently, glycerol was prohibited by the World Anti-Doping Agency (WADA) because it was thought to be a way for cheating athletes to mask the physiological responses to blood doping.[20] However, effective January 1, 2018, WADA removed glycerol from their prohibited substances list because of additional research showing that it minimally affects parameters of the Athlete Biological Passport, which is an electronic record that's used to monitor biomarkers of doping in athletes. Even though it's now legal, glycerol is known to cause gastrointestinal side effects like nausea and bloating if it's taken in concentrated dosages over a short period of time, which is why it should be mixed and consumed with fluid over an hour or so.[21] Certain individuals should also avoid taking glycerol for health reasons, including (but not limited to) pregnant women and those with cardiovascular diseases, diabetes, kidney disease, migraines, and liver disorders. Finally, it's important that fluid isn't overconsumed during exercise when using glycerol ingestion as a pre-exercise fluid-loading strategy, as the combination of the two can cause hyponatremia.

Beyond glycerol, there's another fluid-loading approach that might be worth a try: taking in more sodium. As mentioned earlier, a drop in blood sodium is one of the stimuli that sparks urine production when you consume a large volume of plain water, and by ingesting a good bit of sodium with water, reductions in blood sodium are blunted and urine output is curtailed. While only a handful of studies have examined whether this strategy impacts exercise performance, there's reason to feel somewhat positive about it. In a study led by exercise physiologist Stacy Sims, pre-exercise ingestion of roughly 25 ounces of water containing a large amount of sodium (about 3,700 milligrams per liter) allowed runners to exercise longer at 70 percent of VO$_2$max in a hot environment as compared to ingesting low-sodium water (230 milligrams per liter).[22] A second study by Sims found a similar result when female cyclists consumed either high-sodium or low-sodium beverages before cycling to exhaustion in 90°F conditions.[23] One caveat to both of these studies is that the athletes weren't allowed to drink fluid during exercise, which may have exaggerated the performance benefits.

To summarize, pre-competition fluid loading may enhance body water storage and decrease the need for fluid ingestion during exercise, at least in sweltering conditions. This may allow you to consume a smaller, more gut-friendly volume of fluid during exercise without becoming dehydrated. However, the interactions between fluid loading and fluid ingestion during exercise haven't been well studied, so the idea that you need to drink less during exercise when you've fluid-loaded is based on theoretical grounds, and any athlete trying this approach should be careful not to overdrink during exercise (because of the risk of hyponatremia). Both glycerol and sodium-rich beverages are viable options for pre-exercise fluid loading, but the wider availability of sodium-rich beverages makes them the more practical choice for most athletes. If you ultimately decide to consume a concentrated sodium drink to fluid load, you should start consuming the beverage about two hours before competition, taking a 3-to-4-ounce serving every 10 minutes for about one hour. You can make your own beverage, but be aware that table salt (sodium chloride) is only 40 percent sodium by weight. Alternatively, you could purchase a pre-formulated version from companies like Osmo or The Right Stuff.

FLUID TEMPERATURE

Ultimately, anything that retards emptying from your stomach could contribute to fullness, bloating, and nausea, so it's important for you to consider how the foodstuffs you ingest affect this process. As it relates to fluids, one factor that impacts stomach emptying is beverage temperature. In a study that fed people orange juice at different temperatures, 30 percent of juice kept at 39°F had left the stomach 12 minutes after ingestion, contrasted against 45 percent of the juice that was kept near body temperature.[24] On the other hand, people usually opt to consume more fluid while exercising in the heat if a beverage is cool or cold, and chilled fluids delay the rise in body temperature and prevent premature fatigue during exercise in hot conditions.[25] Given these benefits, is reduced stomach emptying from a colder beverage really something you should be concerned about in terms of gut comfort or distress?

The short answer is that beverage temperature is unlikely to profoundly impact gut symptoms. Once they reach your stomach, chilled beverages are warmed to near body temperature within 5–10 minutes, making the effects on gastric emptying short-lived.[26] Indeed, the same investigation that found hindered stomach emptying 12 minutes after cold juice ingestion also found no differences in emptying between the cold and warm juices at later time points. And while studies comparing the consumption of fluids kept at different temperatures have frequently neglected to collect information on gut symptoms, the fact that cool fluid ingestion has often improved exercise capacity in these studies suggests that any increase in symptoms is either negligible or not severe enough to impact performance.

VOLUME AND FREQUENCY OF DRINKING

Other than fluid temperature, the frequency and volume of fluid ingestion can also affect stomach emptying. It's long been recognized that large volumes of fluid held in the stomach elicit the fastest rates of emptying, but as fluid leaves the stomach, emptying begins to slow.[27] This means that the rate of emptying falls exponentially over time. So, if you continually drink, say, every 10–15 minutes, with the goal of keeping your stomach topped off with fluid, that should result in a superior rate of fluid delivery to your small intestine. Consequently, exercise science textbooks sometimes recommend that athletes consume fluid every 10–15 minutes during prolonged exercise in order to maintain a high rate of gastric emptying.

On a practical level, however, it's questionable whether this modest increase in emptying and fluid delivery leads to better exercise performance because, as I explained earlier, drinking above the dictates of thirst hasn't been consistently shown to improve performance and can actually hinder performance if it causes gut discomfort. In addition, the frequency with which an athlete drinks often depends on the constraints of the sport, and in some sports (e.g., professional soccer), drinking every 10–15 minutes might not be feasible.

SUMMARY

FLUID AND HYDRATION

In some athletes, a loss of body water resulting in a body mass loss of greater than 2 percent may impair certain types of exercise performance, particularly prolonged **aerobic exercise** in the heat.

For competitions lasting one to two hours, **drinking based on thirst** likely optimizes gut comfort and performance in most athletes, while for longer exercise bouts, a more structured hydration plan may be warranted in some cases.

Replacing a large percentage of your **sweat losses** (75–100 percent) is likely to cause gut discomfort when sweat rates exceed 34 ounces (1,000 milliliters) per hour.

Pre-exercise fluid loading (with glycerol-containing or sodium-rich beverages) enhances **body water storage** and could, in theory, lessen the need for fluid ingestion during exercise (particularly in the heat) and indirectly prevent gut distress.

Cold beverages may temporarily slow **stomach emptying**, but this doesn't seem to impact gut symptoms or hinder performance.

SODIUM

Sodium is one of those substances—along with fat and sugar—that makes everything taste better. (Have you ever eaten unsalted saltines or nuts? Yech.) Big Food has long known of sodium's ability to favorably augment the taste of otherwise bland foods, which is why food processors haven't hesitated to load up their products with salt. Today, sodium intakes in industrialized societies range from about 2 to 5 grams per day, roughly equivalent to 1–2 teaspoons of table salt.[1] Doing a quick back-of-the-envelope calculation, the total yearly sodium consumption for the entire United States population (about 330 million people) equates to slightly more than the mass of the Empire State Building. That's a heck of a lot of sodium.

The majority of this sodium comes from processed and restaurant foods, so unless a person's diet consists primarily of fresh foods and meals made from scratch, it's likely they are consuming more sodium than they need for optimal health. In fact, while it may seem like a benign substance, sodium may be responsible for over 1.5 million premature deaths across the world every year.[2] Yes, you read that right, over 1.5 million deaths! Sodium's blood pressure–raising effects explain the bulk of these premature demises.

Sodium is one part of table salt; the other part is chloride. When mixed in water, table salt disassociates into positively charged sodium particles and negatively charged chloride particles. Minerals that dissociate into charged particles when mixed into water are what we call electrolytes, and in your body, they allow for the conduction of electrical impulses, help maintain fluid balance, and play a role in enzymatic reactions. The most important electrolyte related to hydration and exercise is sodium, as its concentration in sweat is multiple times greater than other electrolytes, such as potassium and calcium. This is, in part, why sodium supplementation is so popular during exercise, in addition to that fact that athletes often have strong beliefs about the powers of sodium, including that it stops muscle cramps and prevents hyponatremia.

Sodium supplementation is especially common during ultraendurance events; one study involving participants of the 100-mile Western States Endurance Run found that 94 percent of surveyed finishers used a sodium supplement.[3] Is all this sodium doing any good, or is it simply another popular nutrition strategy that's based on lackluster science? And what effects do large doses of sodium have on gut symptoms? We explore these and other questions in this chapter, and as you'll come to find out, sodium supplementation is in many ways one of the most overhyped sports nutrition strategies out there.

SODIUM AND EXERCISE PERFORMANCE

As I covered in the last chapter, consuming a sodium-rich beverage one to two hours before exercise can be an effective method of increasing body water stores. Under the right circumstances, this can stave off dehydration and theoretically allow you to get away with consuming less fluid during exercise. However, a separate issue is whether sodium ingestion *during exercise* influences performance. Several studies have assessed whether sodium ingestion during exercise delays fatigue or improves how fast athletes finish a race. The bad news is that sodium supplementation has, for the most part, elicited few positive performance effects.

In one example, 114 competitors of the Cape Town Ironman triathlon ingested either sodium chloride or placebo tablets during the race;[4] despite consuming an average of about 3.5 grams of sodium, the sodium chloride group didn't fair better in comparison to the placebo group when it came to finishing time, core body temperature, or body mass changes. In another study, nine cyclists completed two 72-kilometer time trials over hilly terrain in New Zealand; one trial was done while ingesting 0.7 grams of sodium chloride per hour, and the other was done while ingesting a placebo.[5] The athletes drank as much fluid as they wished, and despite the fact that sodium supplementation led to greater thirst, more fluid consumption, and better maintenance of blood volume than placebo, performance wasn't different between the interventions. A final example comes from a study that supplemented athletes with 1.8 grams of sodium or cornstarch during treadmill running or cycling.[6] After two hours of exercising at a moderate intensity, treadmill grade or cycling power was increased every minute until the athletes threw in the towel. Each athlete completed two trials while ingesting each treatment, and in the end, none of the outcomes (temperature change, thermal sensation, body weight change, or performance) were influenced by sodium.

In contrast to these three studies, one 2016 experiment did show a possible improvement in half-Ironman triathlon performance when researchers assigned 26 participants to either electrolyte capsules (containing sodium, chloride, potassium, and magnesium) or a placebo.[7] In the end, the electrolyte group finished about 26 minutes (roughly 7.8 percent) faster than the placebo group. While this seems impressive, the sample size was quite small for this type of study (meaning the results are less trustworthy), and because the electrolyte supplement also contained several compounds other than sodium, the benefits could have been from one of these other ingredients.

If supplementing with sodium during exercise likely doesn't impact real-world performance, then why is it included in most sports beverages in moderate amounts (200–600 milligrams per liter)? To be sure, some research does show that including sodium in a beverage confers slight physiological advantages (e.g., maintenance of plasma volume and serum osmolality). These are just the kinds of findings that excite geeky sports scientists making electrolyte drinks, but ultimately, they probably don't translate to tangible benefits on the racecourse or field. Another reason sodium is added to these beverages is that it stimulates the drive to drink; as you'll recall from the previous chapter, most hydration scientists used to believe that more was better when it came to fluid ingestion, even though today we recognize that's often not the case. And last but not least, beverage makers also don't mind it when athletes drink more of their products (for obvious financial reasons), and sodium is one of several ingredients that can increase consumption of said products.

Before concluding this section, I want to be clear that it is important for some athletes to up the sodium content of their diets in order to replace losses through sweating. Athletes can lose several grams or more of sodium each day if they have large total sweat volumes, and for these athletes the standard amount of dietary sodium probably isn't enough. However, this lost sodium can easily be replaced by eating sodium-rich foods and beverages throughout the day. (Hooray for those *salted* Saltines, eh?) That's not to say that consuming an electrolyte-containing drink during exercise is a poor choice; instead, I'm saying athletes shouldn't expect to improve their performance by consuming sodium during exercise itself.

After cutting through the hype, the data underpinning the supposed benefits of sodium supplementation during exercise are quite weak. While some studies show that body weight, blood volume, and blood sodium levels are slightly better maintained with sodium supplementation, these physiological changes haven't consistently translated into meaningful performance advantages. That being said, ingesting a sodium-rich beverage *before exercise* is a potentially viable strategy for enhancing endurance performance in hot/humid conditions, especially when fluid availability is limited during competition.

SODIUM AND CRAMPING

If you've ever experienced a muscle cramp during a race or game, you probably know that the pain can be excruciating. In some cases, it seems as if an invisible force is tightening the muscle beyond what is possible through human will. Marathon spectators can plop themselves around mile 20 and watch as dozens of runners pass by as they try, sometimes in vain, to work out the cramps in their legs. Muscle cramps in cyclists and swimmers are also fairly common and can even be dangerous if they hit suddenly and unexpectedly. While quite rare, occasionally a swimmer will drown after suffering from a muscle cramp that they can't relieve.

Strategies for preventing exercise-associated muscle cramps include making sure you taper your training volume going into competition and—for endurance races, specifically—that you don't start out of the gate too fast. Still, muscle cramps can hit even the best prepared athletes, and at that point, many turn to stretching and massage. Beyond these mechanical remedies, athletes, coaches, and practitioners often believe that dehydration and electrolyte imbalances are leading causes of exercise-associated muscle cramps. This widespread belief has grown out of media reports and a few observational studies, such as an investigation that showed five footballers who had a history of cramps lost twice as much sodium in their sweat during a training camp as teammates with no history of cramping.[8]

Initially, these correlational studies gave credence to the hypothesis that electrolyte imbalances play a role in exercise-associated muscle cramps. As such, foods and beverages rich in electrolytes have been regularly consumed by athletes seeking relief from muscle cramps. One sodium-rich beverage, pickle juice, has received an inordinate amount of attention as a surefire way to alleviate cramps. In one well-documented instance, the 2000 Philadelphia Eagles supposedly fought off muscle cramps in 100°F conditions by using pickle juice and, in the process, defeated the cramp-laden Dallas Cowboys.[9] (This has since been dubbed the "Pickle Juice Game.") Considering the abundance of these sorts of media reports in the early 2000s, it isn't surprising that by 2008 up to one-quarter of athletic trainers were using pickle juice to treat muscle cramps.[10]

Despite the hype, studies on pickle juice and muscle cramping are few and far between. In one well-controlled experiment, however, ingestion of pickle juice did actually curtail cramping as compared to ingesting water.[11] Researcher Kevin Miller and his colleagues had participants exercise until they lost 3 percent of their body mass through sweating, after which toe muscle cramps were induced through electrical stimulation of the tibial nerve. The average cramp duration with water ingestion was 134 seconds, which was reduced by 37 percent with pickle juice. Although this finding would at first glance lend weight to sodium's effectiveness as a cramp reliever, the fluids were ingested immediately after the cramps were induced, meaning there wasn't enough time for the sodium to be absorbed and carried through the participants' bloodstreams to directly impact their cramping muscles.

What, then, could explain pickle juice's positive influence in this study? One leading hypothesis is that something in the pickle juice other than sodium stimulates receptors in the mouth and gut that, when activated, affect signaling between the nervous system and skeletal muscles. If not sodium, what ingredient in pickle juice could be doing this? Our current best guess is that the vinegar in pickle juice is responsible for these cramp-relieving effects. Specifically, vinegar is believed to activate receptors in the mouth and upper gut that quiet the neurons that send signals to your muscles. This is likely why

151

athletes and athletic trainers often describe pickle juice as having a rapid onset of action; it doesn't need to be digested and absorbed to work.

Subsequent studies have revealed that other food ingredients activate these same receptors (referred to scientifically as transient receptor potential [TRP] vanilloids and ankyrins).[12] Ginger, cinnamon, mustard, and chili peppers have all been identified as activators of these receptors, and in a promising series of studies, ingesting mixtures of these types of ingredients reduced muscle cramp severity and cramp thresholds.[13, 14]

Before you go into a state of muscle cramp–relieving ecstasy, be aware that the improvements in these studies were of modest magnitude, so you shouldn't expect to completely prevent all muscle cramps with the use of pickle juice or other TRP activators. Even so, with these scientific developments, we're beginning to learn that the old anecdotes about pickle juice and muscle cramping are partially true. However, the common belief that sodium is responsible for these benefits is probably unfounded.

GASTROINTESTINAL EFFECTS OF SODIUM SUPPLEMENTATION DURING EXERCISE

When it comes to two of the purported benefits of salt ingestion during exercise—improving performance and preventing muscle cramps—the science doesn't justify spending your efforts on sodium supplementation. Yet many athletes—particularly ultraendurance runners—continue to gobble down sodium tablets and capsules during races. While this practice isn't dangerous, there's some reason to be cautious about over-doing it with the sodium supplements during exercise. In one of the aforementioned studies that examined the effects of sodium supplementation, 2 of 11 athletes reported nausea after ingesting sodium capsules, and one of the athletes quit an exercise test due to nausea and vomiting.[6]

The most plausible explanation for these side effects is a slowing of stomach empty-ing. Similar to his work on dietary fats, scientist John N. Hunt showed that the presence of large amounts of sodium chloride in the stomach impedes emptying.[15] While most sports drinks don't contain nearly enough sodium to have this effect, the quantities found in tablets or capsules could almost certainly do the trick if you consume enough of them. Unfortunately, nearly all the other studies that have supplemented athletes with sodium during exercise didn't attempt to document gut discomfort as a side effect, so we're left with little data on how common a problem this really is. Still, the following recommendations regarding sodium supplementation should help minimize the risks of gut symptoms like nausea, vomiting, and abdominal cramps:

- Athletes considering sodium supplementation should trial it during training in order to minimize the risk of gut intolerance during competition; specific electrolyte products and rates of ingestion should be tested individually.
- If athletes have a goal of replacing sweat sodium losses during prolonged exercise (more than two to three hours), they should start with a target rate of 500–1,000 milligrams of sodium per hour.
- Spread out the intake of electrolyte tablets/capsules during exercise (e.g., one capsule every 15 minutes instead of four capsules once per hour).
- Athletes using electrolyte capsules/tablets should consider purchasing products that contain as few ingredients as possible.
- If an athlete's main goal is preventing or managing muscle cramps, they'd probably be better off trying foodstuffs that activate TRP vanilloids and ankyrins (e.g., pickle juice or a specially formulated product, like HOTSHOT) than supplementing with electrolytes.

153

SODIUM

Most experiments that have supplemented athletes with sodium during exercise have failed to find performance benefits, although some have found better maintenance of **thirst**, **body mass**, and **blood volume**.

Despite occasionally finding **correlations** between sodium losses in sweat and the onset of exercise-associated muscle cramping, most studies refute the role of **sodium depletion** as the primary culprit in this condition.

Foods and beverages that activate **TRP vanilloids and ankyrins** (pickle juice, vinegar, mustard, ginger, etc.) may reduce the duration and/or severity of **muscle cramps**.

Although there aren't many severe risks of taking sodium supplements during exercise, large quantities of sodium can **slow stomach emptying** and induce gut symptoms like **nausea** in a minority of athletes.

TRAINING THE GUT

Your body has an extraordinary capacity to adapt. With endurance training, your heart's chambers enlarge and your blood volume increases, allowing more nutrients and oxygen to be circulated during maximal aerobic exercise. Inside your muscles, the enzymes that speed up certain metabolic pathways increase in quantity, allowing you to produce ATP more rapidly or efficiently. With resistance training, your skeletal muscle fibers enlarge and are able to generate extra force. And as recent research in older adults has demonstrated, even certain regions of the brain adapt to exercise training by enlarging.[1, 2]

To achieve these adaptations, most athletes spend the bulk of their training time slogging away on the pavement, hitting the practice field, or pumping iron in the weight room. All this training stimulates muscle growth, builds muscular strength and endurance, and is the basis for long-term athletic development. There's one type of athlete, however, who focuses less on developing their muscles and heart and more on training their gut. These are the competitive eaters of the world, and as I mentioned in Chapter 1, the world record in hot dog eating is 74 frankfurters and buns in 10 minutes, held by none other than Joey Chestnut. Although genetics likely play a role in determining one's potential to become a high-caliber speed eater, Chestnut and his fellow competitors certainly weren't born entirely capable of choking down dozens of hot dogs in just 10 minutes. No, these athletes train just like any other athlete, except their idea of "keeping fit" involves repeatedly stretching their stomachs by eating masses of food and fluid.

The other giant of the competitive eating world is Takeru Kobayashi, who holds numerous records and dominated Nathan's Fourth of July contest before Chestnut's first victory there in 2007. In a 2015 interview with the online magazine *Vice*, Kobayashi detailed some of the training methods that make him such a prolific devourer of foodstuffs, one example being that he prepares months in advance by drinking slightly more water every day.[3] On the afternoon he was interviewed, Kobayashi planned to drink 3 gallons of water in 90 seconds. (Warning: Chugging water like this can be dangerous because it can lead to hyponatremia.) Other competitive eaters conduct two or three practice eating sessions each week, where they gorge on huge quantities of food.

In contrast to competitive eaters, the performance of cyclists, runners, triathletes, footballers, basketballers, and various other athletes isn't dependent on eating piles of food during competition. Even so, being able to tolerate modestly larger intakes during exercise could be advantageous for athletes looking to push the boundaries of their in-competition nutrition plans. Thus, it's worth pondering how you might be able to train your gut to optimize the digestion, absorption, and delivery of nutrients during exercise.

Amazingly, science tells us that your gut has the capacity to adapt to not only physical training but also to the diet you eat over days and weeks. What's also remarkable is that many of these adaptations are nutrient specific. Just as adaptations to exercise training follow the principle of specificity, so do many of the adaptations of gut training. If your objective is to get stronger, it works best to lift heavy weights. In a similar way, if your objective is to absorb and burn more carbohydrate during exercise, it works best to eat a high-carbohydrate diet. In this chapter, we cover these nutrient-specific adaptations in the gut as well as how they might impact exercise performance and the development of digestive symptoms.

THE GUT'S ADAPTATION TO EXERCISE TRAINING

By now, you should be aware that the redistribution of blood flow during exercise is a way for your body to prioritize the delivery of oxygen and nutrients to your muscles. This additional blood also serves to remove by-products of metabolism that, if left to accumulate, induce fatigue. Blood flow to your skin increases too, particularly in hot/humid environments, which facilitates heat loss and prevents a rapid rise in body temperature.

In nonathletes, cardiac output is equivalent to about 5 liters of blood per minute at rest, of which the gut and liver receive about 20 percent.[4] During maximal aerobic exercise, cardiac output swells roughly fivefold to 25 liters per minute in an average man, with the skeletal muscle receiving the lion's share (roughly 80 percent). While the *absolute amount* of blood flowing to your gut may not decline much during heavy exercise, the *relative percentage* of your cardiac output reaching your gut drops to just a few percent. With fluid losses from sweating, gut blood flow can become even further compromised.[5, 6] Undoubtedly, reductions in gut blood flow help explain the greater occurrence of digestive symptoms reported during endurance events.

157

What effect, if any, does physical training have on these blood-flow impairments of the gut? Well, both animal and human studies demonstrate that long-term exercise training blunts the reduction in gut blood flow that typically occurs with acute exercise.[7] The primary explanation for this adaptation is a reduction in sympathetic nervous system output. As a reminder, the sympathetic nervous system is the fight-or-flight division of your nervous system that readies your body for physical action, and one way that it accomplishes this is by constricting blood vessels in your gut. (Historically, blood flow to the gut wasn't a priority when one was being chased by a lion, was it?) In essence, as you increase your fitness over time, your autonomic nervous system becomes less "fight-or-flight" and more "rest-and-digest" at a given exercise workload. The long-term effects of exercise training on gut blood flow may help explain why several gut symptoms are less common in experienced athletes;[8, 9] these athletes may have trained their guts—through hundreds or thousands of hours of training time—to better maintain blood flow during exercise.

ADAPTATION TO INCREASED CARBOHYDRATE INTAKE

Carbohydrate ingestion—and its subsequent digestion, absorption, and delivery to skeletal muscle—is imperative for maintaining carbohydrate burning during intense exercise that lasts longer than 60–90 minutes. As carbohydrate stores in your body dwindle, rates of energy production and muscular contraction decline because slower-burning fatty acids become an increasingly dominant fuel source. Consequently, ingesting carbohydrate helps maintain higher absolute workloads during intense, prolonged exercise.

There is a natural limit, though, to the amount of carbohydrate you can digest and absorb over any given period. The SGLT1 and GLUT5 transporters located in the intestinal brush border have upper limits as to how quickly they let carbohydrate into your body. If you consume too much carbohydrate, abdominal cramping, diarrhea, and flatulence may develop. To combat this problem of limited absorptive capacity, ingesting a mix of carbohydrate types (fructose and glucose), as opposed to a single source, is recommended—at least when you plan to consume more than 50 grams per hour.

One intriguing question is whether it's possible to train your gut to increase the capacity of these transporters, which would allow you to increase the amount of carbohydrate you absorb and burn during exercise. As discussed in an eloquently written paper by sports scientist Asker Jeukendrup, an abundance of data from animal studies makes it clear that the activity and/or concentration of these transporters can change based on the carbohydrate content of the diet.[10] Simply put, more carbohydrate in the diet equals more of these transporters in the intestinal brush border.

Data directly confirming that this also happens in humans are lacking, in large part because isolating these transporters requires excising a sample of intestine. Even so, there's some indirect evidence that this adaptation also happens in the intestines of humans. Take a study from the Australian Institute of Sport that tested whether feeding a four-week high-carbohydrate diet would increase athletes' capacities to burn carbohydrate eaten during exercise.[11] Athletes assigned to a high-carbohydrate group consumed glucose drinks before and during training sessions while athletes allocated to a moderate-carbohydrate group consumed fat-rich foods (macadamia nuts or a cream drink) after training sessions. Importantly, both diets provided the same total energy. At the start and near the end of the four-week dietary period, the athletes completed a 100-minute cycling test while consuming a beverage containing a special form of glucose that can be traced in the body. The experiment ultimately revealed that the high-carbohydrate diet increased the oxidation of traced glucose by 16 percent, with no apparent change on the moderate-carbohydrate diet. The researchers concluded that enhanced intestinal absorption of glucose was the most likely explanation for this finding. In terms of practical guidelines, studies—albeit using animals—have found that just a few days on a high-carbohydrate diet can upregulate intestinal transporter expression,[10] meaning you probably don't need to crush carbohydrate for weeks straight to see these changes.

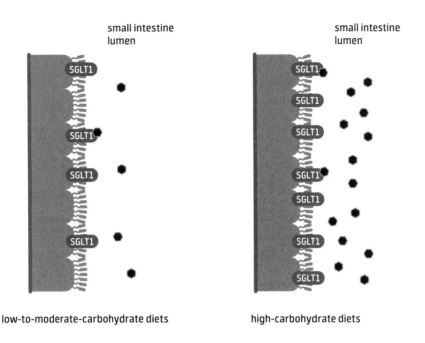

small intestine lumen

SGLT1
SGLT1
SGLT1
SGLT1

small intestine lumen

SGLT1
SGLT1
SGLT1
SGLT1
SGLT1
SGLT1
SGLT1

low-to-moderate-carbohydrate diets

high-carbohydrate diets

figure 9.1. **TRAINING THE GUT FOR GREATER CARBOHYDRATE INGESTION**

Additional carbohydrate added to the diet over several days to weeks promotes the expression of intestinal carbohydrate transporters, which can enhance carbohydrate absorption, reduce gut distress, and perhaps improve performance when an athlete ingests 50-plus grams per hour of carbohydrate during exercise.

While mounting evidence supports the notion that eating a high-carbohydrate diet boosts the quantity and/or activity of intestinal carbohydrate transporters like SGLT1, these adaptations' implications on performance are less clear. In fact, that same study from the Australian Institute of Sport also measured performance and failed to find any differences.[11] One potential reason for this is that the moderate-carbohydrate diet still contained an ample amount of carbohydrate; if the comparison diet had been low carbohydrate, it's possible that even larger differences in carbohydrate burning would have been observed, which could have led to meaningful changes in performance. That said, one recent study conducted by researchers at Monash University in Australia did find improvements in running performance after two weeks of a carbohydrate-based gut-training protocol, and these improvements were likely mediated through reductions in digestive symptoms.[12] Overall, these studies tell us that training your gut to tolerate more carbohydrate during exercise *could* translate to improvements in not only carbo-hydrate burning and digestive symptoms, but also possibly performance (see Figure 9.1). An important caveat to this statement is that it applies to athletes who are planning to push the envelope of carbohydrate ingestion during competition (i.e., more than 50 grams per hour). If you plan to consume 30–45 grams of carbohydrate per hour, there's little reason to do this sort of aggressive gut-training protocol.

Beyond affecting the intestine's capacity for absorption, the carbohydrate content of a diet also influences emptying from the stomach. Specifically, studies supplementing the diet with either glucose or fructose for just a few days have shown the emptying of these sugars to be accelerated.[13-15] The reasons for this adaptation are still being elucidated but almost certainly involve less feedback inhibition from receptors in your small intestine that detect the presence of carbohydrate. This feedback inhibition—originally discussed in Chapter 1—is a way for your body to regulate the amount of sugar being dumped into your small intestine. Interestingly, fasting for several days also slows the emptying of carbohydrate from the stomach,[16] and it's long been known that the dietary restriction typical of anorexia nervosa induces similar delays and that these effects are quickly reversed if adequate nutrition is provided.[17] Slowed stomach emptying might also explain why athletes who heavily restrict energy intake experience more gut problems than their well-fed counterparts.[18]

Again, the practical implication of this research is that if you plan to consume large amounts of carbohydrate during competition, make sure you don't heavily restrict energy intake during the days leading up to competition, particularly from carbohydrate-rich foods and beverages. If you do, emptying of carbohydrate from your stomach might be slowed and could increase the likelihood of symptoms like fullness, reflux, and nausea.

ADAPTATION TO INCREASED FAT INTAKE

Unlike ingesting carbohydrate, eating fat during exercise doesn't improve performance, primarily because most of said fat isn't burned for energy. The major exception to this rule of thumb is for athletes partaking in relatively low-intensity, ultraendurance-type activities that last many hours to days. There's enough time for more of the ingested fat to be digested, absorbed, and utilized during these events, and as an added bonus, relying more on dietary fat in these situations requires carrying less food because fat is such an energy-dense nutrient.

Even though eating significant quantities of fat during high-intensity exercise doesn't make sense from a performance perspective, can the same be said for high-fat diets eaten over the weeks or months leading up to competition? As covered in Chapter 5, long-term high-fat diets may not hinder performance in all sports, especially in ultraendurance competitions that rely heavily on fat oxidation to sustain muscular contraction.[19] In addition, an increasing number of athletes are trying high-fat diets. What, then, can these athletes expect to happen to gut function if they adhere to a diet that's filled with bacon-wrapped avocado fries and almond-butter milkshakes?

Just as eating a high-carbohydrate diet speeds emptying of carbohydrate from your stomach, eating a fat-rich diet seems to do the same for fat emptying. In one study, men ate a high-fat diet (55 percent of total energy) for two weeks, and before and after they were fed a high-carbohydrate meal as well as a high-fat meal in order to assess how the fatty diet affected stomach emptying.[20] Compared to before the diet, emptying of a fatty meal was accelerated after the high-fat diet, while no change was observed for emptying of the high-carbohydrate meal. In another study, eating a fat-rich diet for four days didn't quicken how fast a fatty meal left the stomach, but fat emptying sped up after two weeks.[21] Finally, a third study showed accelerated emptying after just three days on a diet supplemented with 90 grams of sunflower oil, which ended up supplying almost 50 percent of total dietary energy as fat.[22]

One major limitation of these studies needs to be acknowledged before we definitely declare that eating a fat-rich diet accelerates fat emptying from the stomach. While they often included a control diet (usually a low-fat diet), these experiments typically failed to ensure that total energy and food volume were equal between the diets, so it isn't 100 percent clear if the faster emptying was due to the extra fat, specifically, or just a by-product of the additional food and energy. Still, from the thirty-thousand-foot view, it is true that eating a high-fat diet *as a part of a high-energy diet* accelerates the emptying of fatty meals from the stomach.

The impact on your gut of eating an energy-rich, high-fat diet goes beyond stomach emptying. These diets may also shorten the amount of time it takes for fatty foods to

161

travel from your mouth to your large intestine. In one of the same studies that evaluated stomach emptying, eating a high-fat diet for three days shortened the mouth-to-cecum transit time of a fatty meal from 280 minutes to 226 minutes.[22] (The cecum is a pouch that's considered the beginning of your large intestine.) These findings were replicated over a four-week period as well, with transit time dropping from 318 minutes before a high-fat diet to 248 minutes post-diet.[23]

Whether the effects of high-fat diets on stomach emptying and small intestine transit time ultimately impact athletic performance and gut symptoms is unresolved. An obvious downside of consuming a high-fat diet would be a reduction in the absorptive capacity of carbohydrate during exercise. To counter this potential problem, an athlete adhering to a high-fat diet who also plans to consume a substantial amount of carbohydrate during competition may want to temporarily increase carbohydrate intake for at least a couple days before the event.

ADAPTATION TO INCREASED PROTEIN INTAKE

Research examining how the gut adapts to protein-rich diets is scarce, which is probably because extremely high-protein diets aren't that popular among the public. While several popular diets promote elevating protein intake as a way to preserve muscle mass and blunt hunger, it's still pretty uncommon for protein to make up any more than 35–40 percent of energy in these diets. Thus, the possible range of intakes as a percentage of dietary energy is narrower for protein (10–40 percent) than it is for carbohydrate and fat. In comparison, the carbohydrate content of diets can vary wildly from less than 10 percent to more than 70 percent, and the same is true for fat. So there just aren't many situations in which a truly "very high" quantity of protein is consumed.

Logically, this relative lack of variability makes it less likely that changing protein intake (at least within normal dietary patterns) will dramatically impact gut function. Nonetheless, a couple of rodent studies do suggest that eating a high-protein diet quickens stomach emptying of protein.[24, 25] Obviously, rats aren't humans, so we shouldn't assume these results translate across species. As far as I'm aware, no studies in humans have assessed whether long-term high-protein diets influence how quickly protein empties from the stomach. Moreover, even if high-protein diets do accelerate gastric emptying of protein, that doesn't mean you would reap performance gains from it. As with high-fat diets, it's hard to think of a performance benefit that would arise from protein leaving from your stomach with haste. Remember, you typically burn small amounts of protein during exercise, so it isn't a fuel that limits energy production. Finally, if you eat a relatively large percentage of your diet as protein (say, 30 percent), one or both of the other macronutrients (fat and carbohydrate) will probably end up being restricted. On most high-protein diets, carbohydrates are restricted more heavily than fat, and in the end, the carbohydrate restriction that often accompanies high-protein diets could reduce your intestine's capacity to absorb carbohydrate.

163

ADAPTATION TO INCREASED FLUID INTAKE

Maintaining blood volume during prolonged exercise—especially in the heat—is critical to fighting off fatigue. The American College of Sports Medicine recommends attempting to drink enough fluid to prevent body mass losses of greater than 2 percent (if possible),[26] but a major obstacle to meeting this recommendation is that drinking large volumes of fluid during exercise raises gut discomfort to levels severe enough to slow down athletes.[27, 28] This may be precisely why some research shows drinking to thirst is a superior hydration strategy.

Given these facts, you might be asking yourself if it's possible for your gut to adapt to—as is seen with other dietary components—increased fluid intakes. In the first decade of the 2000s, G. Patrick Lambert, a professor at Creighton University, designed a study to figure out if repeatedly drinking large volumes of fluid during 90-minute runs affects stomach emptying and gut comfort.[29] Participants performed six runs at 65 percent of VO_2max, with each run separated by 7–11 days, and from the second to sixth run they drank a 4 percent carbohydrate beverage at volumes that matched their sweat rates. The average volume consumed was nearly 42 ounces, or slightly over 28 ounces per hour. Although the five trials of drinking large fluid volumes didn't speed stomach emptying over time, the participants' perceptions of stomach discomfort were improved. Specifically, stomach discomfort—which was rated on a 1-to-4 scale (1 = very comfortable, 4 = very uncomfortable)—decreased from about 2.3 during run two to 1.7 by runs five and six.

These findings imply that any athlete who's planning to consume more than 15–20 ounces of fluid per hour during competition should repeatedly practice drinking at those higher rates during training. If you decide to try this, it's important that you don't overconsume fluids, which is a risk factor for developing the potentially serious condition hyponatremia. As a general rule, you shouldn't gain weight over the course of an exercise session; if you do, that's a clear sign you're replacing fluid at a rate that's higher than your sweat losses.

Table 9.1 provides an overview of the major nutrition-related adaptations that have been documented in the scientific literature.

table 9.1. **OVERVIEW OF THE GUT'S ADAPTATIONS TO VARIOUS NUTRITIONAL STRATEGIES**

INTESTINE	
Nutrition Strategy	Adaptation
High-carb diet	Increased brush border SGLT1 transporters
High-fat diet	Faster transit of high-fat meals through the intestine

STOMACH	
Nutrition Strategy	Adaptation
Fasting/low-energy states	Slower stomach emptying
Glucose feedings	Faster emptying of glucose and fructose
Fructose feedings	Faster emptying of fructose
High-fat diets	Faster emptying of fat
High-protein diets	Faster emptying of protein*
Large volumes of fluid	Improved perceptual tolerance to large fluid intakes

Both the stomach and small intestine adapt to your diet, particularly as it pertains to the carbohydrate and fat content.
*Not yet convincingly shown in humans

SUMMARY

TRAINING THE GUT

Reductions in sympathetic nervous system activity help explain why gut **blood flow** at standardized exercise workloads is better maintained after long-term exercise training.

Animal studies show that the activity of **SGLT1 transporters** can be manipulated by changing dietary carbohydrate content.

Supplementing your diet with sugars like **glucose** and **fructose** for even a few days can accelerate how quickly these sugars empty from your stomach; if you plan to eat a good amount of **carbohydrate** during competition (e.g., more than 50 grams per hour) but don't want to follow a super high-carbohydrate diet for weeks on end, then this may be a way to train your gut to better tolerate carbohydrate intake during competition.

Eating a **fat-rich diet** speeds the emptying of fat from your stomach; what this means on a practical level for athletes isn't known scientifically, but perhaps it could be advantageous for an athlete who plans to eat more fat than usual during competition (like an **ultramarathoner** competing over many hours or several days).

Repeatedly exposing your stomach to large volumes of **fluid** during training (e.g., 25–30 ounces per hour) may lessen perceptions of stomach discomfort over time, which, in theory, could allow you to **better maintain hydration** when you're sweating heavily (e.g., more than 35 ounces per hour).

10

DIETARY SUPPLEMENTS

It's estimated that 52 percent of Americans take some type of dietary supplement each month,[1] adding up to over $30 billion in sales every year.[2] Similarly high rates of supplement use are common in northern European countries, like Denmark, the United Kingdom, and Norway,[3] as well as in Asian countries, such as South Korea and Japan.[4,5] The reasons people take supplements are quite varied, but the most oft-cited motivation in the United States is improving or maintaining health.[6] Apparently, many Americans believe that taking pills and powders is a path to optimizing well-being. Although I'm not entirely sure how one would measure such a thing, it's often been said that, due to our prodigious supplementation habits, Americans have the most expensive urine in the world.

In America, supplements are regulated much like foods, which is largely the result of the Dietary Supplement Health and Education Act (DSHEA) of 1994. The simplified explanation of DSHEA is that it allows most supplements to be assumed safe until proven otherwise, and if a safety concern arises with a specific product on the market, the Food and Drug Administration (FDA) has the burden of proving the supplement is unsafe in court before it can be removed from shelves.[2] The regulation of supplements in other countries is variable, with some regulating supplements more tightly and others regulating them less strictly. Regardless, many supplements taken by people across the globe are, in reality, of no benefit, at least in high-income countries where fortified and enriched foods serve as a sort of population-wide multivitamin-mineral supplement.

While there are exceptions of supplements that have good science behind them, many are modern-day snake oils.

It would be one thing if most supplements didn't work but were otherwise harmless. Regrettably, that's not always the case, and there are at least three issues to be worried about when it comes to supplements: (1) contamination, (2) poor quality, and (3) side effects. The first issue—contamination—is of particular relevance to elite athletes. Due to a lack of oversight, a significant proportion of supplement makers don't follow the rigorous manufacturing processes needed to prevent contamination of supplements with unwanted ingredients and substances. For instance, a nontrivial percentage of protein supplements—which are popular with athletes and recreational exercisers—contain concerning levels of heavy metals.[7]

For athletes subject to doping tests, another contamination issue is the presence of banned substances in supplements. An athlete's reputation can be instantly destroyed by a doping allegation, so the issue of contamination is no small matter. In one 2004 study, roughly 15 percent of supplements bought from 15 different countries contained anabolic steroids that weren't declared on the label.[8] While this might not be a surprise when it comes to "muscle building" and "sexual enhancement" supplements, this analysis tested products like vitamins, minerals, herbals, and athletic enhancers (e.g., amino acids, creatine, etc.) that weren't specifically marketed as hormone supplements. Most of the supplements that contained an unlisted steroid didn't contain enough to suggest the manufacturers intentionally added these ingredients; instead, the small amounts that were detected points to cross-contamination from a failure to sanitize or clean machines. If you're tempted to think this study is an anomaly, a subsequent analysis of 58 supplements acquired through retail outlets in the United States found that 25 percent contained traces of steroids while 11 percent contained evidence of stimulants.[7] Clearly, any athlete subject to doping tests needs to exercise caution when using supplements, even when there isn't a banned substance listed on the product's label.

A recent high-profile case from the world of swimming serves as a stark example of the problem of supplement contamination. In February 2018, Madisyn Cox, an American swimmer and the 2017 World Championships bronze medalist in the 200-meter individual medley, failed a doping test for trimetazidine, a drug that's used to treat chest pain but that WADA classifies as a stimulant.[9] Cox denied that she took the drug on purpose and originally suspected her positive test was from contaminated tap water. She eventually had the multivitamin she had been taking analyzed, and lo and behold, trimetazidine was detected. This was good evidence that Cox wasn't knowingly taking trimetazidine, and her ban was reduced from two years to six months. Unfortunately, she missed the United States Championships that July and was therefore unable to qualify for the 2019 World Championships.[9]

Like the issue of contamination, poor supplement quality (for example, a lack of labeling accuracy) is another problem facing the supplement industry. In fact, a fairly large proportion of supplements don't contain the actual quantity of ingredients listed on the label and in some cases contain absolutely no trace of a listed ingredient. In one analysis of multivitamins conducted by ConsumerLab.com, 13 of 38 products either didn't contain the amount of nutrients claimed or improperly listed ingredients.[10] While the magnitude of the discrepancies found in this analysis and others like it aren't typically large enough to pose a health threat to consumers, it does exemplify the poor quality-control practices followed by some manufacturers.

Perhaps the worst offenders when it comes to supplement quality are herbals, which in some cases contain diddly-squat of the plant described on the label. In one example, Steven Newmaster, a researcher from the University of Guelph, analyzed 44 herbal products and was able to authenticate only 48 percent of them based on DNA barcoding, a technique that identifies plant materials based on short, standardized gene sequences.[11] What's more, his group's analysis found that 21 percent contained known filler ingredients like rice, soy, and wheat, even though they weren't listed on labels. While some of these supplements may have been accidentally contaminated with fillers, some of the manufacturers were probably using these ingredients as cheap substitutes for the real deal. The scientific article published by Newmaster and his colleagues caught the attention of the *New York Times*, which published its own story in 2013.[12] Ultimately, this story prompted the New York State Office of the Attorney General to conduct an investigation into supplements being sold in the state, which culminated in cease-and-desist letters being sent to four major retailers (GNC, Target, Walgreens, and Walmart).[13]

In addition to herbals, there's another popular supplement that suffers from widespread quality-control issues: fish oil. After multivitamins/minerals and calcium, fish oil is the third most popular supplement in the United States.[6] People have all sorts of beliefs about the virtues and benefits of fish oil, ranging from preventing heart attacks to treating arthritis to alleviating depression. While there are grains of truth behind some of these claims, others aren't supported by high-quality clinical trials or, in many cases, the magnitude of benefit isn't nearly as big as advertised. Take for example the prevention and treatment of heart disease, which is probably the most common reason people take fish oil. While several trials in the first decade of the 2000s found small reductions in coronary events or premature death in patients with preexisting cardiovascular disease, at least three recent large fish oil trials found no benefits in patients with recent heart attacks or individuals at elevated risk of cardiovascular events.[14]

Several reasons have been put forth to explain why fish oil has failed to reduce cardiovascular events in these trials. One explanation is that risk factors like high blood pressure and LDL cholesterol are managed better today through improved public screening and higher rates of medication use. Another explanation—albeit unproven—is that the poor quality of many fish oil products offsets any benefits. Analyses of fish oil products have found that substantial proportions of them contain high amounts of oxidized lipids;[15, 16] when lipids are oxidized, it interferes with their normal functioning in the body and may have harmful health effects if consumed over prolonged periods. The chemical structure of omega-3 fatty acids—the main fats found in fish oil—makes them particularly prone to being oxidized during processing.

A second problem with the oxidation of fish oil is that it reduces the amounts of the two omega-3 fatty acids (EPA and DHA) thought to be responsible for fish oil's benefits. An analysis of 32 fish oil supplements marketed in New Zealand, for example, revealed that only three contained quantities of EPA and DHA that were equal to or higher than what was listed on the labels.[15] The researchers speculated the low levels of EPA and DHA were due to high oxidation rates. You might be hoping this is just an isolated problem with supplements sold to our Kiwi friends, but a similar analysis found that of 47 omega-3 supplements purchased in the United States, more than 70 percent didn't contain declared amounts of EPA or DHA.[17]

If contamination and poor quality aren't big enough reasons to give you pause before using supplements, then you may also want to consider the potential for adverse and potentially serious side effects. Unfortunately, there's no comprehensive national system in the United States that accurately quantifies the harms of supplements. The

FDA oversees a voluntary reporting system called MedWatch, but the adverse events reported to this system only represent a small fraction of the total number. In addition, because supplements don't undergo rigorous testing prior to marketing, we have little information regarding the expected rate of side effects for any given product. The double-blind clinical trials required for the approval of pharmaceutical drugs are oftentimes unavailable for supplements, and even when they are, the quality of many of these trials is questionable, and most don't comprehensively document side effects.

171

The limited data we do have about potential adverse events associated with supplements are concerning, at least for certain types of products. In a 2015 study published in the *New England Journal of Medicine*, physician Andrew Geller and his colleagues estimated, using nationally representative data from 63 emergency departments, the number of annual visits stemming from supplements.[18] After crunching the numbers, they estimated that about 23,000 emergency room visits were attributable to supplements each year. The most dangerous products seemed to be herbal/complementary nutritional supplements, as roughly two-thirds of visits (after excluding unsupervised ingestion of supplements by children) were attributable to these products. Weight-loss and energy supplements were the major contributors to adverse events among the herbal/complementary supplement users, making up more than half of the events for that category. What's more, the types of adverse events experienced from taking herbal/complementary products were quite different from those that occurred from taking standard vitamins and minerals—heart palpitations, chest pain, and tachycardia (a fast heart rate) were much more likely to occur if a person came to the emergency room after taking weight-loss or energy supplements.[18]

The fact that weight-loss and energy supplements cause adverse cardiovascular effects isn't surprising in light of the fact that they often contain stimulants. In addition, the FDA has issued numerous recalls for products that fall within these categories because of reports of liver damage, stroke, kidney failure, and death.[19] In one well-known case, Baltimore Orioles pitcher Steve Bechler died after collapsing during spring training, with the coroner ultimately determining that an herbal stimulant he was taking could have contributed to his death.[20] Although ephedra—the stimulant in the supplement Bechler was using—has since been banned by the FDA, weight-loss and sports-enhancement supplements often remain on the market for years after being recalled for containing banned substances and, more often than not, still contain these banned substances after being recalled.[21]

This discussion on the safety and quality of supplements is meant to give you pause before buying and consuming any product straight off the shelf. At a minimum, you should spend time evaluating the product and the manufacturer making it. Consider the following questions:

- ◉ Has the manufacturer ever had a recall and, if so, for what reason?
- ◉ Does the product make outlandish and unrealistic claims, especially when it comes to weight loss, boosting energy, or building muscle?
- ◉ Does the product advertise itself as an alternative to prescription drugs or anabolic steroids?
- ◉ Is the product marketed in a foreign language? (The FDA has issued advisories listing this as a possible warning sign.)

Beyond asking yourself these questions, you might consider only using supplements that have been tested through organizations like NSF International, United States Pharmacopeia, Informed-Choice, and ConsumerLab.com. While these third-party testing certifications don't provide an ironclad, 100 percent guarantee that every bottle of a product is free of banned substances and contaminants, they do provide some reassurance for athletes who decide to use supplements.

Next, we turn our attention to some of the supplements that affect gut function during exercise. The purpose of this discussion isn't to endorse any particular supplement; instead, my goal is to provide an overview of the supplements that could affect an athlete's gut during training and on competition day. At the end of the day, each athlete needs to weigh the potential benefits and risks of using a specific supplement.

PROBIOTIC SUPPLEMENTS

People sometimes associate all bacteria with infection and disease, but it's becoming apparent that the microscopic critters living in your gut are critical to your health and well-being. Some of these bacteria, for example, provide a barrier against harmful pathogens traveling through your gut, while others aid in the digestion of otherwise indigestible nutrients or play a role in regulating your immune system.[22]

Over the past three decades, scientists have tried manipulating these bacterial populations to influence health and gut function. The main strategy used to alter the gut microbiome has been supplementing probiotics, which are, according to the World Health Organization's definition, "live microorganisms that, when administered in adequate amounts, confer a health benefit on the host."[23] Probiotics have been tested in a laundry list of health disorders, including gastrointestinal infections, inflammatory bowel diseases, IBS, asthma, respiratory tract infections, eczema, and mood disorders.[24] Despite hundreds of experiments, it's extremely difficult—if not impossible—to provide a simple message about the effects of probiotics, as they depend on a host of factors, like the species/strains and dosage used, as well as the health and diet of the person taking them.

Specific to athletes, perhaps the most frequent type of malady probiotics have been used for is upper respiratory tract infections (URTIs). It may seem odd that bugs in your gut can impact your respiratory tract, but the presence of certain microorganisms in your gut leads to an uptick in the production and activity of immune cells and compounds that offer protection from respiratory infections. In fact, more than a dozen trials have tested the effects of probiotics on various respiratory parameters in trained individuals,[25] and enough of these studies have shown reductions in the duration or severity of URTIs to suggest there are real—albeit modest—immune benefits.

In contrast, studies supplementing probiotics in athletes as a way to reduce undesirable gut symptoms are less plentiful. One of the first of these studies came out of Finland in 2007.[26] For the study, 141 runners who were participating in the Helsinki City Marathon received a drink containing a specific probiotic (*Lactobacillus rhamnosus* GG) or a similar probiotic-free drink for three months before the race. Participants filled out questionnaires about gut symptoms during the three-month pre-marathon supplementation period and for two weeks after the race. Overall, there were no meaningful differences in the percentages of runners in each group who experienced gut-symptom episodes during the training period or during the two weeks following the marathon. However, the average duration of gut-symptom episodes during the two weeks following the marathon was less in the probiotic group (1.0 versus 2.3 days). In a similar but

173

smaller study of marathoners, four weeks of supplementing with several *Lactobacillus* and *Bifidobacterium* probiotics reduced gut symptoms during the last third of a marathon.[27] Although findings from these studies are generally positive, results from others have been more conflicting or have even shown a slight worsening of symptoms.[28] These inconsistencies highlight just how complex the effects of probiotics can be and are in agreement with other studies in nonathletes showing that some strains, if taken in large doses, can worsen flatulence, bloating, and loose stools.[29, 30]

Beyond looking just at subjective symptoms, a handful of studies have evaluated how probiotics influence gut permeability during exercise. As I mentioned in Chapter 4, intense or prolonged exercise causes the narrow spaces between your intestinal cells to open, resulting in increased gut permeability. This gut leakiness permits the passage of potentially harmful substances, such as endotoxins, into your body and may raise the risk of exertional heat illnesses. Interestingly, a study of endurance-trained men revealed that supplementing with a multispecies probiotic reduced a marker of gut permeability after 14 weeks in comparison to a placebo.[31] Unfortunately, this study didn't examine gut permeability during or after exercise specifically. Another trial published two years later did happen to examine gut permeability after exhaustive running in the heat and found that four weeks of supplementing with a multispecies probiotic tended to reduce the amount of endotoxin appearing in the blood.[32] Although the mixtures of probiotics used in these studies were somewhat different, both included *Lactobacillus acidophilus*, *Bifidobacterium lactis*, and *Bifidobacterium bifidum*.

In summary, the simple notion that probiotics effectively reduce gut symptoms in otherwise healthy athletes isn't strongly supported by current evidence. Indeed, probiotics may reduce, have no effect on, or even worsen some symptoms. One positive effect on the gut that probiotics may have is reducing gut leakiness with exercise. Beyond the gut, it's worth keeping in mind that individuals partaking in heavy training may reduce their odds of catching URTIs, or at least reduce the severity of URTIs, by consuming probiotics such as *Lactobacillus rhamnosus* GG, *Lactobacillus casei*, and *Lactobacillus fermentum*. Although more studies in athletes are undoubtedly needed, this benefit has been observed in nonathletes as well, which increases the likelihood that a true respiratory immune boost is to be gained from these microbes.[33] If an athlete decides to give probiotics a whirl, there are several considerations they should keep in mind:[25, 34]

- The effects depend on the strain, species, and dosage used, so careful evaluation of a probiotic product should be undertaken before using it for a given purpose.
- In terms of types of probiotics, *Lactobacillus* and *Bifidobacterium* varieties are the most commonly used and have the strongest track records of providing benefits across a range of applications.
- Foods like yogurt, kefir, kombucha, and sauerkraut can be good sources of probiotics, but there may be some advantages to using supplements, namely that you can better target the dose and strains you want.
- Yogurt is the most popular probiotic-containing food; if relying on yogurt to get a good dose of daily probiotics, look for a seal on the container that says "Live and Active Cultures."
- In the United States, the FDA currently requires manufacturers to list probiotic supplement dosage by weight on the Supplement Facts label, although most manufacturers also choose to list a more useful quantity called colony-forming units, a measure of viable cell numbers.
- There is no minimum dosage that has been shown to be effective for all probiotics, but using one that provides at least one billion colony-forming units per day is often recommended. (Note: If using a multistrain probiotic, each strain should provide at least one billion colony-forming units.)
- Exposure to heat, light, moisture, and oxygen can take a toll on the viability of many of the bacteria found in probiotics, so it's usually advised that they be stored in a refrigerator and used by their expiration date.
- Benefits typically cease soon after stopping supplementation, so if athletes seek sustained effects, they should continue taking probiotic supplements.
- A trial period of at least one to two weeks should be used to determine whether a specific probiotic will cause mild gut side effects (gas, bloating, loose stools, etc.).
- The benefits on respiratory and gut health are likely to be modest, so other strategies that reduce the chances of URTIs and gut infections (e.g., hand hygiene, cooking foods to appropriate temperatures) should also be prioritized.
- Although probiotics have a solid safety record, individuals whose immune systems are severely compromised should avoid them unless advised otherwise by their healthcare provider.

175

BOVINE COLOSTRUM

Most people probably don't remember their first days on this planet, but like other newborn mammals, they likely received colostrum from their mother. Colostrum contains relatively low amounts of natural milk sugar (lactose), but within the first few days after delivery, lactose concentrations in human breast milk increase substantially, and after several weeks, a full transition to what's considered mature milk occurs.[35] While it's occasionally just thought of as a precursor to mature breast milk, colostrum is rich in immune components (e.g., antibodies and white blood cells) and growth factors that are critical to an infant's ability to fight infections and develop optimally.[35] These immune and growth components are also what drive interest in colostrum as a supplement, not only for infants and children, but also for fully grown adults.

As with humans, our pasture-loving bovine friends also produce colostrum, and this version is the most popular supplemental form of colostrum sold in most countries. The thought of ingesting another human's colostrum as an adult is a turnoff for most consumers, so even beyond the regulatory issues of capturing and selling human colostrum, it shouldn't be surprising that supplement makers usually choose the bovine version for production purposes.

Similar to probiotic use, one of the reasons people supplement with bovine colostrum is that they believe it will boost immunity. Indeed, a handful of small trials conducted in athletes seem to confirm the anecdotal accounts of bovine colostrum's cold-fighting powers; specifically, a 2016 analysis of five placebo-controlled trials reported that the number of days with upper respiratory symptoms was reduced by 44 percent with bovine colostrum supplementation.[36] Because athletes are more susceptible to acquiring URTIs during heavy training periods as well as after multihour competitions, supplementing with bovine colostrum represents a relatively low-risk strategy (assuming the supplement is third-party tested for quality) to boost respiratory immune defenses and lower the chances of acquiring a training-killing infection.

Another common reason athletes take bovine colostrum is for its purported ability to improve performance, speed recovery, and enhance body composition. According to a scientific review written by Mathias Rathe, a researcher at Odense University Hospital in Denmark, slightly more than a dozen trials (as of 2013) had put the performance-enhancing claims behind bovine colostrum to the test, and just under half of these trials displayed some sort of the benefit.[37] While more than half a decade has passed since Rathe's review was published, the weight of evidence supporting bovine colostrum hasn't changed all that much. It is worth considering that most of these studies used small numbers of volunteers, and consequently, a clear endorsement of bovine colostrum for performance enhancement probably isn't warranted at this time.

A final alleged benefit of bovine colostrum—and the one most relevant to the focus of this book—is its ability to prevent the leaky gut phenomenon (for a review, see Chapter 4). Bovine colostrum contains several growth factors that may help repair damaged gastrointestinal tissue after an injurious event such as grueling exercise in the heat. When eaten alone, these growth factors are susceptible to digestion in the stomach and are unable to reach the small intestine intact, where they elicit some of their positive effects. However, when combined with the other components in bovine colostrum, their breakdown is largely prevented. At least a half-dozen studies have evaluated whether bovine colostrum can blunt the typical rise in gut permeability that occurs with acute exercise or with chronic heavy training, and all told, three trials have found reductions in gut permeability,[38-40] two have found no changes,[41, 42] and one has actually found an increase in permeability.[43] One potential reason for the inconsistent findings is that the concentrations of bioactive compounds in bovine colostrum supplements often vary due to natural between-animal variations, the timing of collection, and postcollection processing.[44]

All in all, the evidence behind bovine colostrum can be described as mixed. The most consistent value of supplementation seems to be reducing the number of days an athlete is affected by URTI symptoms. When it comes to improving the health and function of the gut, there's certainly reason to think that bovine colostrum might be of benefit under certain circumstances. Of studies done with athletes, about half have shown improvements in gut barrier function, which, in theory, could reduce the risk of heat-related illness or experiencing unpleasant gut symptoms during prolonged exercise. Unfortunately, these two latter proposed benefits remain unverified.

If you decide to supplement with bovine colostrum, you should be cognizant of several things:

- There have been occasional reports of digestive disturbances—nausea, flatulence, diarrhea, abdominal discomfort—from taking bovine colostrum,[37] so taking it immediately prior to or during an important training session or competition isn't advisable unless you know from experience it won't cause problems.

- Bovine colostrum contains several growth factors—including insulin-like growth factor 1—that are prohibited by organizations such as WADA, and even though studies have failed to find consistent increases in blood levels of insulin-like growth factor 1 after colostrum supplementation, WADA still recommends against using it.[45]

- Very few specific colostrum products have been independently verified for quality and/or purity by organizations such as NSF International, United States Pharmacopeia, or Informed-Choice; practically speaking, this makes it difficult to find a product that you could have a high level of confidence in, particularly if you're an athlete undergoing doping tests.

- The amounts of bovine colostrum used in studies on respiratory and gut function have varied quite a bit, but doses of 10–20 grams per day are common.

- Colostrum powders are probably more practical for reaching the typical dosage (10–20 grams per day), as capsules often only contain 0.5–1.0 grams each.

- Compared to many other sports supplements (creatine, whey protein), bovine colostrum isn't particularly cheap, and someone supplementing at the low end of the dosage spectrum (10 grams per day) would likely spend around $1 to $2 per day; with that in mind, using colostrum in a more targeted fashion (during periods of heavy training and when the risk of infections is high) is more cost-effective.

GLUTAMINE

Glutamine is the most abundant amino acid circulating in your blood and found within your skeletal muscles.[46] Although it's technically a nonessential amino acid (meaning that your body can make it), your body's demand for glutamine can outpace its ability to manufacturer it during extreme stress (e.g., trauma, severe infection). This inability to make enough glutamine during times of extreme stress means that you need to consume some in order to optimize the function of several organ systems, including your gut. Consequently, glutamine is what's known as a conditionally essential amino acid.

Glutamine has many vital functions, such as playing a role in the regulation of blood glucose and acid-base balance, but the most important one that's covered here relates to the functioning of your gut. Studies in humans tell us that much of the glutamine you eat is sequestered and metabolized in your gastrointestinal cells. Compared to other nutrients that are readily passed on to your liver and other parts of your body, a smaller proportion of the glutamine you ingest leaves the cells in your gut. In one study, 54 percent of ingested glutamine never entered systemic blood, indicating it was locked up by gut tissue.[47] And importantly, it seems the bulk of this sequestered glutamine is burned for energy by intestinal tissues.[48]

Your gut's appetite for glutamine isn't exclusive, as other rapidly proliferating cells in your body also crave it.[49] Rapidly proliferating tissues are those that replace cells in a short time span; the epithelial cells of the gut are believed to have one of the most rapid turnover rates in adult mammals, with a time frame of two to six days.[50] While other cells (such as lymphocytes and reticulocytes) also experience rapid cell turnover, the size of your gut makes it one of the most important sites of glutamine metabolism.

Knowledge of glutamine's role as an energy source for rapidly proliferating intestinal and immune cells has spurred researchers to evaluate how feeding this amino acid affects people experiencing extreme stress. Clinical trials in critically ill patients, for example, have shown that glutamine administration lowers rates of hospital-acquired infections.[51] Part of this reduction in infections among the gravely ill is believed to occur through maintenance of intestinal barrier integrity, which prevents the passage of harmful pathogens from the gut into the bloodstream. Alternatively, the reduced rates of infection could also stem from glutamine's ability to stimulate the proliferation of immune cells such as lymphocytes.

While glutamine may offer benefits under the extreme circumstances of a life-threatening illness, you might be wondering if any of this is generalizable under the milder (relatively speaking) conditions of exercise. In 2011, a panel of leading scientists authored a position statement on the topic of immunity and exercise that included recommendations related to glutamine supplementation.[52] Even though this group of experts recognized the importance of glutamine as a fuel source for immune cells, they ultimately recommended against supplementation because the best placebo-controlled experiments have failed to show benefits on markers of immune function in the context of exercise. The most likely reason for the lack of benefits is that the body's storage pool of glutamine may not be sufficiently depleted by exercise to impair immune defenses. These conclusions were largely reaffirmed by a more recent consensus statement on the topic.[53]

Specific to gut function and exercise, there's a small but growing body of research documenting glutamine's capacity to act as a gut barrier enhancer. One of the most recent of these investigations was conducted by researchers at Liverpool John Moores University in the United Kingdom. The study, led by Jamie Pugh, examined the dose-response effects of glutamine on exercise-associated increases in gut permeability.[54] Ten men ran on a treadmill for 60 minutes on four occasions, and two hours before each run they consumed one of four glutamine dosages: 0, 0.25, 0.5, or 0.9 grams per kilogram of lean body mass. To give some context, a participant weighing 165 pounds who had a body fat of 20 percent would have ingested 15, 30, and 54 grams before the three glutamine trials. Since sweltering conditions worsen gut leakiness, each run was carried out in a special chamber that created stifling environmental conditions (86°F and 40–45 percent relative humidity). While all three doses of glutamine modestly reduced gut permeability, the effect seemed to be the greatest with the largest dose. This observation that glutamine mitigates increases in gut leakiness during and following exercise aligns with other studies on the topic.[55-57]

Before you decide to start gobbling down glutamine, you should consider a couple of caveats to this research. First, Pugh and his colleagues failed to find differences in gut symptoms between when runners consumed glutamine and when they consumed a placebo. Thus, although glutamine may make your gut somewhat less leaky, those improvements may not translate into a reduction in uncomfortable symptoms. It's possible that glutamine would have lessened symptoms during a longer run, but alas, we don't have that data. The second—and more important caveat—is that the referenced exercise studies showing a benefit of glutamine on gut barrier function didn't use energy-matched placebos.[54-57] As covered in Chapter 4, carbohydrate ingestion during exercise can quell gut permeability, even above and beyond the effects of fluid alone, and adding glutamine doesn't prevent gut permeability any better than a carbohydrate beverage alone.[58]

Looking at the big picture, it's worth keeping in mind that carbohydrate-containing beverages are cheaper than glutamine supplements and also improve endurance. To me, the use of glutamine supplements to prevent gut leakiness during exercise seems largely superfluous, at least until additional research shows it's better than carbohydrate beverages. This also applies to other supplements (curcumin, L-citrulline, etc.) that reduce biomarkers of gut damage or leakiness during exercise but that probably have minimal impact on performance or gut symptoms.[59, 60]

Should you decide you want to try glutamine supplementation despite the above-mentioned caveats, the following is a list of considerations to keep in mind:

- Glutamine supplements are often labeled with the term *L-glutamine*, which is the particular chemical form of glutamine the human body uses.
- Doses used in studies on exercise and gut function have ranged considerably but fall somewhere between 15 and 50 grams.
- Although the above doses have resulted in few adverse effects in short-term studies, there's an absence of long-term data, and it's unclear whether using glutamine at such high doses is safe over months and years.
- As was the case with bovine colostrum, powders are the more practical option for reaching the typical dosage used (it would require taking dozens of capsules to hit a 15-to-50-gram dose).
- If using a single acute dose of glutamine prior to exercise, it is usually taken one to two hours beforehand.
- People with liver failure or cirrhosis should avoid glutamine supplements because they can increase blood ammonia levels.

GINGER

The *Zingiber officinale* plant (otherwise known as ginger root) is thought to have originated in Southeast Asia several thousand years ago and later became an important article of trade during the reign of the Romans.[61] Ginger continued to be traded heavily for centuries, even after the fall of the Roman Empire, at which time much of its trade into Europe was controlled by Arab merchants. Today, the largest producers of ginger are China, India, and Nigeria.

Ginger has been used medicinally for centuries, and although we still have much to learn about its effects, there's currently enough science to appreciate why so many historical cultures jumped on the ginger bandwagon. Ginger contains numerous active compounds, so it's difficult to say for sure exactly which ones are responsible for its effects. However, a combination of test tube studies, animal experiments, and human clinical trials points to a series of phenolic ketone compounds. These compounds— referred to as gingerols, shogaols, and paradols—influence the body's inflammatory mediators that not only cause swelling and pain but that also affect gut function.[62]

The list of sicknesses historically treated with ginger is extensive, ranging from minor concerns like colds, indigestion, and aches and pain to more serious conditions like cancer and diabetes. Despite not having the tools of modern science to evaluate ginger's physiological effects, our predecessors were clearly onto something with their use of ginger. Indeed, experiments have borne out at least some of what traditional Chinese, Arab, and Roman cultures suspected about ginger's therapeutic properties. Clinical trials in patients with osteoarthritis, for example, have shown ginger to be a modestly effective pain reliever.[63] These pain-relieving effects may extend to athletes, as a few experiments have demonstrated that ginger modestly reduces exercise-induced pain.[64]

Specific to the gut, ginger ingestion has long been used as a remedy for nausea and vomiting originating from such culprits as chemotherapy, pregnancy, and stormy seas. The television show *MythBusters* even tried out this age-old remedy by having seasick-prone cohost Adam Savage and sidekick Grant Imahara consume ginger before sitting in a rotating chair. For both of these *MythBusters* men, ginger pills effectively prevented motion sickness, although knowingly ingesting ginger obviously could have induced a placebo effect. Nonetheless, the results of their testing generally align with what's been observed in double-blind trials, which is that ginger is moderately effective for reducing the severity of nausea.[65]

Because nausea is frequently encountered in all kinds of sports, ginger's antibarf properties may be of special interest to athletes. Ultraendurance runners are particularly well acquainted with the desire to spew during races; in one large study, nearly 40 percent of 100-mile trail race competitors reported experiencing nausea and/or vomiting, and it was the leading reason for DNFs.[66] Likewise, anyone who's done a 400-meter dash or ran a mile as fast as possible is probably familiar with the urge to vomit that often appears afterward. While taking ginger before an ultraendurance race or before repeated sprinting makes some logical sense, all the evidence supporting its anti-nausea properties comes from studies of nonathletes. That doesn't mean it's ineffective for managing exercise-induced nausea; it just simply means we can't know for sure if it works because the studies haven't been done. If you ever decide to give ginger a try before intense or prolonged exercise, be aware that despite its potential anti-nausea properties, it can increase the incidence of other gut symptoms, particularly heartburn.[63] It's therefore advisable for any athlete using ginger to consume it well before the start of exercise so that it has time to empty from the stomach.

Ginger isn't a one-trick pony when it comes to the gut. Beyond its anti-nausea properties, ginger may offer protection from gut-damaging substances such as alcohol and NSAIDs. Studies in animals demonstrate that ginger reduces stomach wounds that normally develop after exposure to gastro-erosive substances, and these effects are possibly due to reductions in gastric acid secretion.[67] Likewise, a study of people with osteoarthritis found ginger extract to be as effective as diclofenac (an NSAID) for pain management while also causing less gut pain and increasing stomach mucosa prostaglandins, compounds that protect the stomach.[68] While more research is undoubtedly needed, the evidence we have indicates that, in comparison to NSAIDs, ginger is perhaps a more gut-friendly option for managing pain.

The following are practical considerations when it comes to supplementing with ginger, whether it be for managing nausea, pain, or something else:

- Even though it's typically thought of as being safe when taken over several weeks or months, we're short on studies documenting ginger's long-term safety.
- People who have bleeding disorders or take blood-thinning drugs should consult with their physicians before using ginger because of its propensity to affect blood clotting.

- Dosage-wise, studies that have used ginger as an anti-nausea remedy have typically administered 1–2 grams per day (if taken for several days) or an equal amount about an hour before an expected nausea-provoking event.
- Taking large dosages of ginger (more than a few grams per day) is associated with a greater incidence of gastrointestinal symptoms like heartburn and mild stomach upset.
- Because the content of gingerols largely determines the physiological activity of ginger, it's probably worthwhile to obtain a supplement that is standardized to contain a known or minimum amount (e.g., 5 percent) of these compounds.
- Many premade foods containing ginger (ales, snaps, etc.) don't contain enough gingerols to quell nausea or pain; if you're looking to get a real physiological effect, it's best to go with a supplement or to make your own beverage or food, which allows you to control the amount of ginger added in.
- The active compounds in ginger degrade over time, so it's a good idea to use a ginger supplement or powder within 6 to 12 months of purchasing it.

SUPPLEMENTS THAT CAN CAUSE GUT DISTURBANCES

As you've learned thus far, there are a handful of supplements that might positively impact gut function and symptoms. Even so, there are plenty of supplements with digestive side effects that athletes should be aware of. Let's start with one of the most popular sports supplements in the world: caffeine. I should acknowledge at the outset that caffeine—whether it's taken in the form of a pill, coffee, or energy drink—delivers impressive performance-enhancing benefits. Truly, no other (legal) ingestible substance on earth improves athletic performance in so many different contexts.[69]

Despite a mountain of data supporting caffeine as a performance enhancer, its gut-related effects are something you should consider. Anecdotally speaking, coffee drinkers know that a cup of Joe in the morning helps to open the metaphorical freeway that is their gut. A 1998 experiment confirmed these anecdotes by showing that caffeinated coffee simulates colon activity more than water and decaffeinated coffee.[70] And while obviously not completely generalizable to humans, a study of domestic canines (hound dogs, to be precise) found that intravenous injections of caffeine increased colonic motility in a dose-dependent manner.[71] In some of my own research with triathletes,

I found that higher morning caffeine intakes were correlated with worse lower gut symptoms during the running leg of a 70.3-mile triathlon.[72]

To be clear, I'm not arguing that caffeine should necessarily be avoided as a performance aid; there's just too much scientific evidence documenting its benefits. Instead, these studies simply serve as a reminder that gut function—primarily colon activity—is affected by caffeine and that you should integrate this knowledge with your own experiences to determine the timing and dose of caffeine that works best for you. As an example, you could keep track of your caffeine intake over a few days or a week to see if there's a predictable time span between when you consume caffeine and when you experience urges to empty your bowels.

Another evidence-based—although certainly less popular—performance-enhancing substance that can impact gut function is found in most people's kitchens: Baking soda, or sodium bicarbonate, is a substance that neutralizes acids. It has many domestic usages (cooking ingredient, household cleaner, etc.), but it can also be used to improve high-intensity anaerobic exercise capacity. Short bursts of high-intensity activity produce metabolic by-products that turn the local environment in your muscles acidic, which ultimately interferes with muscular contraction. Extra bicarbonate in your blood helps manage this rise in acidity by increasing the efflux of these metabolic byproducts (lactate and hydrogen ions) from your muscle to your blood. Put simply, sodium bicarbonate allows you to keep the pedal to the metal for a little bit longer. Indeed, a scientific review by researcher Peter Christensen and colleagues found that sodium bicarbonate improved high-intensity exercise performance (lasting from 45 seconds to 8 minutes),[73] and the observed improvement with sodium bicarbonate was roughly the same magnitude as with caffeine.

Despite its potential benefits, few athletes utilize sodium bicarbonate before competition. A major reason is because of its propensity to cause digestive disturbances. Upper gut symptoms like fullness/bloating, belching, and nausea/vomiting predominate for 30-60 minutes after ingestion, while flatulence, urges to defecate, and diarrhea start to become more of a problem 90-120 minutes after ingestion. The severity of symptoms varies tremendously between athletes, but an average rating of 2 on a 0-to-10-point scale is typical.[74] Undoubtedly, experiencing severe forms of these symptoms—particularly vomiting and explosive diarrhea—is enough to stop any athlete dead in their tracks.

185

Thankfully, several strategies can maximize the benefits of sodium bicarbonate while minimizing gut problems. In terms of timing, peak cumulative gut distress typically occurs about 60–90 minutes after commencing sodium bicarbonate ingestion, while its beneficial acid-buffering effects are usually maintained for two and a half to three hours.[75] Consequently, consuming sodium bicarbonate about two hours before competition is a prudent tactic that can minimize gut disturbances during competition. Another easy method of reducing sodium bicarbonate's gut symptoms is to ingest carbohydrate-rich foods with it; around 100 grams of carbohydrate from foods such as toast, cereal, or bars should do the trick.[75] Lastly, an alternative approach to single-dose pre-competition supplementation is to take sodium bicarbonate over several days leading up to competition.[76, 77] This would involve consuming it daily for five or six days (about 40 grams per day spread over several doses) and then ceasing supplementation the day before competition.

On a final practical note, sodium bicarbonate should always be taken with fluid, either by mixing baking soda with water or by consuming fluid with pill or capsule forms of sodium bicarbonate. Probably the most frequently used dose is 0.3 grams per kilogram of body mass (roughly 20 grams for a 150-pound athlete) along with 15–20 ounces of fluid. Care should be taken when measuring out sodium bicarbonate, as large amounts can be toxic. In addition, individuals with kidney or metabolic disorders should avoid supplementing with it or at least consult with their physicians beforehand.

The final supplement covered in this chapter is ketones, which are molecules produced during starvation or when a person follows a very-low-carbohydrate diet. Under normal circumstances, your body burns a mixture of fat and carbohydrate to fuel your activities. However, during extreme carbohydrate restriction, large quantities of fatty acids are liberated from your body's fat stores, causing a change in the way fatty acids are used for energy. Ordinarily, fatty acids are broken down into a molecule called acetyl-CoA, which combines with another molecule called oxaloacetate to form citrate. However, when very large quantities of fatty acids are broken down into acetyl-CoA (such as when a person is on very-low-carbohydrate diet), the normal system of metabolizing fat becomes flooded, causing some of the acetyl-CoA to be converted to ketones.[78]

Starvation and heavy carbohydrate restriction aren't usually a recipe for success in most sports, so companies like the San Francisco–based start-up H.V.M.N. have developed supplemental ketones that are designed to elicit a state of ketosis without having to restrict dietary energy or carbohydrate. Part of the notion behind why ingesting ketones is supposedly beneficial for exercise performance is that they serve as a "fourth fuel" for energy production (carbohydrate, fat, and protein are the other three fuels).[79] In theory, ketone ingestion could also indirectly improve exercise performance by shifting how other fuels are metabolized, one example being the sparing of muscle glycogen stores.[80]

187

Despite some bold claims, there are little data showing that ketone supplements meaningfully improve exercise performance, and the findings to date were nicely summed up in a recent scientific review on the topic:

> " At present there are no data available to suggest that ingestion of ketone bodies . . . improves athletes' performance under conditions where evidence-based nutritional strategies are applied appropriately.[81]

What's more, a pair of studies published in 2017 found that ketone supplementation led to worse exercise performance![82, 83] Upon closer examination, it was apparent in one of these studies that gut distress was the main reason for the athletes' lackluster showings.[83] The most common symptom reported was nausea, which ranged from mild to dry retching. Notably, both studies that showed detrimental performance effects of supplemental ketones used relatively brief endurance tests (less than one hour), so whether ketones work for other types of competition—such as ultra-races where the average exercise intensity is lower—remains to be seen.

Overall, ketones remain an intriguing supplement because they've shown some ability to alter metabolism during exercise. However, these metabolic changes haven't clearly led to better performance and probably don't outweigh the risks of gut distress that can accompany ketone ingestion. If you ever decide that ketone supplementation is something worth trying, going with the ester and salt forms is often recommended, owing to the fact that the free-acid form isn't effective at inducing ketosis.[83] While there are claims that ketone esters cause fewer gut side effects than ketone salts (supposedly making them a better choice for athletes), several studies say otherwise, particularly when ketone esters are taken in large doses.[83, 84]

DIETARY SUPPLEMENTS

If a **safety concern** arises with a supplement sold in the US, the FDA has the burden of proving the supplement is unsafe before it can be removed from the market.

Contamination and **poor quality** are common problems affecting a disconcertingly large percentage of supplements.

In terms of quality, **herbals** are near the top of the list of worst offenders.

Athletes subject to **doping tests** should only use supplements that have been independently tested by organizations like NSF International and Informed-Choice.

Because they often contain ingredients with **stimulant-like properties,** weight-loss aids and energy boosters are some of the most **dangerous** products.

Probiotics and **bovine colostrum** may reduce the incidence and/or severity of URTIs in athletes.

Probiotics, **bovine colostrum**, and **glutamine** may all be capable of reducing gut permeability with exercise, though carbohydrate beverages are probably equally as effective and cheaper.

Although **ginger** has documented anti-nausea properties for motion sickness, chemotherapy, and pregnancy, its ability to prevent nausea and vomiting during and after exercise has yet to be evaluated.

Caffeine and **sodium bicarbonate** are performance-enhancing substances, but they can also cause unpleasant gut symptoms in some athletes.

The gut symptoms associated with sodium bicarbonate ingestion can be **minimized** by taking it with carbohydrate two hours before competition or by using a multiday supplementation protocol.

Although **ketone supplements** are becoming popular, they haven't been shown to improve endurance performance in most situations, which may largely be due to their propensity to cause nausea and other gut symptoms.

PSYCHOLOGY
AND THE ATHLETE'S GUT

11

STRESS
AND ANXIETY

Pre-game nerves. Race-day jitters. Unabating thoughts of choking. A thumping heart. These are all manifestations of competition stress and anxiety, and many athletes—from recreational ballers to Olympic champions—experience these symptoms regularly. The effects of competition anxiety undoubtedly extend to the gut. As an example, one of the more common symptoms associated with stressful competition (or anxiety from a job interview, first date, etc.) is butterflies in the stomach, a ticklish or fluttering feeling in the abdomen. (The exact physiology behind this fluttering is a mystery, but it may have to do with changes in gut blood flow and nervous system activity.) Athletes nervous about an upcoming game or race are known to be stricken by other gut symptoms like nausea/vomiting, abdominal cramping, and unrelenting urges to use the privy.

While the gut is often thought of as being distinctly separate from the brain, the connections between these two parts of your body run deep. As I detailed in Chapter 1, your gut is home to between 100 million and 600 million neurons, which is one reason it's referred to by many scientists as the body's "second brain." These connections allow important information about what's happening in your gut to be relayed to your central nervous system. Likewise, information flowing in the opposite direction—from your central nervous system to your gut—allows your body to prioritize how resources such as blood and oxygen are utilized during times of stress. Like any elegant system, your gut-brain connection is prone to glitches. Experiencing too much stress, excessive anxiety, or a traumatic event can muck up this intricate system.

Before we dive into the science on gut-brain-mood connections in sports, I want to reiterate that I'm not a psychologist or neuroscientist. I have degrees in dietetics and exercise physiology and am a credentialed registered dietitian. So why, then, did I decide to devote an entire section of *The Athlete's Gut* to these gut-brain-mood connections? The main impetus for including this information is that I have personally experienced glitches in these mind-gut connections, both in the context of sports and in everyday life. Like many people, I have mild general anxiety, but my most impactful run-ins with anxiety have been in performance situations. In high school, these symptoms were most severe during basketball season. Performing in front of a crowd, in combination with a fear of letting down other players on my team, were the roots of my anxiety. My uneasiness wasn't usually intense enough for others to notice, but I sometimes found myself overthinking decisions during games, which is generally not advantageous during fast-paced sports like basketball.

My competitive sporting days are largely a thing of the past, but there are still occasions when I have to perform professionally (scientific conferences, media interviews, etc.). Most of the time I come off sounding calm and collected (so I've been told), but that's not always the case underneath the surface, particularly in the moments leading up to these performances. As one saying goes, people are a lot like ducks, calm on the surface, but paddling like the devil underneath. I sometimes experience the gastrointestinal symptoms that accompany anxiety in these situations, including indigestion and mild abdominal cramping; however, it's the cardiovascular and respiratory manifestations of my anxiety—along with my distorted thoughts—that are most unsettling. A slight tightness in my chest, feeling mildly short of breath, and a thumping heart are the physical expressions, while thoughts like "What happens if I can't control these symptoms?" pop into my head, which ultimately exacerbates my physical symptoms. Ninety-nine times out of a hundred these physical symptoms and thoughts abate once the performance begins, but on a couple of occasions they've gotten the better of me, leading to a less-than-stellar presentation. Over the years I've learned to deal with my performance anxiety through a combination of strategies, but I still occasionally struggle with it. The fact is, I will probably always have some of these thoughts and symptoms leading up to professional performances.

As someone who conducts scientific research, I'm fully aware that having firsthand experience with something doesn't automatically make you an expert on that topic. Case in point, there are scores of internet "experts" and "gurus" selling nutrition products and services based on their personal stories. Many of the claims made by these modern-day charlatans are devoid of science. That said, my own encounters with anxiety prodded me to explore the scientific links between the gut and the mind, and because of my established interest in sports science research, I eventually ended up combing through the literature in an attempt to find studies documenting exactly how anxiety and stress influence gut function before and during sporting competition. Although I came across a plethora of research on competition-related anxiety, I found, to my utter surprise, few studies that directly examined how mood states and gut symptoms are connected in athletic competition. To me this was shocking given all the anecdotes of competition-related nerves propelling athletes to puke before games or make frequent trips to the loo.

193

A recent high-profile anecdote of this sort of experience comes from a professional American football player named Brandon Brooks, a guard for the Philadelphia Eagles. In a 2018 *Los Angeles Times* piece written before the 52nd Super Bowl between Brooks's Eagles and the New England Patriots, columnist Bill Plaschke described Brooks's struggle with competition-related anxiety. In addition to stating that Brooks usually pukes before every game, Plaschke wrote:

> *There was a time this fear triggered vomiting all day and night, causing him to miss the game. He has been sick enough for teammates to surround him in prayer, and for team doctors to send him to a hospital where he would watch those teammates on TV with his head stuck in a bowl.*[1]

After missing several games and taking a trip to the hospital, Brooks was diagnosed with an anxiety disorder, which he revealed to the world despite the tough-man culture ingrained in American football.

Brooks's incidents with anxiety and vomiting are obviously on the extreme end of the spectrum of possibilities, but he's by no means the first pro athlete to deal with competition-related anxiety powerful enough to induce vomiting. NBA legend Bill Russell purportedly vomited before almost every game of his professional career, and during one playoff game, Celtics coach Red Auerbach allegedly demanded his team leave the court during warm-ups and return to the locker room because he hadn't yet heard Russell toss his cookies.[2] NFL Hall of Famer Steve Young also reportedly suffered from anxiety-induced vomiting. Although Young was the league's defending Most Valuable Player in 1993, he found himself vomiting before a game against the Atlanta Falcons, which largely stemmed from his fears of disappointing others and replacing the legendary Joe Montana.[3]

Ultimately, the goal of the third part of this book is to explore what's behind a case like Brandon Brooks's, as well as the gastral misfortunes of countless other lesser-known athletes who have dealt with an angry gut that's the by-product of competition-related stress and anxiety. In this chapter, I review the concept of stress and how it relates to health, athletic performance, and gut function, which is followed by a discussion of the connections between anxiety and these same outcomes.

STRESS

Stress is a fundamental, inevitable part of life. Yet for many of us, the word *stress* evokes mostly negative connotations. It's true that too much stress can be harmful to your health and performance, but it's important to remember that stress is your body's response to any demand placed on it. This generalized, purposefully vague definition of stress was first proposed by Hans Selye, an Austro-Hungarian endocrinologist considered to be the father of the modern biomedical stress concept.[4] Selye's thoughts on stress can be succinctly summarized with an oft-used quote from his thousand-plus-page doorstopper, *Stress in Health and Disease*:

> ❝ *Stress is not something to be avoided. Indeed, it cannot be avoided, since just staying alive creates some demand for life-maintaining energy. Even when man is asleep, his heart, respiratory apparatus, digestive tract, nervous system and other organs must continue to function. Complete freedom from stress can be expected only after death.*[5]

As with most sweeping theories, not everyone agrees with Selye's take that stress is best viewed as a nonspecific response.[4] Regardless, there is universal agreement that stress is a necessary part of life. What's also true is that persistent elevations in certain types of stress are damaging to health and performance. For example, heightened psychological stress in the workplace or stress that's a result of a traumatic life event have been linked to ailments such as stroke, type 2 diabetes, and obesity.[6-8]

In athletes, the acute psychological stress that bubbles up before and during competition is ubiquitous but doesn't necessarily have a predictable relationship with performance. Among other reasons, this is because of differences in how stress is defined and measured in studies as well as the variability in how individual athletes appraise the manifestations of stress. As an example, one athlete might perceive a pre-game elevation in heart rate as a positive signal that their body is prepping itself for the challenge to come, while another athlete may view this same response as a disturbing lack of control over their bodily functions.

Despite the inconsistent associations between acute competition-related stress and performance, long-term elevations of stress—especially if they're perceived by an athlete to be negative—are dependably linked with injuries and overreaching syndromes.[9] These connections are so reliable that in 2006 the American College of Sports Medicine (in conjunction with several other medical organizations) published a consensus paper with the following statement about the impact of stress on injury:

> ❝ *Personality factors (e.g., introversion/extroversion, self-esteem, perfectionism) and other psychological factors (e.g., a supportive social network, coping resources, high achievement motivation) alone do not reliably predict athletic injury risk. . . . However, there has been a consistently demonstrated relationship between one psychological factor—stress—and athletic injury risk.*[10]

So even though *direct* relationships between stress and athletic performance are rather unpredictable, it's obvious that an injured or sick athlete is one who can't perform at her peak. Thus, it behooves coaches and practitioners to pay close attention to sources of stress in their athletes' lives.

It's not completely understood how psychological stress contributes to injuries in athletes, though there's no shortage of hypotheses. One possibility is that stressed athletes aren't paying close enough attention to what's going on in the midst of competition, which, in sports like American football and rugby, could lead to being blindsided by an opposing player. To a certain extent, this hypothesis is supported by experiments showing that under stressful conditions, athletes tend to have wandering eyes, and they fixate more on unimportant cues in their visual fields.[11]

An alternative proposed mechanism involves hormone fluctuations, particularly in cortisol, a steroid-type molecule produced in your adrenals. As an anatomy refresher, your adrenal glands sit atop your kidneys and look curiously similar to the bicorne hat that Napoleon once donned. Undoubtedly, cortisol is the hormone that most of the public associates with stress, and the internet is saturated with articles with alarmist-sounding titles like "Cortisol: Why the 'Stress Hormone' Is Public Enemy No. 1."[12] Despite its poor public reputation, cortisol's functions are notoriously difficult to generalize about, as they often depend on the health of the individual, the tissue targeted by the hormone, and how much of (and for how long) it is secreted. What's more, cortisol levels vary with your circadian rhythm, which is a phrase used to describe any biological process that displays an entrainable 24-hour pattern. Cortisol rises upon wakening in the morning, followed by a nadir in the evening. When you also consider that cortisol secretion can vary markedly from day to day in the same person, it's easy to understand why it's so difficult to establish a baseline blood cortisol level for someone. Think of traffic patterns as an analogy; clearly, it would be foolish to assume that the flow of traffic on a freeway at 8:00 a.m. is reflective of what traffic is like at 10:00 p.m.

To address this cortisol measurement conundrum, researchers can take multiple blood or saliva samples from a person, but that's particularly challenging to do in large studies that aim to understand the links between exposures (such as cortisol) and diseases/injuries that develop over weeks, months, or years. Scientists have begun to work around this obstacle by analyzing samples from tissues that are believed to reflect long-term cortisol levels (i.e., human hair), but even with this improvement in analytical methods, relationships between cortisol and health aren't always straightforward. Take the findings of a comprehensive review published in *Psychoneuroendocrinology*, which concluded that although hair cortisol levels were higher among individuals living with chronic pain, depression, and a history of major life events (suggesting they experience more chronic stress), levels among people with anxiety and post-traumatic stress disorder (PTSD) were often lower than in healthy subjects.[13]

Exactly why people with chronic anxiety and PTSD would have diminished cortisol levels is uncertain, but one possibility is that they've developed an overly sensitive feedback response.[14] The hypothalamus and pituitary gland are the prime regulators of cortisol production by your adrenal glands, and when your cortisol levels get too high, your hypothalamus and pituitary gland respond by pumping the metaphorical brakes on its production. This pumping of the brakes—known as negative feedback inhibition— contains your stress response and prevents it from spinning out of control. Under situations of prolonged, elevated stress, however, the hypothalamus and pituitary may become overly sensitive to cortisol, leading to excessive braking and a state of chronic hypocortisolism (low cortisol levels). While this is a workable hypothesis, another conceivable explanation for the links between hypocortisolism and PTSD and anxiety is that low cortisol levels predispose people to developing these conditions. Long story short, the connections between cortisol and health are surprisingly complex.

With that tangent about the measurement of cortisol out of the way, let's return to the more relevant question at hand. Do elevated cortisol levels predict injuries in athletes? The short answer is no. The more complicated answer is that we don't yet fully know, as few longitudinal studies have looked at this question.[15] Considering the totality of evidence, however, there's little reason to believe that excessive cortisol secretion is directly responsible for the development of most injuries and illnesses in athletes.

So if cortisol doesn't clearly explain the higher rates of injuries and illnesses among chronically stressed athletes, then what does? As a scientist, I'm trained to recognize that it's foolhardy to expect a simplistic explanation for a complex phenomenon. This certainly rings true to me when it comes to explaining injuries and illnesses in sports. With this caveat in mind, there's at least one convincing explanation for the greater risk of one type of "injury" in stressed-out athletes: suppression of the immune system. Even in nonathletes, it's been recognized for at least 50 years that chronic stress and major life events often precede the onset of respiratory tract infections and other minor ailments,[16, 17] but it wasn't until years later that scientists began to understand the specific immune changes that occur in response to sustained stress. I won't go into the specifics of these immune changes, but there are loads of studies showing that almost every aspect of immune function is affected by chronic stress. As one scientific review that assessed three decades of research put it, "The most chronic stressors were associated with the most global immunosuppression, as they were associated with reliable decreases in almost all functional immune measures examined."[18]

This state of immunosuppression helps explain why stressed-out athletes often have the sniffles or reoccurring colds. It might also explain why these athletes often don't return from physical injuries as quickly as expected, as the immune system is directly involved in healing.[19] In one frequently referenced study, two small wounds were made on the roofs of the mouths of dental students, the first of which was timed during a low-stress period (summer vacation), while the second was timed during a high-stress period (three days before the students' first exam of the term).[20] Even though both wounds were the same size to start, it took the students 40 percent longer to heal during the exam period. Of course, there are other potential explanations for the different healing rates (diet, exercise, sleep, etc.), but additional studies have produced similar findings in other populations, bolstering the case that chronic stress impairs healing.[21]

In contrast to the prolonged kind, psychological stress that lasts minutes to hours can actually boost immune function, a point articulated by Firdaus Dhabhar, esteemed stress researcher at the University of Miami. Dhabhar thoroughly outlined the evidence for this immune-boosting effect of acute stress in a paper published in *Immunologic Research*, arguing that it makes sense from an evolutionary perspective for the body to prioritize immune function during and after stressful situations because they often (at least thousands of years ago) resulted in wounds, injuries, and infections.[19] Dhabhar reasoned that the process of evolution would be unlikely to select for a system that would allow a person, in his words, "to escape the jaws and claws of a lion only to succumb to wounds and pathogens."

To summarize, a simple way to think about psychological stress is that, when it's experienced in sufficient doses over multiple days, weeks, and months, it can impair health, healing, and physical recovery. Contrary to what is often reported in media stories, cortisol isn't the most important culprit responsible for many of the harms associated with stress. In reality, there are likely several ways by which sustained stress negatively affects your health and recovery, one of the most important being the suppression of your immune system.

STRESS AND GUT FUNCTION

199

One of the most powerful ways that exercise affects your digestive tract is by constricting gut blood flow. Both intense and prolonged exercise result in a profound shift in blood flow away from your gut, toward your skeletal muscles and—especially in hot and humid environments—toward your skin. **As it turns out, psychological stress can also redirect blood flow away from your gut.**[22, 23] (Although if it's only mild in nature, stress has little impact on gut blood flow.[24])

Over the past few decades, advancements in ultrasound technology have allowed scientists to noninvasively probe how gut blood flow changes with a variety of stressors, including those that are psychological in nature. However, you might be surprised to learn that these shifts in gut blood flow were documented almost two hundred years ago. In 1822, a Canadian fur trader named Alexis St. Martin was accidently shot with a musket, resulting in a hand-sized wound that, once healed, still left an opening large enough that a person could see directly inside St. Martin's stomach.[25] William Beaumont—the physician stationed at the site of the accident—initially treated St. Martin but didn't think he would survive. St. Martin did manage to pull through, and Beaumont saw an extraordinary opportunity to study what had long been out of the reach of scientists: the inner workings of human digestion.

Of course, Beaumont's dreams of studying the mysteries of digestion and becoming a world-renowned gastric physiologist hinged on St. Martin's willingness to serve as more or less a human guinea pig. Fortunately for Beaumont, St. Martin was unable to pay his hospital bills and agreed to work and live in Beaumont's home as an indentured laborer. As a part of this *Odd Couple*-like arrangement, St. Martin allowed Beaumont to conduct more than two hundred gastral experiments on him over roughly a decade. Among other things, Beaumont inserted and extracted small muslin bags filled with various foods into and from St. Martin's stomach and even stuck his tongue inside the hole in St. Martin's side. (How else would you figure out how the inner coating of the stomach tastes?) Beaumont's mini-studies—the results of which were published in his book *Experiments and Observations on the Gastric Juice and the Physiology of Digestion*—were pioneering in that few others had successfully probed the process of digestion in humans.[26] Beaumont's book paints St. Martin as somewhat of a cantankerous figure, although if you keep in mind that he was subjected to hundreds of mildly unpleasant experiments, you can hardly blame St. Martin for his irritability. This may also help explain why St. Martin was prone to overindulging in alcoholic beverages on occasion. In one entry, Beaumont writes:

> St. Martin has been in the woods all day picking whortleberries. . . .
> Stomach full of berries and chymifying ailment, frothing and foaming like
> fermenting beer or cider; appears to have been drinking liquor too freely.[26]

Among the discoveries that arose from his experimentation on St. Martin, one of Beaumont's most interesting revelations was that a person's psychological state influences how much blood flows to their stomach. Specifically, Beaumont observed that "fear, anger, or whatever depresses or disturbs the nervous system—the villous coat becomes red and dry, at other times, pale and moist."[26] These changes in appearance from red to pale (and vice versa) were almost certainly the result of alterations in blood flow to St. Martin's visceral organs. In St. Martin, Beaumont had, quite literally, a gastric window into the man's state of mind.

Over the next 150 years, other cases of patients with permanent openings into their digestive tracts corroborated Beaumont's observation that mood state impacts gut blood flow. One such patient, a man known as Tom Little, had an artificial opening into his stomach surgically created after his esophagus was permanently damaged from swallowing scalding hot clam chowder at the age of 9. In 1941, a pair of physicians, Stewart Wolf and Harold Wolff, convinced the then 56-year-old Little to serve as a subject in a series of tests focusing on psychosomatic changes and gastric function. Stewart Wolf later recalled the following about their experimentations on Tom Little:

❝ *The exposed gastric mucosa of Tom made it possible to observe the vascularity of the stomach. . . . In Tom and in other fistulous subjects . . . we found that fright, depression, and attitudes of being overwhelmed were associated with pallor of the mucosa.*[27]

When you pair the information gleaned from historical cases like Alexis St. Martin and Tom Little with the revelations from contemporary studies, it's impossible to deny that an individual's psychological state influences blood flow to the gut.

201

Aside from its effects on gut blood flow, psychological stress can also influence smooth muscle activity in the gut, otherwise known as motility. In particular, stress can tone down stomach motility,[28] and one of the first scientists to document these alterations was Walter Bradford Cannon, a leading American physiologist of the early 20th century. During some of his experiments, Cannon noticed that young male cats were restive when restrained while older female cats remained mellow, and that these differences in temperament corresponded to differences in stomach activity. He further observed that "by covering the cat's mouth and nose . . . until a slight distress of breathing is produced, the stomach contractions can be stopped at will."[29] In an experiment conducted years later, Cannon went so far as to place a barking dog near a restrained cat and then proceeded to take blood samples from the cat to see what effect the "excited blood" had on a strip of intestinal muscle. (It caused a relaxation, or a reduction in motility.[30]) As it relates to athletes, attenuated stomach motility could exacerbate upper gut problems like nausea, fullness, bloating, and reflux, especially when they're trying to consume sizeable quantities of food or fluid in and around the time of competition.

In contrast to the dampening of stomach activity, stress can result in a livelier colon. Early experiments undertaken by physician Thomas Almy at New York Hospital in the 1940s and 1950s documented that simply discussing emotional topics could abruptly throw the colon into spasm. In a 1949 article, Almy describes measuring colon motility in patients as the researchers led them through discussions of unsettling life events.[31] Almy used a latex balloon placed in the colon to measure pressure changes, which gave him an indication of muscle activity. In a constipated German housewife, for instance, colon contractions intensified when, as the researchers put it, she "expressed resent-ment over her husband's ability to have regular bowel movements." (Of all the things you could take umbrage at your spouse for, focusing on his propensity to defecate seems peculiar.) In another case, the colon of a 26-year-old man went into a frenzy after he revealed that a woman he had been seeing "humiliated and scorned him for his inability to satisfy her sexually."[31]

In another article, Almy and his colleagues describe going to even greater lengths to manipulate colon function in an unlucky medical student referred to simply as L. L.[32] After positioning a proctoscope in L. L.'s lower colon, the researchers carried out an elaborate deception to make him believe he had a potentially cancerous lesion. The researchers told L. L. that they had to take a biopsy (even though they never took one), and during this time the motility of L. L.'s colon became progressively more intense. After 20 minutes of dupery, the researchers finally fessed up and told L. L. the procedure was fake. In the associated paper, Almy and his coauthors state that L. L. accepted their reassurances that nothing was truly wrong and that L. L. held no "resentment for the . . . anguish he had been through." Despite Almy's proclamation, something tells me L. L. wasn't completely bitter-free about this skullduggery.

The effects of stress on colon motility observed in Almy's eccentric experiments have largely been confirmed in more contemporary studies.[33, 34] To put it plainly, psychological stress can make the colon go wild. It's somewhat puzzling, then, that the symptoms arising from a more active colon vary drastically. In many cases, cramping and urges to go numero dos are stimulated. In others, constipation and bloating are more prevalent. Thinking about it logically, one would assume that frequent and strong contractions of smooth muscle would translate to a heightened urge to poo, but it really depends on whether those contractions are coordinated and propulsive or of a spastic variety. (Experiencing spastic, uncoordinated smooth muscle contractions in your colon could mean you're headed for constipationville.) That said, anecdotes about having to defecate before stressful competi-tion seem to be reported with more regularity than constipation.

Interestingly, humans have the power to consciously override nerve-induced urges to poop in many situations, but animals that are of a less-inhibited nature are much less capable. As it turns out, rats are particularly inclined to poo when stressed, and, anecdotally, exposing a rat to a new environment (such as a maze or a living space) is a good way to get said rat to empty its bowels. If you're not big on anecdotal evidence, you're in luck, as an experiment carried out in the 1930s found strong correlations between rats' emotional responses (measured via their willingness to eat in a strange enclosure) and their proclivities for defecating.[35] Much like rats in a cage, the psychological stress and anxiety experienced by athletes before endurance races is undoubtedly one reason lines for Porta-Johns are often as long as those for the latest and greatest ride at Disney World. Unlike rats, though, humans can usually keep it in long enough to avoid making a public mess.

There are a few physiological explanations for why reduced stomach motility and amplified colon activity accompany acute psychological stress. One of the most consistent scientific findings is that a hormone called corticotropin-releasing factor (CRF) contributes to the ebbs and flows of gut activity.[36] Your body responds to stress by secreting CRF from your hypothalamus; CRF then binds with receptors in your brain that modify the activity of your autonomic nervous system, the primarily unconscious part of your peripheral nervous system that helps control gut function. Across a variety of studies, directly administering CRF to animals dampens gastric motility and acid secretion while it also spurs colon motility.[36, 37] The role of CRF in provoking gut symptoms with psychological stress is presented in Figure 11.1.

During times of extreme psychological stress, these motility changes and their associated symptoms become commonplace. Few situations are as stressful as what soldiers experience during combat; in contrast to the run-of-the-mill pre-competition jitters experienced by many athletes, absolute fear is the emotion soldiers often feel before and during combat. In some cases, this fear is associated with spontaneous defecation; in an article in a long tome titled *Encyclopedia of Violence, Peace, and Conflict*, the authors report that one-quarter of World War II veterans admitted to defecating in their pants during combat.[38] In these situations, CRF secretion almost certainly contributes to a colon and rectum that are—to put it in layman's terms—massively overstimulated.

Urgent impulses to poo and the nervous shits are common manifestations of acute severe stress. With respect to the other end of the gut, nausea represents an equally troublesome stress-invoked symptom. The secretion of CRF plays a role in triggering

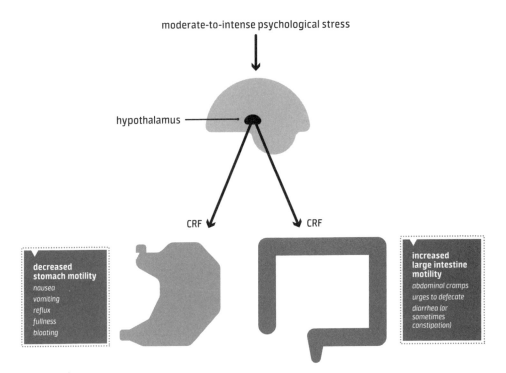

figure 11.1. **HOW ACUTE STRESS AFFECTS THE GUT**

Moderate-to-severe acute stress triggers the release of CRF from the hypothalamus, which modifies gut activity through the fibers of the autonomic nervous system.

said nausea, but there's another hormonal response that may be as equally influential: the release of catecholamines. High-intensity exercise, altitude, and—most directly— injecting catecholamines all increase blood catecholamine levels and can provoke nausea. Although I didn't cover this extensively in Chapter 2, acute psychological stress is also a source of catecholamine secretion. Many studies have demonstrated psychological stress's effect on catecholamine secretion, but I'll focus on one that used what's called the Trier Social Stress Test, a task that's become the gold standard for examining psychosocial stress in the lab. Though variations exist, the Trier Social Stress Test typically subjects participants to a mock presentation in front of a panel (often presented as a job interview), followed by a challenging arithmetic task (e.g., counting backward from a large number by increments of 13). In the example study I'm focusing on, participants had plasma levels of the stress hormone norepinephrine (also called noradrenaline) measured before and after the Trier Social Stress Test, and as expected, norepinephrine levels shot up, with levels ending up about twice as high as they were beforehand.[39]

The Trier Social Stress Test is a reliable method of inducing stress in a laboratory, but it's sometimes criticized because it doesn't reflect the diversity of tense and trying situations that people encounter in everyday life. With this in mind, researchers have assessed the catecholamine response to stress in more naturalistic situations—academic exams, a visit to the dentist's office, even skydiving. Specific to sports, a slew of investigations have evaluated stress responses to real-life competition. Take for example a study that contrasted the stress responses of elite German tennis players under practice and tournament conditions; urine epinephrine (a.k.a. adrenaline) levels were about twice as high two hours before a tournament than in practice.[40]

Despite the fact that elevations in catecholamines are nearly ubiquitous in stressful situations, not all athletes experience nausea before competition. Although the stress response to athletic competition isn't usually potent enough to induce nausea and vomiting in most athletes, there will always be exceptions, as in the cases of Philadelphia Eagles lineman Brandon Brooks and Celtics legend Bill Russell. And of course, the bigger the stage, the more likely an athlete will experience stress severe enough to trigger nauseousness. In *Without Limits*, the definitive running biopic about legendary runner Steve Prefontaine, there's a notable scene in which Prefontaine pukes under the bleachers before the 3-mile race at the 1974 Hayward Field Restoration Meet, which was renamed the Prefontaine Classic after his tragic death. In the scene, Prefontaine laments that he doesn't think he can hang with the likes of Frank Shorter and Gerry Lindgren anymore, even as the crowd chants his name. The scene perfectly sums up what countless athletes have felt in the moments leading up to their biggest competitions.

If you do happen to perpetually suffer from stress-induced nausea, you could consider implementing the following strategies to dial down the magnitude of catecholamine release in the hours leading up to competition:

205

- Shun caffeine and other stimulants.
- Avoid dehydration and hypoglycemia by consuming adequate amounts of fluid and carbohydrate beforehand.
- Consult with a sports psychologist or other qualified mental health professional, as they can help you implement a variety of strategies— from breathing exercises to meditation to cognitive behavioral therapy—that could blunt catecholamine release prior to competition.

I want to be clear that these strategies are based primarily on indirect evidence. Even so, there are probably minimal risks in trying them.

On a final note, one other gut function change that can stem from psychological stress is heightened gut permeability.[41] While it's transient and relatively harmless in many situations, gut leakiness may, in some cases, contribute to heat illness during and after prolonged exercise. Psychological stress increases gut leakiness via the actions of stress hormones like CRF as well as through its actions on various components of the immune system.[42, 43] Much like with stress-induced nausea, it's conceivable that interventions such as deep breathing and meditation could blunt the stress response to competition and subsequent onset of gut leakiness, though I'm not aware of research that's documented those effects specifically.

ANXIETY

Up to this point, I haven't made a distinction between stress and anxiety. I'm not a psychologist, so I won't pretend that I'm qualified to speak on all the nuances that separate these two psychological phenomena. In general terms, however, mental health professionals tend to make some consistent distinctions between stress and anxiety. Definitions of stress and anxiety abound, but I'll rely on the text that's traditionally thought of as the Bible of psychiatry, the *Diagnostic and Statistical Manual of Mental Disorders* (*DSM-5*), currently in its 5th edition. According to the *DSM-5*, stress and anxiety are defined as follows:

Stress. "The pattern of specific and nonspecific responses a person makes to stimulus events that disturb his or her equilibrium and tax or exceed his or her ability to cope."[44]

Anxiety. "The apprehensive anticipation of future danger or misfortune accompanied by a feeling of worry, distress, and/or somatic symptoms of tension. The focus of anticipated danger may be internal or external."[44]

An important distinguishing feature of anxiety—based on the *DSM-5* definition—is worry, and, notably, this worry stems from thoughts of *future* misfortune. The worries that accompany anxiety can come in many forms—vague and generalized in some cases, extremely specific in others.

For me, worries of being unable to speak effectively sometimes bounce around in my head during the hours preceding an important speaking engagement. When this anxiety is at its worst, my brain envisions and puts me through a series of disastrous possibilities, most of which are amalgamations of a past experience and what I know about the upcoming engagement (the room, the size of the crowd, etc.). In scientific studies, psychologists often refer to this transient anxiety as "state anxiety," or anxiety in the moment. For other people, their worries are less specific, instead encompassing almost every aspect of their lives. This type of anxiety is often referred to as "trait anxiety," which is the anxiety a person tends to experience generally and is thought to be more of a stable characteristic.

As you might expect, people's state and trait anxieties usually correlate strongly with one another.[45] Another way to say this is that people who live with loads of anxiety from day to day also tend to become more psychologically aroused and anxious when they're in stressful situations. Even though they're interrelated, there's a reason for measuring both types of anxiety instead of just one or the other. If you asked me to complete two separate questionnaires regarding my state (in the moment) and trait (in general) anxiety on a Saturday afternoon in the summer, I'm likely to report low levels on both. However, if you ask me to complete these same two questionnaires 30 minutes before a job interview, you're likely to see a divergence between the two, with scores on the state questionnaire spiking more so than scores on the trait questionnaire.

Beyond proximity to a stressful situation, other seemingly insignificant factors impact my state anxiety in performance situations. As an example, being stuck behind an elevated podium makes me feel surprisingly anxious in comparison to when I'm able to move freely in front of a crowd. I'm not sure why elevated podiums make me feel this way, but perhaps my brain interprets the situation akin to being prey that's stuck in a highly visible spot and therefore vulnerable to encroaching predators. Another factor that impacts my anxiety is time of day, and for whatever reason, mornings are worse for me than any other time.

The reason for bringing attention to the distinction between state and trait anxiety is that it may have implications for gut function in athletes. You, for instance, might be like me in that you don't have excessive general anxiety, but when competition time comes around, your nerves spike considerably. As a consequence, you might be more vulnerable to experiencing anxiety-associated gut problems around competition and might benefit from interventions that manage anxiety more acutely. Some of these interventions are listed here:

- Avoid or limit caffeine and other stimulants on the day of competition.
- Avoid dehydration and hypoglycemia before competition by consuming adequate amounts of fluid and carbohydrate beforehand; eating huge amounts isn't needed, but going into competition fasted is likely problematic for some athletes.
- Distract yourself by talking to teammates or competitors at the event.
- Breathe slowly and deeply for 5 minutes within 15–30 minutes of the start of competition.
- Try positive imagery or visualization.
- Practice positive self-talk to control negative thoughts; these statements should be realistic and believable ("I can relax myself" and "I am strong and capable").
- Do a quick progressive muscle relaxation exercise, such as contracting and slowly relaxing several muscle groups one by one.

Obviously, implementing several of these strategies (particularly visualization and self-talk) is more nuanced than described above. If these practices are something you'd like to try, consider reaching out to a sports psychologist or coach who has experience with these techniques. Likewise, there are several good books that detail how to implement these sorts of strategies in sporting situations, including *The Champion's Mind* by Jim Afremow and *How Champions Think* by Bob Rotella.

ANXIETY AND GUT FUNCTION

When it comes to anxiety's effects on gut function, it can be challenging to distinguish them from the effects of psychological stress. This is partly because as the perceptions of one go up, so do the perceptions of the other. Obviously, some people cope better with stress than others and may not experience as much anxiety when stressed, but in general, self-reported stress and anxiety levels typically correlate pretty strongly with one another.

Even with these challenges in teasing out the effects of anxiety and stress on gut function, there is a small body of research that seemingly confirms that inducing anxiety is sufficient to cause some of the aforementioned gastrointestinal changes. In one notable example, volunteers underwent a series of stomach function evaluations after being put through a standardized 10-minute anxiety induction procedure.[46] Specifically, volunteers wrote about events from their pasts that would make them anxious if they recalled them, which were then recorded and played back to them while they sat in a darkened room. To further spark feelings of anxiety, fearful facial expressions were projected in front of the volunteers on a screen. The researchers measured gastric pressures and volumes using an inflatable bag inserted through the mouth into the stomach. In comparison to looking at neutral facial expressions and listening to a neutral personal story, the anxiety-inducing procedure led participants to report discomfort at lower gastric volumes (489 milliliters versus 630). This means they were less able to tolerate stuff in their stomachs, and for an athlete this would potentially equate to more fullness and discomfort when eating before and during competition. Indeed, in another part of the study, the volunteers consumed a liquid meal during the 10-minute anxiety procedure, and in comparison to the neutral condition, listening to anxiety-provoking stories and looking at fearful faces aggravated the severity of fullness and bloating by roughly 25–45 percent.

It's interesting to note that a similar experiment from the same group of researchers failed to find that this type of anxiety-provoking experience impacts colorectal function.[47] Still, other studies consistently show that psychological stress intensifies colonic motor activity, not to mention the innumerable anecdotes that abound of people losing control of their bowels during war, high-level sporting competition, and other extremely stressful situations. In the end, whether anxiety impacts the functioning of your colon may come down to what it is that's inducing the anxiety and whether the anxiety borders on fear. Sitting in a lab while reflecting on a distressful event from the past, for example, may simply not be potent enough to impact colon function, whereas being faced with possible death or thinking about playing in front of sixty thousand screaming fans is enough to do the trick.

SUMMARY

STRESS AND ANXIETY

Prolonged elevations in **psychological stress** predict injuries and illnesses in athletes.

There are several ways **sustained stress** negatively affects your health and recovery as an athlete, one of the most important being **suppression** of your immune system.

Acute psychological stress can reduce gut blood flow, slow stomach emptying, increase colon motor activity, and increase **gut leakiness**, all of which may contribute to a greater incidence and/or severity of gut symptoms before and during competition.

The changes in gut function associated with psychological stress result, in part, from the secretion of **CRF** and **catecholamines**.

In theory, engaging in stress-reducing activities and avoiding **stimulants** (including caffeine), **dehydration**, and **hypoglycemia** on competition day could reduce the severity of stress-induced gut symptoms.

12

MANAGING STRESS AND ANXIETY

If you've ever strolled through the aisles of your local bookstore or library, there's a decent chance you came across a section devoted entirely to books on stress management. Similarly, a quick Google search using the phrase *stress management* returns a dizzying assortment of websites that offer all kinds of schemes for reducing stress. The purpose of this chapter isn't to cover every conceivable intervention for managing stress and anxiety; instead, I detail the strategies that have also been used to reduce gut dysfunction.

There's one important qualifying point to keep in mind regarding much of the science discussed in this chapter, and that is most of the studies I reference were carried out in people experiencing gut symptoms because of underlying gastrointestinal disorders. As much as I'd like to say these strategies have a proven track record of alleviating gut symptoms that arise from competition stress and anxiety, I have an obligation to be completely transparent about what the science really says. And unfortunately, there's little to no research available to tell us how well these strategies work for dealing with competition anxiety or its associated gut problems. On the bright side, most of these interventions come with minimal serious risks, although some (such as prescription drugs) have side effects and require oversight from a healthcare provider.

BREATHING

Manipulating one's breath has been used for millennia—often in conjunction with other practices like mindfulness and prayer—to achieve a sense of oneness or spiritual enlightenment. In recent decades, breathing exercises have become mainstream, having made their way from Buddhist temples into health clinics. Indeed, interventions that manipulate the breath have become increasingly utilized in the management of a growing list of health problems—anxiety, depression, panic disorder, asthma, heart disease. There are numerous styles of breathing to choose from: slow and deep; fast and shallow; in through the nose, out through the mouth; focusing on breathing with the belly. Each of these means can lead to disparate ends, making it tricky to generalize about the effects of breathing interventions. When it comes to improving gut problems, though, slow deep breathing has the most scientific oomph behind it.

Although I didn't discuss motion sickness in Chapter 2, nausea is universally recognized as one of its most common and debilitating symptoms. And because motion sickness is so easy to induce (try slowly spinning in a chair if you don't believe me), it makes for a convenient model of studying how various interventions impact nausea. Interestingly, slow deep breathing is one of many interventions that scientists have trialed as a motion sickness remedy. The physiological basis for thinking that slow deep breathing would mitigate nausea has to do with its effects on the autonomic nervous system. At rest, the parasympathetic (rest-and-digest) branch of your autonomic nervous system is more active than the sympathetic (fight-or-flight) branch. At the onset of motion sickness, there's a reduction in parasympathetic activity along with a parallel uptick in sympathetic activation.[1] What's more, larger decreases in parasympathetic activity correlate with greater severities of motion sickness.[2]

Based on these facts, it is logical to think that anything that prevents a shift from parasympathetic to sympathetic dominance has the potential to relieve motion sickness. And in fact, experiments do show that slow deep breathing consistently increases parasympathetic activity[3] and seems to lessen the severity of motion sickness.[4-6] In one illustrative study, college students spent 10 minutes wearing 3-D goggles that simulated stormy seas.[5] Sounds like fun, right? Half of the participants practiced slow deep breathing during the simulation while the other half observed themselves and their environment. Participants rated nausea on a 1-to-4 scale, and by the 10th minute, those in the slow deep breathing group rated their nausea at 1.5, while those in the attentional control group rated nausea roughly 30 percent higher.

How exactly can these findings be applied to athletes? That's a difficult question to answer, as nausea induced in a laboratory isn't necessarily the same as nausea that arises because of pre-game nerves or from sprinting or ultraendurance exercise. Theoretically, though, slow deep breathing could help manage any form of nausea that's exacerbated by excessive sympathetic nervous system activation. As such, pre-competition queasiness associated with extreme levels of stress and anxiety seems like a form of nausea that's likely to benefit from slow deep breathing, and this was even mentioned as a strategy that Brandon Brooks planned to use before Super Bowl LII.[7]

215

Other than nausea, several gut symptoms have the potential to be managed through the practice of slow deep breathing. Take for example functional dyspepsia, a cluster of chronically occurring symptoms that includes fullness after eating, premature satiation, epigastric (upper abdomen) pain, and epigastric burning.[8] Although many people are only vaguely aware of it, the worldwide prevalence of functional dyspepsia is between 11.5 percent and 29.2 percent.[9] Sympathetic-parasympathetic nervous system balance is often disturbed in patients with functional dyspepsia,[10] which provides an underlying rationale for how slow deep breathing could improve its symptoms. Unfortunately, few studies have tested the effectiveness of slow deep breathing in patients with functional dyspepsia, although one experiment found that, compared to a control group that did nothing, daily slow deep breathing for five minutes improved quality of life and increased the amount of soup that patients could tolerably consume in one sitting.[11]

Similar to functional dyspepsia, IBS is another prevalent gut disorder that's associated with a state of sympathetic nervous system predominance.[12] Even though studies have included breathing exercises as a part of multicomponent interventions (e.g., yoga) for IBS, few of them isolated the effects of slow deep breathing. As a result, it's not clear what effect slow deep breathing has on quality of life and gut symptoms in people with IBS.

In sum, research has clearly documented the power of slow deep breathing to manipulate sympathetic-parasympathetic nervous system activity. However, further research is needed to truly confirm or refute whether slow deep breathing offers significant relief for athletes and to determine what protocols are most practical, efficient, and effective. Still, for athletes who are troubled by gut symptoms arising from psychological stress or anxiety, slow deep breathing is one tactic that they could give a shot. A simple daily protocol to follow is to target four to six breaths per minute, with exhalations lasting slightly longer than inspirations, for 10–15 minutes total.

MINDFULNESS

The practice of mindfulness involves focusing your attention on the present moment. It can include monitoring your thoughts, emotions, and bodily sensations, as well as being more aware of your surroundings. Focusing on your breath, noticing the way your feet feel against the ground, and lingering over the tastes and textures of food are all examples of practicing mindfulness. In essence, mindfulness is a form of meditation.

Mindfulness interventions have been tested in a broad range of health conditions, but mood disorders have probably received the most attention. The results of several comprehensive analyses of mindfulness interventions suggest they're efficacious and cost-effective for improving symptoms of anxiety in people diagnosed with anxiety disorders.[13, 14] Exactly why mindfulness seems to boost mood and diminish anxiety isn't entirely clear, but one possibility is that it might limit the ruminating and worrying thoughts that are so common in people living with anxiety and depressive disorders.[15]

Albeit to a lesser extent than with slow deep breathing, there's some evidence that being mindful can increase parasympathetic nervous system activity,[16, 17] and as is the case with slow deep breathing, modulation of the autonomic nervous system could explain why a number of experiments have found reductions in symptoms when patients with chronic gut disorders implement mindfulness-based interventions.[18, 19] That said, most of these trials were done in patients with IBS, and mindfulness was often just one component of a multipronged treatment approach. As a result, it's hard to say what effect mindfulness training would have in athletes other than those diagnosed with IBS.

While there are many ways to practice mindfulness, it might be particularly effective to combine it with slow deep breathing. You can do this by noticing how it feels as the air passes in and out of your nose or how your chest and abdomen rise and fall with each breath or by counting breaths until your reach a certain number (e.g., 50).

EXERCISE TRAINING

Acute exercise can bring about a multitude of annoying—and sometimes even debilitating—gut symptoms. One might assume, then, that long-term exercise training does the same. In most cases though, this is not the case. In fact, experiments reveal that exercise training blunts the typical reductions in gut blood flow that occur during acute exercise,[20] and these findings are bolstered by studies demonstrating that seasoned runners typically suffer from fewer gut symptoms while exercising than their novice counterparts.[21-23]

What remains unclear is the extent to which declines in anxiety are responsible for these reductions in gut symptoms over time with exercise training. Overall, aerobic training[24, 25]—as well as resistance training,[26] yoga,[27] and Tai Chi[28]—seem to modestly dampen anxious thoughts and feelings. The question, then, is whether these reductions in anxiety translate to fewer anxiety-related digestive problems. Regrettably, these studies didn't collect information on gut symptoms. Perhaps the most promising evidence tying long-term exercise training to decreases in anxiety-related gut symptoms comes from studies of IBS patients, many of whom deal with anxiety issues. In at least two trials, increasing physical activity lessened gut symptoms in people with IBS.[29, 30] Similarly, the results from a half-dozen trials suggest that yoga improves quality of life and eases gut symptoms in IBS.[31]

HYPNOSIS

Ritualistic ceremonies and practices bearing a resemblance to modern-day hypnosis have been performed throughout recorded history. The Egyptians, for instance, supposedly induced sleeplike trance states millennia before European physicians started dabbling in practices similar to hypnosis.[32] Today, hypnosis is often considered by traditional healthcare practitioners as an alternative medicine that should be reserved for situations where modern treatments fail to elicit favorable responses. Nevertheless, millions of people—even in Western societies—try hypnosis every year. In the 1990s, a survey of Americans found that roughly 1 percent of adults had used hypnosis over the previous year.[33] More recent surveys put these estimates closer to 0.1–0.2 percent, indicating that hypnosis may be falling out of favor, at least in the US.[34]

Hypnosis is notoriously difficult to study, in large part due to the varied techniques that can be utilized to induce hypnotic states as well as the high likelihood of placebo/ expectation effects. Bear in mind, it's essentially impossible to blind research participants to the fact that they're being hypnotized. This reality, in combination with the fact that many hypnosis experiments are of poor methodological quality, makes it challenging to glean useful insights from the research on hypnosis and anxiety.[35]

These caveats aside, clinical trials of patients with IBS provide some thin evidence that hypnosis can diminish gut symptoms in comparison to no intervention or usual medical management.[36, 37] Exactly how hypnosis would achieve improvements in gut discomfort and other forms of pain remains mostly a mystery, even in an age when we can probe the brain noninvasively. While it's unequivocal that hypnosis modifies brain activation patterns, the particular regions involved frequently differ between studies.[38]

Like with many of the other interventions that are presented here, there's essentially no research available to tell us how hypnosis influences psychologically induced gut symptoms in sports. Thus, any athlete who uses hypnosis in an attempt to alleviate gut symptoms from competition nerves is doing so largely in the absence of concrete evidence. Lastly, it's important to keep in mind that, although hypnosis is thought to be relatively safe, it isn't completely risk-free.[39]

MUSIC

Nowadays, the sight of athletes wearing headphones as they walk off their team bus or enter a stadium is ubiquitous. The image of Michael Phelps listening to music before his swimming events during the 2016 Rio Olympics (while also giving rival South African swimmer Chad le Clos the death stare) is an iconic example of this sort of pre-competition routine. At the Winter Olympics, it's not uncommon to see snowboarders pull out a pair of earbuds just as they finish a run down the half-pipe. American snowboarding legend Shaun White's 2018 Olympics playlist on Spotify included motivational tracks like "Iron Man" by Black Sabbath and "Immigrant Song" by Led Zeppelin. In contrast, Japanese silver medalist Ayumu Hirano shared that one of his favorite jams to listen to around competition time is Bob Marley's "Three Little Birds" because of its calming effects.[40]

Beyond these anecdotes, studies substantiate the idea that many athletes listen to music before competition to get a psychological boost. A study of 195 collegiate athletes from the United Kingdom found that 24 percent listened to fast, upbeat music on the day of competition, while another 21 percent listened to slow, soft music.[41] In a similar survey of 252 Swedish athletes, the pre-competition period was the most popular time for athletes to listen to music, surpassing other periods like training and competition itself.[42]

For athletes who rely on music to calm their nerves, what's the evidence that it does any good? Surprisingly, few studies have addressed this question in detail or in the realm of real-life competition. In one example, a group of college athletes listened to a three-minute selection of self-chosen music prior to actual competition while a control group went sans music.[43] Although the music listeners reported higher self-confidence levels after the intervention, these ratings were collected roughly 30–105 minutes before competition, so it's unclear whether their self-assuredness persisted into competition.

In another study, undergraduate students were told they would be partaking in a skills competition and—to induce more anxiety—that there may be an audience present or that they might be filmed.[44] Then the students were assigned to a relaxing-music condition, a nonrelaxing-music condition, or a no-music condition, and each was applied for 10 minutes before the students threw beanbags at a 1-meter hoop on the floor that was 7 meters away. Although some of the data were suggestive of a benefit of relaxing music on anxiety, there were no clear, unambiguous differences between the groups. Furthermore, average performance on the beanbag-throwing task was similar in all groups.

Even though there isn't much direct evidence that relaxing music reduces anxiety before sporting competition, studies looking at music listening in other stressful situations support the notion that it can calm a person's worries and dampen physiological arousal. Combined data from 19 scientific publications reveal that music eases self-reported anxiety in healthy adults,[45] and similar benefits have been found in individuals undergoing medical procedures like cardiac catheterizations.[46, 47] These findings—in addition to the ardent beliefs that many athletes have about the power of music—provide justification for its application as a potentially valuable tool to be used in and around the time of competition.

In terms of gut function before or during competition, very little is known about the effects of music. Unlike some of the other interventions that have been discussed so far, there isn't much research on how music impacts conditions like IBS and functional dyspepsia. Although some studies have used music as a part of a larger relaxation intervention for these disorders, the independent effects of music remain unknown.

COGNITIVE BEHAVIORAL THERAPY (CBT)

As opposed to more antiquated forms of psychotherapy—such as Freud's psychoanalysis—cognitive behavioral therapy (CBT) is backed by literally hundreds of clinical trials. The basic idea behind CBT is that a person's maladaptive thoughts, beliefs, and attitudes contribute to mood disturbances and cause them to engage in unhelpful behaviors. An example would be a woman who thinks she always comes off as being awkward at social gatherings (a maladaptive thought), which causes her to avoid those situations to the detriment of her psychological health (an unhelpful behavior). The anxiety that often accompanies these maladaptive thoughts can trigger physical symptoms, including gut woes.[48] Consequently, various forms of CBT have been used not only in the treatment of mood disorders but also IBS and functional dyspepsia.

When someone undergoes CBT, a variety of exercises and techniques are used to help root out and address the thoughts and behaviors that are causing problems for them. Journaling is frequently involved, as it can help link thoughts, beliefs, and behaviors to identify patterns and tendencies that can be targeted for therapy. Then a therapist may ask a client to work on challenging or restructuring the maladaptive thoughts and beliefs that were identified through journaling. A client might also start engaging in other pleasant or enjoyable activities that can improve mood or function (relaxation, meditation, exercise, etc.).

Overall, CBT is at least moderately effective for treating all kinds of anxiety disorders,[49, 50] and therapist-guided, self-guided, group-based, and internet-delivered variations are all viable options. Given the obvious role that people's thoughts play in determining their mood states, it's not surprising that CBT can dampen anxiety and improve mood. What may come as a surprise is just how effective CBT can be for taming the *physical* symptoms experienced by people living with IBS and functional dyspepsia. A 2013 article in *Clinical Gastroenterology and Hepatology* found that CBT reduced symptoms or improved quality of life in about 90 percent of 30 studies that included people with functional gut disorders (IBS, dyspepsia, etc.).[48]

Given how effective CBT is for improving both anxiety and gut symptoms in individuals living with disorders like IBS, it seems like a no-brainer that CBT could help hyperamped athletes manage pre-competition nerves. One form of CBT—known as rational emotive behavior therapy (REBT)—has been applied in sports ranging from triathlon to archery to golf. Martin Turner, a senior lecturer at Staffordshire University in the United Kingdom, has been involved with numerous case studies claiming that REBT not only diminishes anxiety and irrational beliefs but also boosts athletic performance.[51] Unfortunately, large experiments with control groups testing the effectiveness of REBT and other forms of CBT for easing anxiety and improving performance in athletes are few and far between, and the same is true when it comes to CBT's role in ameliorating competition-induced gut symptoms.

ACCEPTANCE AND COMMITMENT THERAPY (ACT)

Although CBT is the most studied form of psychotherapy in the treatment of gut disorders, it's by no means the only game in town. Steven Hayes, a psychologist and professor at the University of Nevada, Reno, is widely credited as the founder of a psychotherapy technique known as acceptance and commitment therapy (ACT).[52] Even though ACT and CBT are both behavioral-based therapies and share several features, there are some distinctions to be made between these two contemporary psychotherapies. One of the main goals of CBT is to change maladaptive thoughts to more constructive cognitions. Instead of changing these thoughts and feelings, ACT teaches people to accept them without judgment.[53] This process of accepting negative thoughts and feelings means that a person should learn to observe them more passively and respond to them less reactively. In essence, it's designed to help people deal with the natural ups and downs of life.

The evidence base supporting ACT for anxiety disorders is fairly strong, with improvements reaching similar levels as CBT.[54] However, in comparison to CBT, less research has been devoted to the use of ACT in gut disorders, and although there are some initial promising results, more work in these populations is needed.[55] Likewise, there isn't much we can say, scientifically speaking, about the utility of ACT for managing competition-related anxiety and its associated gut symptoms.

221

PHARMACEUTICAL DRUGS

The treatment of mood disorders prior to the advent of pharmaceutical drugs was often ineffective, unpleasant, and sometimes even deadly. Examples from the pages of history include the lobotomy, bloodletting, poison-induced vomiting, and even being burned alive.[56] As the 1950s came around, a number of new drugs started to be used in patients with depression, one of the first of these being iproniazid. Interestingly, iproniazid wasn't originally intended to be used as an antidepressant but rather as a tuberculosis remedy. However, clinicians using it in tuberculosis patients noticed "side effects" such as euphoria and improved sleep, and these observations prompted a group of researchers to test the drug in psychiatric patients. The results of that study, published in 1957, showed that 70 percent of patients demonstrated at least some mood improvements while on iproniazid.[57] Soon thereafter, several hundred thousand people with depression were taking iproniazid until it was removed from the market in 1961 because of reports of liver toxicity.[56]

Around the same time that iproniazid was being tested as an antidepressant, another drug called imipramine was developed as an antipsychotic. Imipramine has a chemical structure similar to chlorpromazine, an antipsychotic drug that was introduced as a treatment for psychiatric patients in the mid-1950s.[58] A Swiss drug company asked a psychiatrist named Roland Kuhn to test a number of novel but chemically similar compounds they thought would have similar effects as chlorpromazine, including imipramine.[59] Although imipramine didn't end up exhibiting antipsychotic effects in schizophrenics, Kuhn observed that it elevated mood in patients who were also suffering from major depressive symptoms. Subsequent studies confirmed the antidepressant effects of imipramine, and today it's still occasionally used for treating depression.

In the two decades that followed the introduction of iproniazid and imipramine, numerous other antidepressants hit the market. Yet virtually all these new drugs were of the same class as either iproniazid, a monoamine oxidase inhibitor, or imipramine, a tricyclic antidepressant. It wasn't until the introduction of selective serotonin reuptake inhibitors (SSRIs) in the 1980s that a new generation of antidepressants was made available. Today, SSRIs and serotonin-norepinephrine reuptake inhibitors (SNRIs) are the most popular types of antidepressants in the world. In addition to their widespread use for depression, SSRIs and SNRIs are commonly used in anxiety disorders, and along with CBT, they're viewed by many as the first treatment options.[60, 61]

Interestingly, poor mood isn't the only target of these drugs. Functional dyspepsia and IBS also respond to some types of antidepressants. In one meta-analysis of placebo-controlled trials, IBS patients who were given placebo pills were more likely to show no improvement in symptoms than those given the real SSRIs (67 percent versus 45 percent).[37] Similar results were found for tricyclic antidepressants, with 64 percent of those given a placebo nonresponding versus 43 percent of those given the active drug. On the downside, more of the patients given the antidepressant drugs had side effects, although most of them were considered minor. In reference to functional dyspepsia, only tricyclic antidepressants have shown consistent positive effects on gastrointestinal symptoms.[62]

I'm sure this is beginning to sound all too familiar, but we currently know next to nothing (scientifically speaking) about how antidepressants affect an athlete's gut. Obviously, if an athlete is diagnosed with IBS or functional dyspepsia, the use of antidepressants will hopefully translate to fewer gut symptoms throughout the day as well as during training and competition, but that is yet to be verified in controlled experiments.

A FEW OTHER INTERVENTIONS

I've covered some of the most popular interventions used to manage disorders associated with excessive stress and anxiety as well as IBS and functional dyspepsia. There are numerous other treatments and approaches out there, and it would be impractical to cover every one of them in detail. A sampling of other interventions is summarized below.

Acupuncture. The practice of acupuncture, which usually involves inserting needles into specific points (a.k.a. acupoints) on the body, probably originated in China several thousands of years ago.[63] According to a meta-analysis, acupuncture does a superior job of treating IBS in comparison to sham procedures or usual care.[64] (In case you're wondering, sham acupuncture involves placing needles in non-acupoints or touching them to the skin without penetrating it.) For functional dyspepsia, there are some positive data suggesting a benefit, but because many of the studies have been of low quality, strong conclusions about acupuncture's effectiveness aren't currently warranted.[65]

223

Biofeedback. Dysregulation of bodily systems contributes to a host of medical maladies, including mood disorders. The presence of an anxiety disorder, for instance, is associated with inadequate parasympathetic nervous system activity.[66] Biofeedback is a technique that helps a person gain control over this physiological dysregulation for the purpose of improving health and/or performance. During biofeedback training, a person is connected to an instrument capable of monitoring physiological responses, allowing them to observe in real-time how various interventions (relaxation, deep breathing, etc.) can be used to manipulate these responses. Physiological parameters commonly monitored include breathing rate, heart rate, muscle activity, brain activity, temperature, and electrical conductivity of the skin.[67] Given all the bodily systems that can be monitored—as well as all the different forms of training that can be used to manipulate these systems—it's challenging to make straightforward conclusions about biofeedback training and anxiety symptoms. Even so, enough positive evidence is available to say that biofeedback training is a viable option in the armamentarium of treatments for anxiety.[67, 68] There's limited research on the use of biofeedback in isolation for conditions like IBS and functional dyspepsia, but some preliminary data suggest it could be helpful.[69, 70]

Probiotics. It may seem like a fantastically weird idea that microorganisms in your gut can impact your mood, but evidence from numerous studies (albeit mostly using animals) does in fact show this to be true.[71] Exactly how these microbes could influence mood is still being investigated, but some of the likely pathways include activation of neuronal circuits in the gut and modulation of the hypothalamic-pituitary-adrenal axis, which is the body's primary stress response system. In light of these discoveries, researchers have begun testing probiotics for improving anxiety and depressive symptoms in humans. Unfortunately, the combined results from 12 clinical trials (with more than 1,500 participants) indicate that probiotics aren't particularly effective at alleviating anxiety.[72] This analysis, published in *Depression and Anxiety*, reported that 3 of the 12 studies did find a benefit; however, these trials had smaller samples and there were no shared characteristics among them in terms of the strain or dose of microorganisms used. Despite the lackluster findings related to anxiety, probiotics are able to ease gut symptoms in some individuals living with IBS.[73]

MANAGING STRESS AND ANXIETY

Slow deep breathing, mindfulness, and listening to relaxing music all have the power to dampen sympathetic nervous system activity and promote parasympathetic activity. Consequently, these interventions might be helpful for reducing pre-competition anxiety, though no research has tested whether they have benefits when it comes to mitigating gut distress arising from competition stress and anxiety.

Both **CBT** and **ACT** can be utilized to effectively manage anxiety problems, though when it comes to treating gut disorders like IBS and functional dyspepsia, CBT has more evidence behind it. Neither of these two psychotherapies have been scientifically tested to reduce gut symptoms in athletes.

Today, **SSRIs** are the most popular class of drug used to treat depression and anxiety disorders, and they are also sometimes used to tackle certain gut disorders, particularly IBS. When it comes to functional dyspepsia, **tricyclic antidepressant**s are probably more effective than SSRIs. Very little is known about how these drugs impact gut symptoms in athletes during training and competition.

A variety of other interventions, from **acupuncture** to **hypnosis**, have been trialed as remedies for functional gut disorders, and although there are some positive findings, the quality of many of the studies has been lackluster.

225

APPENDIX A: GASTROINTESTINAL DISORDERS

Even before the advances of modern medicine revealed the inner workings of the gut, the ancient Greeks knew of its importance. As Hippocrates famously said, "All disease begins in the gut." While Hippocrates obviously wasn't right in an absolute sense, his millennia-old thought still represents contemporary thinking on the role of the gut in many diseases.

Although the primary objective of *The Athlete's Gut* is to help you understand the causes of gut disturbances that arise with training and competition, the fact is, many athletes end up suffering from some type of acute or chronic gut disorder during their lifetime. Consequently, I would be remiss if I ignored the role of these disorders in athletes' gut problems. As such, this appendix provides an overview of common maladies known to impact the gastrointestinal system. You'll have seen many of them mentioned earlier in specific contexts, but here I'll provide more focused detail. Remember, the material covered here is for informational purposes only and isn't intended to diagnose, treat, or cure any medical condition. If you're personally experiencing persistent or bothersome gut symptoms, you should seek the counsel of your healthcare provider.

CELIAC DISEASE

Upward of 1 percent of people live with celiac disease,[1] a condition characterized by damage to the small intestine from ingesting gluten, a protein found in wheat, barley, and rye. Diarrhea, pain, and bloating are common gut manifestations of celiac disease, although it can impact the body in additional ways—weight loss, fatigue, headaches, and softening of the bones, to mention but a few. Some people with celiac disease have mild symptoms, which is why it's common for there to be an extended delay before it's diagnosed. In fact, the majority of people living with celiac disease don't even know they have it. Although it can be difficult to diagnosis and often goes unrecognized for years, there are predisposing risk factors that make it more likely for someone to develop celiac disease, including being female, having close relatives with the disease, and having a diagnosis of other immune-driven disorders.[2]

The intestinal injury characteristic of celiac disease is mediated through the immune system, which is thought to be overreacting to the presence of gluten. This reaction to gluten damages the finger-like villi distributed throughout the small intestine, causing poor absorption of nutrients. In turn, this malabsorption of nutrients leads to many of the signs and symptoms of celiac disease. Left untreated, it can lead to osteoporosis, infertility, and gastrointestinal cancers.[3]

Sadly, there's no cure for celiac disease, so complete removal of gluten from the diet is the only direct treatment. For newly diagnosed athletes, removing gluten from their diet can seem daunting, especially if they're accustomed to eating lots of bread, cereal, pasta, crackers, and the like. While there are plenty of carbohydrate-rich alternatives available (fruits, starchy vegetables, rice, beans, potatoes, quinoa, etc.), some athletes find the transition difficult and end up underconsuming energy and carbohydrate. These athletes would likely benefit from consulting with a registered dietitian with expertise in both sports nutrition and celiac disease.

Because diarrhea and nutrient malabsorption are common in newly diagnosed cases of celiac disease (and in longstanding uncontrolled cases), deficiencies of key vitamins and minerals that impact performance should be evaluated. Some of the key nutrients when it comes to athletic performance are iron, calcium, and vitamin D. Poor iron and vitamin D status can harm physical performance, while shortfalls in calcium and vitamin D can negatively impact bone mineralization. Blood tests (ferritin for iron, and a marker called 25(OH)D for vitamin D) can be a first step to establishing whether supplementation is needed; in the case of bone health, a DEXA scan (short for dual-energy X-ray absorptiometry) may be used to quantify bone density. Because celiac patients are often deficient in several other micronutrients, gluten-free multivitamin-mineral supplements are often prescribed, at least initially while they work to adapt to a gluten-free diet.

GLUTEN SENSITIVITY

Starting around 2006, Google searches for *gluten free* began to rise and outpace queries for *celiac disease*.[4] Although up to 1 percent of the world's population has celiac disease (based on blood tests, anyway), most of these people are unaware they have the condition. So, given that fewer than 1 million of 325 million Americans have a diagnosis of celiac disease, what explains the exploding interest in gluten-free foods over the past decade?

Increased awareness of celiac disease among the public is one obvious reason for this trend. In addition, growing numbers of Americans believe that a gluten-free diet is superior regardless of whether they have celiac disease. When surveyed, many say that a sans-gluten diet is simply healthier or that it accelerates weight loss or improves digestive health. This trend is also occurring in athletes, with one large 2013 survey finding widespread belief that a gluten-free diet enhances performance, reduces illness, and improves body composition.[5] Remarkably, 41 percent of the 910 athletes from this survey followed a gluten-free diet at least half the time, even though none of them had a diagnosis of celiac disease. In one of my own studies that surveyed 422 marathoners, a gluten-free diet was the third most common eating regimen, trailing only vegan/vegetarian diets and Paleolithic diets.[6] In addition, the percentage of respondents who followed a gluten-free diet (3.5 percent) was well above the prevalence of celiac disease. Even elite athletes like quarterback Drew Brees and tennis great Novak Djokovic have reportedly gone without gluten at some time or another.[7]

It's obvious many people are following a gluten-free diet because they believe in its power to improve health and performance. However, another important reason for the growth in gluten-free eating is the rise in people who believe they have non-celiac gluten sensitivity, or gluten sensitivity for short. The concept of gluten sensitivity has been described since at least the early 1980s, but it didn't take off in the medical literature until about 10 years ago.[8] Descriptions of gluten sensitivity vary, but it is commonly defined as experiencing gastrointestinal and/or extraintestinal symptoms (i.e., outside the gut) upon ingestion of gluten-containing grains, with symptom improvement once gluten is removed from the diet.[9] Importantly, celiac disease and wheat allergy need to be ruled out before gluten sensitivity can be diagnosed.

Unfortunately, there are no laboratory tests that can, with a high level of accuracy, diagnose someone as gluten sensitive. Instead, clinicians ask patients to remove gluten from their diet and then observe what happens to their symptoms. Alternatively, if a patient is already following a gluten-free diet, a clinician may ask the person to eat a certain amount of gluten-containing foods for a specified period; if symptoms return, gluten sensitivity would be suspected. Because of its varying definitions and the fact that gluten sensitivity is largely a diagnosis of exclusion, some researchers question whether it's a distinct entity. These concerns are bolstered by studies that show more than 80 percent of people with a suspected gluten sensitivity cannot be formally diagnosed after performing a gluten challenge in a blinded, placebo-controlled fashion.[10]

When you consider these findings, why do so many people with a suspected gluten sensitivity respond favorably to a gluten-free diet outside of the confines of controlled studies? One explanation is the placebo effect. Simply put, if you expect a diet to work, chances are it'll improve your symptoms. Alternatively, a portion of people who believe they have gluten sensitivity may be reacting to other things found in wheat-containing grains. Late in 2017, a study published in *Gastroenterology* received heaps of press when it reported that fructan, a type of carbohydrate found in not only wheat but also foods like asparagus, garlic, and onions, was the more likely culprit responsible for symptoms in people who were suspected of having gluten sensitivity.[11] In a blinded fashion, volunteers were assigned to three seven-day diets supplemented with bars containing gluten (6 grams), fructan (2 grams), or neither (placebo). By the study's end, the volunteers completed all three diets, and overall they had more severe symptoms—particularly bloating—on the fructan diet than when they were on the gluten diet. Moreover, there were no differences in symptoms between the gluten-bar and placebo-bar diets.

In reality, it's likely that some people do suffer from gluten sensitivity. That being said, some people who believe they're sensitive to gluten don't react to gluten when challenged in a blinded manner. For these people, another component of wheat-containing products—such as fructan—could be responsible for their troubles. This information isn't intended to discount the experiences of people who have had success on gluten-free diets; rather, it's meant to serve as a reminder that studying the causes of food reactions, in the absence of a straightforward diagnostic test, is incredibly challenging since almost all foods contain hundreds, if not thousands, of distinct components.

CROHN'S DISEASE

Crohn's disease is an inflammatory disorder that can affect any portion of the intestinal tract, although it's often found in the distal part of the ileum (the very end of the small intestine).[12] The precise etiology of Crohn's disease is still being elucidated, but regardless of its underlying causes, its symptoms are well documented: chronic diarrhea, abdominal pain, and weight loss, which are often accompanied by nonintestinal symptoms like fever, loss of appetite, and malaise.[13] Although it's not that common (less than 0.3 percent in most industrialized countries),[14] Crohn's disease often profoundly impacts the lives of those who suffer from it.[15] This is largely because it is a lifelong condition that, for many, recurs despite medical management. What's more, up to 80 percent of patients require at least one surgery in their lifetime.[16]

Given the rarity of Crohn's, few studies have evaluated exactly how it affects exercise training and competition in athletes. However, a number of pro athletes have opened up about the struggles they've dealt with while living with Crohn's. Larry Nance Jr., a basketballer who has played for the Los Angeles Lakers and Cleveland Cavaliers, wrote in 2015 about the symptoms he experienced in high school before being diagnosed:

> ❝ *I loved basketball . . . but I felt too sick and exhausted to put in the necessary work. . . . I even was benched on my freshman team because the coaches said I lacked energy.*[17]

Another athlete who has dealt with Crohn's is Matt Light, a three-time Super Bowl champion who played for the New England Patriots from 2001 to 2011. In 2004, Light had 13 inches of his intestines removed during the off-season, with hopes of returning for the start of training camp.[18] But because of complications from surgery, Light ended up in the hospital for a month and lost more than 50 pounds. He eventually went on to have a long, stellar career, but not all athletes living with Crohn's are able to keep competing at such a high level. One reason is that a condition known as short bowel syndrome can develop in people who have undergone surgeries to remove portions of their small intestine. The nutrient malabsorption and persistent diarrhea that stem from short bowel syndrome make it incredibly challenging—if not impossible, in some cases—to maintain the rigors of training required to be an elite athlete.

Similar to celiac disease, Crohn's can lead to the malabsorption of nutrients critical to an athlete's performance and health. Iron deficiency, poor vitamin D status, and reduced bone mineral density are all possibilities, though deficiencies of folate, vitamins B_6 and B_{12}, zinc, and selenium are also common.[19] Further, some of the medications (like corticosteroids) used to treat Crohn's can also reduce bone density, so skeletal health is a particularly relevant issue to be aware of. In the long run, this means that taking a multivitamin-mineral supplement is probably a sound idea, though athletes should talk to their healthcare providers about whether individual vitamin or mineral supplements are needed to address any specific deficiencies.

Finally, if an athlete experiences an acute flare of their Crohn's symptoms, they may need to make dietary adjustments to avoid exacerbating the situation. This can include eating small, frequent meals; avoiding high-fiber and spicy foods; drinking plenty of fluids; and saying no to alcohol.

FRUCTOSE MALABSORPTION

Fructose is a sugar naturally present in fruits, vegetables, and honey but is also a component of high-fructose corn syrup, a much-demonized sweetener product made from corn starch. Fructose malabsorption, or dietary fructose intolerance, as it's sometimes called, is a condition of poor fructose absorption through the brush border of the intestine. While accumulation of fructose in your intestinal lumen may seem like a benign event, it has clear downsides; any unabsorbed carbohydrate—whether it be fructose, glucose, sucrose, or lactose—causes fluid to shift into your gut lumen and leads to loose stools and gas production once it reaches your ileum and colon.

The most common method of determining whether someone is a fructose malabsorber is through hydrogen breath testing.[20] The principle behind hydrogen breath testing is straightforward; bacteria in the latter portion of your gut—particularly your large intestine—produce gases (including hydrogen) as they ferment unabsorbed carbohydrates. Some of this hydrogen gas is then expelled out your back end, but most of it gets absorbed through the intestinal wall into your blood, at which point it's transported to your lungs, where you subsequently breathe it out. Measuring the rise in breath hydrogen can therefore provide an indication of the extent of fructose malabsorption.

Studies that have performed hydrogen breath tests tell us that even people with "normal" fructose absorptive capacities develop symptoms if they're given big doses of fructose.[21] Thus, it's useful to think of fructose malabsorption on a continuum; everyone has some level of malabsorption if they eat enough of this sweet sugar, and people who have a low capacity for absorption are the ones we consider as having the diagnosable clinical condition. What dosage of fructose is used as a reference for determining whether someone has clinically meaningful fructose malabsorption? There's no universal consensus, but 25–50 grams is used in most situations.[20, 22]

A common strategy for dealing with fructose malabsorption—as you probably guessed—is limiting fructose intake. This means that athletes with fructose malabsorption will want to heavily restrict the intake of fructose-rich foods, particularly in the hours before important training sessions or competitions. Full lists of fructose-rich foodstuffs can easily be found online, but some examples include agave syrup, caramel, honey, high-fructose corn syrup, pears, apples, apple juice, mangoes, grapes, melon, and cherries.

A less intuitive strategy for managing fructose malabsorption is balancing the glucose and fructose contents of foods and beverages you eat, or supplementing with glucose when you eat fructose-rich foods. Experiments show that ingesting glucose with fructose enhances fructose absorption, and while it's not entirely clear what the mechanism for this is, it's probably the product of a glucose-stimulated upregulation of intestinal transporters or a passive dragging effect.[21] Practically speaking, an athlete would want to ingest an amount of glucose that's equivalent to the fructose in the food they're eating. For example, a 12-ounce cup of unsweetened apple juice has about 20 grams of free fructose and 10 grams of free glucose, so taking a couple of glucose tablets (which contain 4–5 grams of glucose each) would make up the 10-gram difference.

FUNCTIONAL DYSPEPSIA

Dyspepsia is a modern term derived from the Greek word *dyspeptos*, meaning "hard to digest" (*dys*- is the prefix for "bad" and *peptos* is Greek for "digested"). In olden times, dyspepsia described an array of vague digestive problems, but in today's modern medical world it is considered a diagnosable condition characterized by one or more of the following: fullness after eating, premature satiation, epigastric (upper abdomen) pain, and epigastric burning.[23] Obviously, everyone feels Thanksgiving-level fullness on occasion due to overindulging, but the key element of dyspepsia is that these symptoms are perceived as bothersome by the person and happen at least a few days per week over several months.

There are numerous identifiable causes of dyspepsia, including—but not limited to—GERD, stomach ulcers, gastritis, heavy NSAID use, and intestinal cancers. In many cases, though, evaluation of a person experiencing dyspepsia fails to turn up any signs of a structural/anatomical cause (also sometimes called an organic cause). If an organic cause can't be identified, a diagnosis of functional dyspepsia is made when the person's symptoms have persisted for more than a few months.[23]

234

Functional dyspepsia is divided into two subtypes: epigastric pain syndrome and postprandial distress syndrome. Epigastric pain syndrome—as the name implies—is defined by intermittent pain or burning in the epigastric region, while postprandial distress syndrome consists of bothersome postmeal fullness (even with normal-sized meals) or premature satiety that stops someone from finishing meals.[24] Although some people with functional dyspepsia have features of both subtypes, postprandial distress syndrome is slightly more common.

The worldwide prevalence of functional dyspepsia is somewhere between 11.5 percent and 29.2 percent,[25] and it places a massive burden on health systems. In one analysis of data extracted from US-based employers, employees with functional dyspepsia incurred costs that were $5,138 greater per year than other employees' costs (mostly due to higher medical and prescription drug costs).[26] Beyond economic costs, the pain and discomfort of functional dyspepsia also take their toll on one's life.[27] This burden was concisely summed up in an 1823 letter by the English essayist and frequent dyspepsia sufferer Thomas De Quincey: "Dyspepsy is the ruin of most things: empires, expeditions, and everything else."[28]

The causes of functional dyspepsia are often nebulous, which, given that there aren't any identifiable structural defects associated with it, is unsurprising. Still, some potential suspects are listed here:[23, 24]

- Delayed stomach emptying
- Impaired stomach accommodation (i.e., failure of the stomach to relax and expand in response to eating)
- Hypersensitivity of the nervous system to chemical and mechanical changes in the gut

- Low-grade inflammation of the duodenum
- *Helicobacter pylori* infection or other gut infections
- Anxiety, stress, or depression
- Consumption of high-fat or fried foods

Athletes who have a diagnosis of functional dyspepsia can take a multipronged approach to managing their condition. To some extent, treatment depends on the subtype that an athlete predominantly suffers from. Lifestyle interventions for postprandial distress syndrome include consuming small, frequent meals and avoiding fat-rich foods (say goodbye to Oreo sundaes and cream sauces), while for epigastric pain syndrome, people are often advised to avoid foods and substances that are alleged stomach irritants (e.g., coffee, alcohol, and cigarettes).[23] Although these recommendations are logical, most haven't been tested in rigorous experiments.

Like these lifestyle modifications, choice of drug treatment depends to a certain extent on the subtype of functional dyspepsia. Prokinetics—drugs that stimulate intestinal motility—are often prescribed for those who have symptoms consistent with postprandial distress syndrome. Epigastric pain syndrome, on the other hand, tends to be more responsive to antisecretory drugs, which target gastric acid release.[23] *Helicobacter pylori* infection is responsible for roughly 5 percent of dyspepsia cases, and eradication of this bug with antibiotics is modestly effective at ameliorating symptoms.[29] If none of these medications elicit a favorable effect, an antidepressant drug (usually from the tricyclic class) is sometimes administered.[30]

Lastly, interventions that reduce stress and modify sympathetic-parasympathetic nervous system balance are low-risk and potentially effective for dyspepsia. Good examples include slow deep breathing, meditation, relaxation training, and biofeedback. These interventions could be particularly useful for cases of functional dyspepsia that worsen in the hours leading up to stressful competition.

DIVERTICULOSIS

With aging, the body becomes more susceptible to developing pouch-like formations—called diverticula—in the mucosa and submucosa layers of the colon. Diverticula

235

tend to develop where blood vessels pass through the colon's muscular layer, which is a weak point in the wall. The presence of these diverticula in the colon is known as diverticulosis.[31]

Diverticulosis is classified in several ways depending on the nature of a patient's symptoms as well as clinical and laboratory findings: symptomatic uncomplicated diverticular disease, acute uncomplicated diverticulitis, and complicated diverticulitis.[32] Diverticulitis is a form of diverticulosis characterized by inflammation or infection in one or more of the diverticula. The term *complicated* describes a situation where problems from diverticulitis arise, which can include perforations, abscesses, obstructions, or bleeding. Symptomatic uncomplicated diverticular disease is a form of chronic diverticulosis associated with abdominal pain in the absence of diverticulitis or overt colitis.

Because diverticulosis can be asymptomatic and is often found inadvertently during colonoscopies, it's hard to know precisely what percentage of the population has this structural abnormality. Regardless, it's indisputable that age is a strong risk factor; in one French study, the presence of diverticulosis increased from just over 10 percent in those age 20 to 49 years to nearly 60 percent in those older than 80.[33] Despite the increasing prevalence with age, most individuals remain symptom-free. In fact, only about 20 percent of people with diverticulosis develop a symptomatic version.[31] Family history is another risk factor for diverticulosis, and studies of twins suggest that its heritability is roughly 40 percent (heritability is a statistic used to estimate the degree of variation in a disease that's due to genetic variation).[34]

Diet is a modifiable factor that has, for nearly a half century, been believed to play an important role in the onset of diverticulosis. Two of the most influential researchers who swayed beliefs about diet and diverticular disease were physicians Denis Burkitt and Neil Painter. Burkitt spent much of his early career working as a surgeon in Africa in the 1950s and 1960s, and the observations he made there shaped his beliefs that a lack of dietary fiber was responsible for a host of gut-related diseases in developed countries.[35] His ideas about fiber and health were so pervasive that he eventually earned the moniker The Fibre Man. Neil Painter was more fixated on diverticular disease, the focus of his master's thesis,[36] and he was one of the first to conduct a clinical study on the effectiveness of fiber as a treatment for symptomatic diverticulosis.[37] In 1971, Burkitt and Painter coauthored an article in the *British Medical Journal* that posited that a lack of fiber was largely responsible for the rise of diverticular disease in Western civilization.[38] To support their hypothesis, Painter and Burkitt highlighted data showing strikingly lower rates of diverticular disease in rural Africa and Asia (which had higher fiber intakes) as compared with developed Western countries.

The belief that a diet devoid of fiber elevates a person's risk of diverticulosis was firmly ensconced in the medical field for decades after the observations of Burkitt and Painter. More recently, some research has challenged this long-held notion about the protective role of dietary fiber.[39] This isn't to say there aren't studies—even recent ones—showing that fiber intake is associated with a lower risk of diverticulosis or its various subtypes. Yet, the evidence to support the diverticulosis-fiber hypothesis is inconsistent and comes mostly by way of observational studies that aren't particularly reliable for determining cause-and-effect relationships.[40, 41] Despite the shifting scientific associations between fiber and diverticulosis, there are several other modifiable factors that are more consistently linked with diverticular disease, including smoking tobacco, being overweight, and being sedentary.[42, 43]

Given that age is a strong risk factor for diverticulosis, masters athletes are much more likely to deal with it. For these athletes, treatment approaches for diverticular disease vary with each subtype of the disease. For years, antibiotics were the foundation of treatment for acute diverticulitis attacks, but guidelines from organizations such as the American Gastroenterological Association Institute have shifted to recommending them on a more limited basis due to a lack of evidence.[44] For many initial cases of acute uncomplicated diverticulitis, a physician may recommend rest and a liquid diet until symptoms abate. Notably, once a person has had an acute episode of diverticulitis, they are at greater risk of future attacks. Traditionally, surgical resection of the colon has been a common approach for preventing recurrences of diverticulitis, though nowadays it is becoming less common because the risk-to-benefit profile isn't as favorable as once thought. Finally, fiber and vigorous physical activity may help prevent the reoccurrence of diverticulitis, though the quality of evidence behind this is far from ironclad.[44]

GASTROESOPHAGEAL REFLUX DISEASE (GERD)

Gastroesophageal reflux disease (GERD) is a condition in which someone experiences persistent reflux of acid and other stomach components back into the esophagus. Typical symptoms include heartburn, difficulty swallowing, chest pain, and indigestion but can also include cough, voice changes, nausea, and breathing troubles.[45] While it may seem like a mild annoyance to observers, GERD can really affect one's quality of life, especially if it interferes with sleep.[46] Furthermore, poorly controlled GERD can lead to complications like Barrett's esophagus, an abnormality where the normal lining of the esophagus is replaced with tissue that is more cancer susceptible. And in fact, this is why Barrett's esophagus is associated with a higher risk of esophageal adenocarcinoma, a cancer that typically has a poor prognosis. In North America, approximately 18–28 percent of people have GERD, and similar estimates have been found in most other regions of the world.[47] Factors that raise the risk of GERD or that exacerbate its symptoms include obesity, pregnancy, smoking, and heavy alcohol use.

GERD is probably the most common cause of upper gut symptoms in athletes, and these athletes' peptic problems often worsen during exercise, particularly vigorous exercise. To avoid these issues, athletes with GERD can try avoiding food intake within an hour or two of exercise, especially fat-rich and solid foods. As with dyspepsia, deep breathing, relaxation, and biofeedback are low-risk strategies that could be employed prior to stressful competition. During exercise itself, avoiding concentrated carbohydrate beverages (especially greater than 10 percent) can be helpful.

Outside the context of exercise, lifestyle management of GERD includes losing weight for people who are overweight or obese, avoiding meals two to three hours before bedtime, and elevating the head of the bed for those suffering from nocturnal symptoms. Medical treatments run the gamut, from medication (often proton pump inhibitors, which tone down acid production) to surgical interventions.[46] Other potential strategies for alleviating GERD symptoms (or general reflux for those who experience occasional symptoms) are discussed in the "Reflux, Regurgitation, and Heartburn" section in Chapter 2.

IRRITABLE BOWEL SYNDROME

Irritable bowel syndrome, or IBS, is defined as a cluster of symptoms (cramping, bloating, pain, gas, etc.) and changes in bowel habits (diarrhea, constipation, or both) that occur in the absence of any physical gut damage or disease. One early reference to IBS in the scientific literature comes from a 1950 article in the now defunct *Rocky Mountain Medical Journal*.[48] In the article, titled simply "The Irritable Bowel Syndrome," physician Philip W. Brown describes it as a condition characterized by "diarrhea, either intermittently or chronic, abdominal soreness, gas pains, cramping and varying degrees of ill health and inefficiency" that appears "as life becomes more complex." Brown was by no means the first person to talk of an IBS-like syndrome. In the 1930s, "spastic colon" and "irritable colon" were often used to describe what we know today as IBS. Even before the 20th century, references to gut disturbances that sound uncannily similar to IBS were made by a variety of physicians and philosophers.[49]

Even if you're unaware of it, you almost certainly know someone who has IBS. Between 10 percent and 20 percent of people have it, though estimates from individual countries range widely, from about 3 percent in France to over 30 percent in Nigeria (though Nigeria's rate was based on a single study).[50] Specific to sports, there's scant research to tell us whether IBS is more or less common among athletes. The stressful and anxiety-provoking lifestyles of competitive athletes would suggest—at least intuitively—that IBS may be more common among high-level sportspersons, but then again, physical activity interventions have reduced symptoms of IBS in a few studies.[51] One recent study found that 9.8 percent of runners and triathletes meet diagnostic criteria for IBS,[52] but that doesn't tell us how that compares to nonathletes who are otherwise similar in terms of demographic background. At this point, it simply isn't clear how common IBS is in athletes from a broad range of sports.

One fact that's seemingly agreed on by nearly everyone in the medical community is that IBS is a gut-brain disorder. Remember, your gut contains between 100 million and 600 million neurons, and 90 percent of the fibers in your vagal nerve send information from your gut to your central nervous system. Clearly, there's a deep physical connection between your gut and brain, which provides a strong underlying rationale for why IBS is considered a gut-brain disorder. Furthermore, the overlap between IBS and mood disorders like anxiety and depression is undeniable; in a 2014 analysis of studies, patients with IBS were found to be significantly more likely to have anxiety and depression.[53] As physician Fred Kruse wrote succinctly way back in 1933, a "large proportion of the habitually constipated and irritable colon group are of neurotic constitution."[54]

For athletes who deal with IBS, a range of treatments exist and could include one or more of the following options:[51]

- Antidepressant and anxiolytic medications
- Anti-allergy medications
- Medications that alter gut motility
- A high-fiber diet
- Elimination of trigger foods
- Physical activity
- Psychotherapies such as group therapy, CBT, and relaxation training
- Peppermint oil

There are a couple things to note with this list of treatment strategies. First, the evidence behind many of them is weak or inconsistent, and for a good chunk of people living with IBS, complete symptom relief can be hard to come by even when they're actively treated.[55, 56] Second, the strategy used by a healthcare provider will depend not only on the person's background and personal preferences but also on the subtype of IBS they are diagnosed with: diarrhea-predominant, constipation-predominant, or a mixed form. For example, prescribing a laxative to an athlete with diarrhea-predominant IBS doesn't make a whole lot of sense.

LACTOSE INTOLERANCE

If you're lactose intolerant, it basically means that you kind of suck at digesting and absorbing lactose, a sugar found mostly in the milk (and milk-based products) of mammals. The lactose-challenged among us have less activity of lactase, the enzyme that splits lactose into its two component sugars, glucose and galactose. Although most newborns make enough lactase to adequately digest lactose (which makes sense given a baby's dependence on breast milk), persistence of high lactase activity into adolescence and adulthood varies across the world. In populations that have traditionally practiced cattle domestication, lactase persistence is often above 90 percent (e.g., Scandinavia) while it's below 10 percent in most populations from Asia and Africa.[57]

Ill effects of lactose intolerance include abdominal pain/cramps, bloating, excessive flatulence, and diarrhea.[58, 59] These symptoms occur when undigested lactose reaches the large intestine, where it gets fermented by legions of colonic bacteria and causes fluid to be pulled into the intestinal lumen. The minimum amount of lactose that triggers these symptoms varies, but most people who report suffering from lactose intolerance can actually consume small dosages (5–10 grams, or about 0.5–0.75 cups of milk) with few or no symptoms.[60] The most common way that lactose intolerance is diagnosed is through a hydrogen breath test, which consists of feeding a standardized amount of lactose to a person and subsequently measuring hydrogen expelled in their breath.[61]

For lactose-intolerant athletes, the most obvious solution to what ails them is to eliminate milk-based products, but this may have the unfortunate side effect of lowering diet quality and compounding the risk of certain diseases like osteoporosis. In addition, it may make them more sensitive to the negative effects of lactose, should they ever subsequently consume it. A better approach might be to eat small amounts of dairy foods throughout the day and/or to consume lactase-treated products or dairy substitutes like soymilk. Finally, gradually increasing lactose in the diet over a week or two can lessen symptoms among people who are lactose intolerant.[58] As an example, an athlete could start by drinking 4 ounces of milk two to three times per day and then increase the amount at each serving by 1–2 ounces every few days. This process could be continued until the person experiences noticeable digestive symptoms or until they reach serving sizes of about 12 ounces.

PEPTIC ULCERS

Pepsin is derived from the Greek word for "digestion," *pepsis*. Nowadays, the word *peptic* is commonly used to describe the section of gut that includes your stomach and duodenum. Thus, the phrase *peptic ulcer* is typically used in reference to a painful sore in the lining of this region. For the bulk of the 20th century, surgery was a cornerstone for managing peptic ulcers, and an Austro-Hungarian surgeon named Dragutin (Carl) Schwarz was one

of the first to document its use. In his 1910 article titled "Ueber penetrierende Magen-
und Jejunalgeschwüre" (if you trust Google, it translates to "About penetrating gastric
and jejunal ulcers"), Schwarz reported the results of 14 patients treated with surgical
excision of their ulcers.[62] After observing that ulcers only appeared in areas of the gut
where acid was thought to be secreted, Schwarz wrote a seemingly inconsequential line
of text that ended up as a dictum for decades to come: "Ohne sauren Magensaft kein
peptisches Geschwür" (essentially, no acid, no ulcer).[62, 63]

For the next half century or so, interventions that targeted gastric acid were the
main treatments for peptic ulcers. As an example, physicians started performing
vagotomies, procedures that involve cutting one or more branches of the vagus nerve.[63]
Impulses sent through the vagus nerves reach the stomach, stimulating parietal cells to
release hydrochloric acid; consequently, severing some of these connections blunts acid
secretion. Less invasive approaches included dietary changes and the consumption of
alkaline substances (antacids).[64]

These surgical and nonsurgical approaches remained the pillars of ulcer treatment
until the 1970s, at which point newer drugs that target acid secretion were developed.
The first of these newer drugs was cimetidine, which acts on what are called histamine-2
receptors.[63] (Specifically, cimetidine and other medications in this class prevent histamine from binding to histamine-2 receptors, an integral step in the secretion of stomach
acid.) In the late 1980s, another class of antacid drugs known as proton pump inhibitors
hit the market, and they're currently one of the first-line therapies for treating ulcers.[65]

Possibly the most important—and surprising—cause of peptic ulcers wasn't discovered until the 1980s. For a century prior, a number of scientists speculated that
microorganisms were somehow involved in the pathogenesis of peptic ulcers but were
unable to provide irrefutable evidence to support their suspicions.[63] Then, in 1979, a
pathologist named Robin Warren was working in Australia when he was sent a biopsy of
stomach tissue that showed severe gastritis.[66] Warren saw what he thought consisted
of numerous bacteria, and although he eventually convinced his colleagues that what
he was seeing was indeed microbes, they expressed doubt about the significance of
his findings and challenged him to replicate them with other samples. But even after
collecting additional cases over the next couple of years, few of Warren's colleagues

seemed interested in, or impressed with, his work. By a bit of happenstance, Warren teamed up with a young gastroenterology fellow named Barry Marshall, and their work together ultimately led to winning the Nobel Prize (in Physiology or Medicine) in 2005. In Warren's 2005 Nobel lecture, he recounted the serendipitous circumstances of how he became acquainted with Marshall:

> ❝ *Marshall . . . had been told to find a research project, and since he did not like the one suggested, his superiors sent him to me. . . . He did not seem impressed at first, but he agreed to send me a series of biopsies from apparently normal gastric antrum, to see if the same findings were present.*[66]

The collaboration between Marshall and Warren took off from this fortuitous meeting, and their research together was eventually described in an article in *The Lancet*, in which they report discovering a previously unidentified curved-looking bacteria present in almost all of their patients who had active chronic gastritis or peptic ulcers.[67] Soon thereafter, Marshall decided to take their discovery one step further by infecting himself with this bacteria (later dubbed *Helicobacter pylori*). Marshall later described his self-experimentation in an interview in the *Canadian Journal of Gastroenterology*, an excerpt of which is provided here:

> ❝ *I underwent endoscopy in early July 1984 to confirm that I was negative for H pylori. Three weeks later, I drank the "brew" which was a suspension of two culture plates of the organism.*[68]

Several days after ingesting the special *H. pylori* concoction, Marshall began experiencing bloating, fullness, vomiting, and a lack of appetite. A follow-up endoscopy also showed the presence of severe acute gastritis in his stomach. The scientific paper that detailed Marshall's case experiment was written in the third person,[69] but it later became known that the volunteer was Marshall himself. By 1988, the results of a double-blind clinical trial led by Marshall confirmed that eradication of *Helicobacter pylori* improved ulcer healing and helped prevent relapses.[70]

The discovery that a specific type of bacteria—in this case *Helicobacter pylori*—contributes to ulcer formation was groundbreaking, and extermination of *Helicobacter pylori* infection is now a leading treatment for peptic ulcers. Unfortunately, several key antibiotics (such as clarithromycin and levofloxacin) that have been traditionally used on *Helicobacter pylori* are becoming less effective in many places because of an increasing prevalence of strains that are antibiotic resistant.[71] In fact, the effectiveness of *Helicobacter pylori* eradication with some commonly used antibiotic regimens has fallen from more than 90 percent 20 years ago to less than 70 percent in many countries.[65] Today, treatment for *Helicobacter pylori* often involves the administration of two or three antibiotics plus a proton pump inhibitor.[65]

Another contributor to peptic ulcers—that is particularly relevant to athletes—is popping NSAIDs (e.g., ibuprofen, naproxen). Notably, 15–30 percent of people who regularly take NSAIDs have one or more ulcers upon endoscopic examination,[72] and compared with people who don't regularly use them, frequent users have two to four times the risk of complications from peptic ulcer disease.[65] The toxic effects of NSAIDs on the stomach and duodenum result from the inhibition of cyclooxygenase-1, an enzyme involved in producing substances (prostaglandins and mucus) that protect your stomach from substances like acids and alcohol. Ulcers found in patients who are NSAID users are typically treated by ceasing NSAID use (if possible), switching to a cyclooxygenase-2 inhibitor, adding a proton pump inhibitor, or a combination of these strategies.[73]

Athletes often rely on NSAIDs to deal with the nagging hurt that comes from daily training and competing or for coping with more serious injuries. Occasionally taking an NSAID or two isn't something to worry about, but athletes who are gobbling down NSAIDs are putting themselves at risk of developing ulcers or gastrointestinal bleeding, among several other problems. Instead, they might consider other approaches to managing pain, which can include anything from reducing training volume to mindfulness to trying dietary supplements like ginger, curcumin, omega-3s, and cannabidiol compounds.

Lastly, anxiety and stress have historically been thought to play a role in the onset or exacerbation of ulcers. In a 1921 article, George Eusterman, a physician at the renowned Mayo Clinic, wrote:

> ❝ *Worry or anxiety and mental or emotional strain for any reason greatly retard favorable response to treatment. Whenever necessary the reeducation of the patient, so that his occupation may be carried on with a minimum expenditure of nervous and physical energy, should be carried out.*[74]

However, with the discovery of *Helicobacter pylori* in the 1980s, the role of psychological factors has been seriously questioned. Today, the controversy over whether stress and anxiety influence peptic ulcer formation remains largely unresolved. Although it's true that individuals reporting high levels of stress are sometimes at greater risk for developing ulcers,[75] the stress itself may not be the true instigator. People who are stressed may be more likely to take NSAIDs, smoke tobacco, or engage in other behaviors that are the real culprits, and while the best studies try to mitigate these problems through statistical adjustments to their data, this type of design flaw is inherent to observational investigations.

245

SMALL INTESTINE BACTERIAL OVERGROWTH (SIBO)

As its name implies, small intestine bacterial overgrowth (SIBO) is a situation where the small intestine is overrun with bacteria.[76] Under normal circumstances, microbial density increases along the length of the gut, increasing from a few million total bacteria in the stomach to about 40 trillion in the colon.[77] This lack of microbes in the upper gut is generally a good thing because if too many bacteria lived in your stomach and small intestine, they would ferment much of the carbohydrate you eat before it has a chance to be absorbed.

There are several ways your body prevents the overgrowth of bacteria in your upper gut. Gastric acid makes your stomach a rather inhospitable environment, and other compounds secreted into your intestinal tract, such as immunoglobulins, also prevent microorganisms from flourishing in your upper gut. Similarly, maintenance of normal motility and an intact ileocecal valve (a sphincter that separates your small and large intestines) minimize your small intestine's exposure to bacteria from your colon.[78] It's not surprising, then, that several risk factors for SIBO involve dysfunction of these protective mechanisms; a few examples are achlorhydria (absent or low hydrochloric acid secretion), surgical removal of the ileocecal valve, and motility disorders.

Although SIBO is sometimes asymptomatic, it often causes bloating, flatulence, abdominal cramps, and diarrhea, as well as nondigestive symptoms like weight loss and general malaise stemming from the malabsorption of nutrients.[78] The prevalence of SIBO is hard to estimate because of variability in the tests (and their interpretation) used to diagnosis it. The current gold standard for diagnosing SIBO involves sampling small bowel fluid, followed by a culture and bacterial count,[76] but given the expense, difficulty, and invasiveness of this type of testing, breath testing for gases is typically used in clinical settings instead. Depending on the diagnostic method and criteria applied, SIBO is found in 0–20 percent of otherwise healthy people,[79] though it is more common in people with diseases like IBS, Crohn's, ulcerative colitis, and fibromyalgia.

Very little research on SIBO in athletes exists, so we're left a bit clueless as to how often it plays a role in triggering gut symptoms during training and competition. If an athlete does receive a diagnosis of SIBO, management of their condition will depend on the suspected cause; if possible, treatment of the underlying disease or structural problem is the priority. However, in some situations, like when a person has had their ileocecal valve removed, this isn't feasible.[79] Alternative approaches include antibiotics and dietary changes. Elemental diets (made of predigested nutrients that are rapidly absorbed) and restricting FODMAPs (discussed in Chapter 4) are two popular nutrition interventions. Overall, these diets have shown some success in terms of alleviating symptoms in the short term, but it's unclear how helpful they are for managing SIBO over years.[76] In addition, there's concern about the nutritional adequacy and health consequences of following these restrictive diets for long periods of time. Still, they could be good options prior to important events or competitions.

TRAVELER'S DIARRHEA

Throughout history, infectious gut illnesses have been a terrible menace for the human species. The pages of history are replete with tales of people suffering from the unwanted effects of gut infections. In *Seven Pillars of Wisdom* (an autobiographical account of a British soldier's service during the Great Arab Revolt of World War I), T. E. Lawrence (otherwise known as Lawrence of Arabia) wrote:

> **❝** *Dysentery of this Arabian coast used to fall like a hammer blow and crush its victims for a few hours.*[80]

Well before Lawrence's time, gut infections were blamed for the deaths of an incalculable number of people, from commoners to royalty such as King Henry V. Although advancements in sanitation and the introduction of antibiotics in the 20th century dramatically curtailed the number of people dying from gastrointestinal infections in developed countries, many millions of people throughout history have succumbed to these illnesses. Even today, roughly 1.3 million people around the world—most of them children in low-income countries—die from diarrheal diseases each year.[81]

Gut infections (a.k.a. traveler's diarrhea) are quite common when people travel to international locales with less-than-optimal water and food quality. If you want to get technical about it, traveler's diarrhea is defined as three or more loose-to-watery stools over 24 hours, with or without other symptoms such as cramping, nausea, and low-grade fever.[82] Vomiting and severe cramping accompanied by blood or mucus in the stool can also occur but are less frequent manifestations. The microorganisms typically responsible for traveler's diarrhea are *E. coli*, salmonella, campylobacter, shigella, giardia, norovirus, and rotavirus.[83] Most cases subside within a week without any pharmaceutical treatment, but in a minority of cases, symptoms persist for weeks and can even transform into something that bears resemblance to IBS after several months.[82]

The term *traveler's diarrhea* comes from the fact that these gut infections often occur when people travel outside of their countries of residence. Studies in the 1950s and 1960s led by physician Benjamin H. Kean were some of the first to quantify the incidence of traveler's diarrhea; in one survey of Americans flying to Los Angeles from Mexico, Kean found that 33 percent reported at least one spell of diarrhea if they had spent a week or more abroad.[84] In contrast, only 7.6 percent of Americans returning from Hawaii reported any diarrhea. Kean's findings are consistent with the incidence of traveler's diarrhea experienced by international tourists today. A review published in the *Journal of the American Medical Association* reported that, depending on the destination and the background characteristics of travelers, anywhere from 10 percent to 40 percent of people get traveler's diarrhea during a two-week trip.[83] And according to the Centers for Disease Control and Prevention, it is the leading cause of illness among people traveling from high-income to developing countries and is most endemic in Asia (except for Japan), the Middle East, sub-Saharan Africa, and Central and South America.[85]

In the world of sports, these types of infections can derail the ambitions of athletes going for gold. In 1986, the US swimming team underwhelmed at the World Championships in Madrid, thanks in large part to many of the team's members coming down with a nasty stomach bug. More than 20 years later, several athletes on the US track and field team, including Shalane Flanagan, were reportedly hit with symptoms suggestive of traveler's diarrhea during the Beijing Olympics. Fortunately, Flanagan recovered well enough to medal, but still, these incidents are reminders that years' worth of blood, sweat, and tears can all be for naught when a virulent stomach bug hits.

In order to prevent traveler's diarrhea, it's helpful to be aware of its risk factors, most of which are listed here:

- Travel to a destination where pathogenic microorganisms are endemic in the food and water
- Eating food from street vendors
- Eating food served buffet-style
- Poor hygiene conditions of a food establishment
- Eating in native homes and small restaurants
- Ingesting unpasteurized dairy products or prepeeled fruit
- Drinking tap water or water from an unknown source
- Younger age (possibly because youth are more adventurous and/or eat more food)
- A diagnosis of inflammatory bowel disease

Based on these risk factors, simple strategies for minimizing the risk of traveler's diarrhea include washing your hands with soap and water before every meal, avoiding tap water, only drinking fluids from sealed bottles, only eating food served hot, and shunning raw foods and unpasteurized dairy products. In addition, athletes participating in sports held in natural waters (kayaking, triathlons, etc.) should take care not to swallow water while training and competing.

Supplementing with probiotics is a potentially appealing tactic to prevent traveler's diarrhea because of its simplicity and safety, but, unfortunately, there isn't strong evidence that it's particularly effective.[86] Athletes who suffer from repeated bouts of traveler's diarrhea, or those who cannot tolerate any chance of getting sick (such as an athlete traveling for a once-in-a-lifetime competition), should consider speaking with a physician about prophylactic treatment with antibiotics or other prophylactic drugs prior to traveling to high-risk regions.

ULCERATIVE COLITIS

Crohn's disease and ulcerative colitis are both inflammatory bowel diseases, but unlike Crohn's, ulcerative colitis is limited to the colon. Another feature distinguishing ulcerative colitis from Crohn's is that the inflammation is confined to the mucosa (the innermost layer of the gut), whereas in Crohn's it often infiltrates all layers.[87] Ulcerative colitis can induce an assortment of unpleasant symptoms (chronic diarrhea, abdominal cramps/pain, mucus in the stool), although the main presenting symptom, which is reported by more than 90 percent of patients, is blood in the stool.[88]

The prevalence of ulcerative colitis varies across the world, though the highest rates are found—for partially unknown reasons—in developed countries.[14] In the United States, the number of people living with ulcerative colitis is similar to that of Crohn's. In one study done in Minnesota, the annual incidence of ulcerative colitis from 2000 to 2010 was 12.2 cases per 100,000 persons, which was only slightly higher than the estimate for Crohn's (10.7 cases per 100,000).[89] By extrapolating these numbers to the entire population, it's estimated that roughly 785,000 Americans have Crohn's and that 910,000 have ulcerative colitis.

The strongest risk factor for ulcerative colitis is having a close relative with the disease. If you have a parent or sibling with it, your risk is 10 to 15 times greater than normal.[88] While diet seems like a logical contributing factor to the onset of ulcerative colitis, the studies done up to this point have largely been inconclusive. There's some evidence that omega-3 fats and fiber offer mild protection, but these data are based almost entirely on observational studies.[90] Surprisingly, nonsmokers and people who have quit smoking seem to have higher chances of developing ulcerative colitis than smokers.[88] It's not exactly clear why this is, but it's one of the only positive benefits ever to be documented with smoking. Obviously, the other problems that arise from smoking still make it one of the worst behaviors you can do for your overall health.

Anecdotally, ulcerative colitis can profoundly affect an athlete's ability to train and compete. Take for example the case of Fernando Pisani, a pro hockey player who competed for the Edmonton Oilers for five seasons. In 2005, Pisani was diagnosed with ulcerative colitis, but it wasn't until 2007 that his symptoms really started to have a profound impact on his life. Recounting his ordeal in an article for *The Hockey News*, Pisani wrote:

> *I was going to the bathroom 20–30 times a day, losing a lot of blood and a lot of weight. I could barely leave the house and when I did, I had to know where the nearest bathroom was.*[91]

Pisani was in such bad shape that he lost roughly three quarts of blood and even developed a transitory case of diabetes because of the medications he was initially put on. Eventually Pisani started taking the drug Remicade, which reversed his symptoms and allowed him to resume his hockey career. Clearly, any athlete suffering from ulcerative colitis needs to work closely with their healthcare provider to come up with a treatment strategy that takes their individual circumstances into account. Thankfully, with appropriate medical management, people living with ulcerative colitis are often able to maintain their physical activity and physical fitness despite occasionally going through periods of reduced activity.[92]

When a healthcare provider develops a plan to treat ulcerative colitis, they need to consider not only the severity of the patient's disease (location and extent) but also the age at onset, history of relapse, previous medications, and any extraintestinal symptoms the patient is experiencing.[93] Medication and surgery are mainstays of treatment, but with each passing decade, new and better drugs are added to the armamentarium of treatment choices for the disease, which has resulted in declining numbers of patients requiring surgeries.[94] Still, many people end up requiring surgery at some point over the course of their disease.[95]

Besides medication and surgery, athletes living with ulcerative colitis often ponder whether it's worthwhile to try complementary treatments like dietary supplementation, biofeedback, hypnosis, and acupuncture. They should be aware that most of these treatments remain scientifically untested or have shown little to no benefit specific to ulcerative colitis. One exception, however, is a probiotic dubbed VSL#3, which has been used extensively in ulcerative colitis. It comprises eight different strains of lactic acid–producing bacteria, and based on trials that have included hundreds of patients, VSL#3 lowers the risk of relapses when added to conventional therapy.[96] As with any medication or supplement, patients with ulcerative colitis should consult with their physicians before using VSL#3 or any other probiotic.

APPENDIX B: MEDICATIONS AFFECTING THE GUT

The following tables provide an overview of many of the medications known to impact the gut. Some are used to manage gut disorders while others have no direct role in managing these disorders but cause unpleasant gut-related side effects (opioids and selective and nonselective NSAIDs). For each class of medications, the typical indications for use, physiological mechanisms, and potential side effects are described. In addition, specific considerations for athletes using each class of medications are reviewed. (Note: For drug classes with unfamiliar or impenetrable names, I have added basic descriptions of what they're used for in parentheses.)

This appendix isn't meant to be an exhaustive review of every medication on the planet that impacts the gut. That said, it can serve as an initial source of information for athletes who are taking, or are considering taking, over-the-counter or prescription medications. As always, you should consult with a healthcare provider before deciding to take any of these medications.

5-HT$_3$ RECEPTOR ANTAGONISTS (ANTI-NAUSEA MEDICATIONS)

Examples: ondansetron, granisetron, dolasetron, alosetron, palonosetron	
Typical indications	• Nausea and vomiting from medical interventions such as chemotherapy, radiation, surgery, and anesthesia[1] • Sometimes used off-label for morning sickness • IBS[1]
Physiological mechanisms	• Reduce nausea severity by dampening activation of vagal sensory nerve fibers and the chemoreceptor trigger zone • Work by blocking the binding of 5-hydroxytryptamine (a.k.a. serotonin) with 5-HT$_3$ receptors[2]
Side effects	• Headaches, constipation, and dizziness[1] • Cardiac rhythm changes[1]
Considerations for athletes	• In a small study of 21 runners who were administered ondansetron for nausea and/or vomiting during ultrarunning races, two-thirds thought the medication was effective.[3] • Race medical services often keep ondansetron on hand as an anti-nausea/anti-vomiting drug.[4] • No published randomized trials have tested the effectiveness of these drugs for exercise-associated nausea and vomiting.

ANTACIDS

Examples: calcium carbonate, sodium bicarbonate, aluminum hydroxide, magnesium hydroxide, alginate	
Typical indications	• Symptomatic relief from GERD, occasional heartburn, and indigestion
Physiological mechanisms	• Most antacids work by chemically neutralizing gastric acid without significantly impacting gastric acid secretion. • Alginate creates a gel that floats on top of stomach contents, providing a physical barrier that blocks the acid from irritating the proximal stomach and esophagus.[5]
Side effects	• Taking large amounts of sodium bicarbonate and magnesium hydroxide can induce diarrhea, whereas aluminum hydroxide and calcium carbonate can induce constipation.
Considerations for athletes	• Athletes using antacids for heartburn should be cognizant of their gut side effects (diarrhea, constipation, etc.). • Beyond its role as a gastric acid neutralizer, sodium bicarbonate is an effective performance enhancer for high-intensity exercise if its ingestion is timed appropriately in relation to competition.[6]

ANTIBIOTICS

Examples: penicillin, amoxicillin, cefotaxime, cefprozil, clarithromycin, erythromycin, azithromycin, ciprofloxacin, levofloxacin, ofloxacin, tetracycline, gentamicin, trimethoprim	
Typical indications	• Treatment or prevention of bacterial infections, including respiratory tract infections, skin infections, gut infections, urinary tract infections, sexually transmitted infections, and bacterial sepsis • Note: Upward of 30% of outpatient oral antibiotic prescriptions in the US may be unnecessary (e.g., for common colds), which is contributing to the growth of antibiotic-resistant infections.[7]
Physiological mechanisms	• Varies depending on the type; examples include targeting the cell wall of bacteria, inhibiting the synthesis of proteins important to the bacteria's function, and interfering with DNA copying
Side effects	• Antibiotics often disturb the normal balance of bacteria in the gut, leading to diarrhea and other gut side effects[8] • Vary with different classes of antibiotics, but most can cause diarrhea, nausea, vomiting, abdominal pain, bloating, and rashes
Considerations for athletes	• Co-administering probiotics (particularly *Lactobacillus* strains) with antibiotics may reduce the incidence and/or severity of antibiotic-associated diarrhea.[9,10] • Although routine prophylactic treatment with antibiotics isn't advised when traveling abroad, athletes who suffer from repeated bouts of traveler's diarrhea might consider speaking with a physician about prophylactic treatment prior to traveling to regions where the risk of gut infections is high.[11]

ANTIDIARRHEALS

Examples: loperamide, diphenoxylate-atropine, bismuth subsalicylate	
Typical indications	• Traveler's diarrhea, nonspecific acute diarrhea, chemotherapy- or radiation-induced diarrhea, and certain forms of chronic diarrhea
Physiological mechanisms	• Antidiarrheals generally work to treat diarrhea by reducing fluid secretion into the gut and/or lessening peristalsis. • Loperamide stimulates opioid receptors in the periphery and gut, which reduces peristalsis and secretion of fluid and electrolytes into the lumen.[12] • Diphenoxylate-atropine blunts the secretion of fluids into the lumen and reduces gut motility.[13] • Bismuth subsalicylate has antimicrobial properties and reduces the secretion of fluid and electrolytes into the lumen.[14]
Side effects	• Loperamide can cause constipation, dizziness, nausea, abdominal cramps, and, in rare cases, ileus and fecal impaction.[15] • Because diphenoxylate-atropine crosses the blood-brain barrier, central nervous system side effects like confusion, lethargy, and dizziness are possible.[13] • Bismuth subsalicylate can cause tongue discoloration, dark or black stools, constipation, and nausea.[16]
Considerations for athletes	• There aren't sufficient clinical trial data to say whether loperamide is helpful for exercise-induced diarrhea, but endurance race medical services often keep it on hand.[4] • Loperamide is often used for mild cases of traveler's diarrhea and as an adjunctive treatment with antibiotics for moderate or severe cases.[17] • Bismuth subsalicylate can help prevent traveler's diarrhea, so athletes traveling to international destinations might consider asking their physician about prophylactic treatment.[17] • Diphenoxylate's central nervous system effects and atropine's ability to inhibit sweating make diphenoxylate-atropine a poor choice for the treatment of exercise-induced diarrhea.

256

DOPAMINE-RECEPTOR ANTAGONISTS (ANTI-NAUSEA MEDICATIONS)

Examples: perphenazine, prochlorperazine, metoclopramide, domperidone	
Typical indications	• Nausea and vomiting from surgery, anesthesia, and chemotherapy[18]
Physiological mechanisms	• Reduce nausea by blocking the binding of dopamine with dopamine receptors in the chemoreceptor trigger zone[19] • May also enhance upper gut motility and stomach emptying, which would indirectly reduce nausea[19]
Side effects	• Side effects depend on dosage and specific drug. • Among other side effects, cardiac arrhythmias, tardive dyskinesia (involuntary movements of the face, trunk, and extremities), akathisia (feeling of inner restlessness), sedation, and low blood pressure upon standing are possible.[18]
Considerations for athletes	• Anecdotally, metoclopramide has been used to successfully treat nausea in ultraendurance competitors.[4] • No published randomized trials have tested the effectiveness of these drugs in the treatment of exercise-associated nausea and vomiting.

H₁ ANTIHISTAMINES (ANTI-NAUSEA MEDICATIONS)

Examples: 1st generation: dimenhydrinate, diphenhydramine, meclizine, promethazine. 2nd and 3rd generations: cetirizine, desloratadine, fexofenadine, levocetirizine, loratadine	
Typical indications	• Nausea or vomiting that arises during pregnancy, chemotherapy, and motion sickness, as well as after surgery[20] • Only 1st generation H1 antihistamines effective for nausea • Also used for allergies, itching, and as sleep aids
Physiological mechanisms	• Reduce nausea by dampening activation of the vomiting center in the brain • Block or counteract the action of histamine on H_1 receptors in the brain[20]
Side effects	• Side effects depend on dosage and specific drug. • Among other side effects, sedation, drowsiness, fatigue, headache, and cardiac arrhythmias are possible.[20] • 2nd and 3rd generation versions typically have fewer side effects than 1st generation because they don't cross the blood-brain barrier or only do so in small amounts; on the flip side, they may not be as useful for managing nausea.[20]
Considerations for athletes	• There's no research available to describe their effectiveness or safety in the treatment of exercise-induced nausea and vomiting.

H$_2$ ANTAGONISTS (GASTRIC ACID REDUCERS)

Examples: cimetidine, ranitidine, nizatidine, famotidine	
Typical indications	• GERD, peptic ulcer disease, functional dyspepsia, and Zollinger-Ellison syndrome (excessive acid secretion due to tumors)
Physiological mechanisms	• Reduce gastric acid secretion by blocking the action of histamine on H$_2$ receptors found in the stomach
Side effects	• Headaches, diarrhea, drowsiness, and dizziness[21]
Considerations for athletes	• H$_2$ antagonists can reduce episodes of acid reflux during exercise as measured through probes, but these reductions don't always translate to less subjective heartburn.[22] • They may reduce the risk of gut bleeding with ultraendurance running but not with shorter distances.[23, 24]

LAXATIVES (ANTICONSTIPATION MEDICATIONS)

Examples: lactulose, magnesium oxide, polyethylene glycol, sodium picosulfate, bisacodyl	
Typical indications	• Chronic constipation, constipation-predominant IBS, and preparation for bowel procedures (e.g., colonoscopies)
Physiological mechanisms	• Osmotic laxatives (lactulose, magnesium oxide, polyethylene glycol) are made of nonabsorbable molecules that draw water into the intestinal lumen.[25] • Stimulative laxatives (sodium picosulfate and bisacodyl) cause the intestines to secrete water into the lumen.[25]
Side effects	• Diarrhea, abdominal cramps, flatulence, rectal pain, dehydration, dizziness, fainting, low blood pressure, electrolyte disturbances, and acid-base disturbances[26]
Considerations for athletes	• Although relatively uncommon, some athletes (particularly distance runners, gymnasts, dancers, jockeys, wrestlers) use laxatives as an unsafe way to control their weight.[27] • The side effects of chronic/heavy laxative use (dehydration, dizziness, low blood pressure, electrolyte disturbances, etc.) have the potential to interfere with training and impair performance.

MUSCARINIC CHOLINOCEPTOR ANTAGONISTS
(ANTI-NAUSEA AND ANTICRAMPING MEDICATIONS)

Examples: hyoscine, atropine	
Typical indications	• Postoperative nausea/vomiting, motion sickness, and abdominal cramping
Physiological mechanisms	• Block activity of muscarinic acetylcholine receptors, which are present in the brain stem and peripheral nervous system and play a role in regulating nausea/vomiting[19] • Reduce abdominal cramping by relaxing smooth muscle and decreasing motility in the stomach and intestines[28]
Side effects	• Dry mouth, blurred vision, sedation, accelerated heart rate, itching, and reduced sweating[19]
Considerations for athletes	• Although hyoscine effectively minimizes the symptoms of seasickness and motion sickness,[29] there's no research on its effectiveness for treating exercise-induced nausea and vomiting. • Side effects such as sedation, impaired sweating, and fast heart rate would be unfavorable changes for many athletes; thus, use of these drugs for exercise-induced gut symptoms is often discouraged.[30]

259

NSAIDS, NONSELECTIVE (ANTI-INFLAMMATORIES)*

Examples: naproxen, ibuprofen, diclofenac	
Typical indications	• Pain and inflammation management
Physiological mechanisms	• Block actions of cyclooxygenase-1 and cyclooxygenase-2 enzymes, reducing the production of prostaglandins and other inflammatory molecules[31]
Side effects	• NSAIDs raise the risks of heart attack, stroke, peptic ulcers, gastrointestinal bleeding, and kidney disease.[31] • Although taking NSAIDs for even a few weeks can raise the risks of cardiovascular events, higher doses taken for longer time frames seem to be associated with the most risk.
Considerations for athletes	• Increase gut permeability during exercise[32] • Associated with abdominal cramps/pain and race dropout during endurance competition[33] • May raise the risk of hyponatremia during prolonged exercise[34] • May blunt exercise training adaptations when taken in high doses[35, 36] • Can induce asthma attacks in people with asthma[37]

* NSAIDs have no direct role in managing gut disorders but cause unpleasant gut-related side effects.

NSAIDS, SELECTIVE (ANTI-INFLAMMATORIES)*

Examples: celecoxib, meloxicam	
Typical indications	• Pain and inflammation management
Physiological mechanisms	• Block actions of cyclooxygenase-2 enzymes, reducing the production of prostaglandins and other inflammatory molecules[31]
Side effects	• Fewer gut problems compared to nonselective NSAIDs, but more adverse cardiovascular events[31] • Note: Other specific drugs from this class (rofecoxib, valdecoxib) have been removed from the market because of cardiovascular dangers.
Considerations for athletes	• Induce less gut permeability than nonselective NSAIDs[38] • May have similar risks as nonselective NSAIDs when it comes to hyponatremia during exercise[39] • May have similar effects as nonselective NSAIDs on training adaptations, though more research is needed to verify this.[40]

* NSAIDs have no direct role in managing gut disorders but cause unpleasant gut-related side effects.

OPIOIDS*

Examples: hydrocodone, oxycodone, tramadol, codeine, morphine, fentanyl, alfentanil, methadone, buprenorphine, meperidine	
Typical indications	• Acute and chronic pain
Physiological mechanisms	• Activate opioid receptors on nerve cells • The analgesic effects are mediated by a variety of opioid receptor subtypes (mu, kappa, delta).[41]
Side effects	• Sedation, dizziness, slowed breathing, and physical dependence[42] • Constipation (reported by a majority of opioid users)[43, 44] • Nausea, abdominal pain, and gas (reported by a minority of opioid users)[43]
Considerations for athletes	• Some athlete groups (such as former professional American footballers) are more likely to use and abuse opioids.[45, 46] • The International Olympic Committee consensus statement on pain management cautions against the long-term use of opioids (>10 days) because of their serious risks and lack of evidence for long-term benefit.[47] • Opioid use around the time of competition is generally considered ergolytic (performance harming) because it detrimentally impacts cognition, respiratory function, neuromotor function, and reaction time.[47]

* Opioids have no direct role in managing gut disorders but cause unpleasant gut-related side effects.

PROSECRETORY DRUGS (ANTICONSTIPATION MEDICATIONS)

Examples: linaclotide, lubiprostone, prucalopride	
Typical indications	• Chronic constipation and constipation-predominant IBS
Physiological mechanisms	• Help ease the passage of stools by increasing secretion of fluid, electrolytes, and other molecules from the gut wall into the gut lumen[25]
Side effects	• Diarrhea, abdominal pain, abdominal distension, flatulence, nausea, and headache[48, 49]
Considerations for athletes	• No studies have investigated effects specifically in athletes. • Although there are likely fewer gut side effects than with laxatives (p. 258), the side effects from prosecretory drugs could theoretically interfere with training and impair performance in some situations.

261

PROTON PUMP INHIBITORS (GASTRIC ACID REDUCERS)

Examples: omeprazole, dexlansoprazole, pantoprazole, rabeprazole, esomeprazole, lansoprazole	
Typical indications	• GERD, peptic ulcers, functional dyspepsia, and Zollinger-Ellison syndrome
Physiological mechanisms	• Block actions of the gastric hydrogen-potassium ATPase pump, which is responsible for acid secretion[50]
Side effects	• There are few serious short-term adverse effects, but long-term use may increase the risk of fractures, certain infections (C. difficile), and pneumonia in specific populations (e.g., elderly and hospitalized patients).[51]
Considerations for athletes	• Appear to reduce the risk of gut bleeding with ultrarunning[52] • Can reduce episodes of acid reflux during exercise as measured through probes, though these reductions don't always translate to less subjective heartburn[53]

SELECTIVE SEROTONIN REUPTAKE INHIBITORS (IBS MEDICATIONS)

Examples: citalopram, fluoxetine, paroxetine, sertraline, escitalopram	
Typical indications	• IBS, when used for gut disorders • Major depressive disorder, generalized anxiety disorder, social anxiety disorder, panic disorder, and eating disorders
Physiological mechanisms	• Can reduce gut symptoms in some IBS patients, though it's not entirely clear how • May work by reducing somatization (when psychological issues are expressed as physical symptoms)
Side effects	• Agitation, sexual dysfunction, sleepiness, weight gain, weight loss, dry mouth, insomnia, fatigue, nausea, diarrhea, and tremors[54-56]
Considerations for athletes	• Although SSRIs can improve symptoms of IBS,[57] it's unclear whether they specifically reduce gut symptoms that occur during exercise in athletes with IBS. • There's currently no clear consensus as to whether long-term SSRI use impacts exercise performance or endurance.[58, 59]

TRICYCLIC ANTIDEPRESSANTS (IBS AND DYSPEPSIA MEDICATIONS)

Examples: imipramine, nortriptyline, desipramine, amitriptyline, doxepin, protriptyline, trimipramine	
Typical indications	• IBS and functional dyspepsia, when used for gut disorders • Major depressive disorder, generalized anxiety disorder, panic disorder, attention deficit hyperactivity disorder, and insomnia[60]
Physiological mechanisms	• Similar mechanisms as SSRIs but also block histaminic, cholinergic, and adrenergic receptors, leading to more undesirable side effects (weight gain, dry mouth, drowsiness, dizziness, and constipation)[61]
Side effects	• Sedation, dry mouth, fatigue, blurred vision, constipation, weight gain, difficulty urinating, sexual dysfunction, headache, dizziness, agitation, tremor, low blood pressure upon standing, and cardiac arrhythmias[59, 61] • May increase the risk of cardiovascular disease including myocardial infarction and stroke[62] • Note: Due to their higher incidence of side effects, tricyclic antidepressants are usually reserved for situations where SSRIs aren't well-tolerated or are ineffective.
Considerations for athletes	• Tricyclics likely reduce symptoms of IBS,[57] but it's unclear whether they specifically reduce gut symptoms that occur during exercise in athletes with IBS. • Although they haven't been studied specifically in athletes, several side effects of tricyclic antidepressants (such as extreme sedation, weight gain, and cardiac arrhythmias) would obviously be problematic for many athletes.[59]

ACKNOWLEDGMENTS

I relied on hundreds of sources of information during the two years it took to write *The Athlete's Gut*. I've done my best to acknowledge each of these sources in the text and the Notes section. Still, a few of these works deserve a special acknowledgment because of the extent to which I relied on them or because of the inspiration they gave me. *The Gastrointestinal System: Gastrointestinal, Nutritional and Hepatobiliary Physiology* edited by Po Sing Leung (Springer, 2014) was incredibly helpful when it came time to describe the nitty-gritty details of the digestive system; it's one of the more comprehensive, yet accessible textbooks on the gut. I wish to recognize the editor and chapter authors for creating a wonderful resource for understanding the mysteries of the gut.

Another source that was incredibly valuable to me was *Gulp: Adventures on the Alimentary Canal* by science writer Mary Roach (Norton, 2013). If you're not familiar with Roach's writing, I strongly encourage you to dive into her book catalog. There are few authors who can take otherwise prosaic scientific topics and make them as accessible and entertaining as Roach does. Her books are filled with hilarious (and sometimes disturbing) anecdotes, bringing the subject matter to life. In Chapter 1 of *The Athlete's Gut*, I describe a 23-year-old model with bulimia who died after eating 19 pounds of food in one sitting, which is a story I first learned of from reading *Gulp*. Roach's account of that fateful meal inspired me to go down the virtual rabbit hole of PubMed to find other stories of people keeling over from overeating. Likewise, Roach's interviews with flatulence researchers (particularly Michael Levitt from the Minneapolis VA Health Care System) prompted me to include sections of text on farts and the subjective rating of said farts. (Remember that study I mentioned in Chapter 2 that had two people eject flatus up their noses? I learned about that from *Gulp*.) *Gulp* is without a doubt the most entertaining book I've read about the gut, and if you haven't had your fill of digestive science after reading *The Athlete's Gut*, you should definitely give *Gulp* a try.

263

The book *My Age of Anxiety: Fear, Hope, Dread, and the Search for Peace of Mind* by Scott Stossel (Alfred A. Knopf, 2014) inspired me to share some of my own issues with anxiety as well as seek out anecdotes of athletes suffering from anxiety-induced gut problems. In *My Age of Anxiety*, Stossel weaves together information from scientific research, historical accounts, and his own experiences to vividly depict the toll that anxiety can have on the human body and the gut. He pulls no punches when it comes to sharing his own struggles with anxiety, and several of his anecdotes involve severe anxiety-induced gut distress. One of these is a humiliating yet hilarious toilet-clogging incident at the Kennedy Compound in Hyannis Port, Massachusetts. Stossel was there to do research for a book he was writing on Sargent Shriver when he was stricken with severe anxiety while out and about. He rushed back to the house and proceeded to clog the guest bathroom, ruining his pants in the process. This all happened with Arnold Schwarzenegger, Bill Clinton, and Ted Kennedy around. If you're a glutton for these types of stories and writing that mixes science, self-deprecating humor, and history, I'm sure you'll appreciate *My Age of Anxiety*.

Beyond these written sources, several people deserve my sincerest thanks for helping to bring *The Athlete's Gut* to life. I cannot thank VeloPress enough for taking a chance on an author like me who is accustomed to writing dull scientific articles. Casey Blaine and, in particular, Andy Read pushed me to make my writing more accessible and engaging for the reader. Andy did a magnificent job of helping me to shape and focus the narrative of the book without compromising the scientific integrity of the information. I'd also like to thank Managing Editor Sarah Gorecki for her efforts to keep the editing process on schedule. My appreciation also goes out to copyeditor Marjorie Woodall, who went through the manuscript with a fine-tooth comb to find all the inevitable typos and errors that come with writing a book of this magnitude and scope, as well as to proofreader Carolyn Sobczak. A final thank you goes out to the individuals involved in the illustrations, artwork, and cover design—Vicki Hopewell, Andrew Nilsen, Corey Hollister, and Erin Farrell.

NOTES

Introduction

1. E. P. de Oliveira, R. C. Burini, and A. Jeukendrup, "Gastrointestinal Complaints During Exercise: Prevalence, Etiology, and Nutritional Recommendations," *Sports Medicine* 44, no. 1 (2014): 79–85.
2. J. N. Pugh et al., "Gastrointestinal Symptoms in Elite Athletes: Time to Recognise the Problem?" *British Journal of Sports Medicine* 52, no. 8 (2018): 487–488.

Chapter 1

1. W. V. Nascimento et al., "Gender Effect on Oral Volume Capacity," *Dysphagia* 27, no. 3 (2012): 384–389.
2. C. S. Lear, J. B. Flanagan, and C. F. Moorrees, "The Frequency of Deglutition in Man," *Archives of Oral Biology* 10, no. 1 (1965): 83–89.
3. "Choking Prevention and Rescue Tips," National Safety Council, https://www.nsc.org/home-safety/safety-topics/choking-suffocation.
4. T. J. Song et al., "Correlation of Esophageal Lengths with Measurable External Parameters," *The Korean Journal of Internal Medicine* 6, no. 1 (1991): 16–20.
5. J. N. Blackwell et al., "Radionuclide Transit Studies in the Detection of Oesophageal Dysmotility," *Gut* 24, no. 5 (1983): 421–426.
6. "Blue whales," NOAA, Alaska Fisheries Science Center, https://www.afsc.noaa.gov/nmml/education/cetaceans/blue.php.
7. A. Geliebter and S. A. Hashim, "Gastric Capacity in Normal, Obese, and Bulimic Women," *Physiology and Behavior* 74, no. 4–5 (2001): 743–746.
8. M. S. Levine et al., "Competitive Speed Eating: Truth and Consequences," *American Journal of Roentgenology* 189, no. 3 (2007): 681–686.
9. G. M. Edwards, "Case of Bulimia Nervosa Presenting with Acute, Fatal Abdominal Distension," *The Lancet* 1, no. 8432 (1985): 822–823.
10. A. Usui et al., "A Case Report of Postmortem Radiography of Acute, Fatal Abdominal Distension After Binge Eating," *American Journal of Forensic Medicine and Pathology* 37, no. 4 (2016): 223–226.
11. T. Maruyama, Y. Yoshioka, and S. Suzuki, "Abdominal Aortic Blood Flow Disturbance Due to Binge Eating," *Journal of Gastrointestinal Surgery* 22, no. 12 (2018): 2182–2183.
12. M. Elsharif et al., "Abdominal Aortic Occlusion and Vascular Compromise Secondary to Acute Gastric Dilatation in a Patient with Bulimia," *Annals of The Royal College of Surgeons of England* 96, no. 8 (2014): e15–e17.
13. T. L. Halton and F. B. Hu, "The Effects of High Protein Diets on Thermogenesis, Satiety and Weight Loss: A Critical Review," *Journal of the American College of Nutrition* 23, no. 5 (2004): 373–385.
14. E. B. Chang and P. S. Leung, "Gastric Physiology," in *The Gastrointestinal System: Gastrointestinal, Nutritional and Hepatobiliary Physiology*, ed. P. S. Leung (New York: Springer, 2014).
15. M. Hosseinpour and A. Behdad, "Evaluation of Small Bowel Measurement in Alive Patients," *Surgical and Radiologic Anatomy* 30, no. 8 (2008): 653–655.
16. H. F. Helander and L. Fändriks, "Surface Area of the Digestive Tract—Revisited," *Scandinavian Journal of Gastroenterology* 49, no. 6 (2014): 681–689.
17. E. B. Chang and P. S. Leung, "Pancreatic Physiology," in *The Gastrointestinal System: Gastrointestinal, Nutritional and Hepatobiliary Physiology*, ed. P. S. Leung (New York: Springer, 2014).
18. S. J. O'Keefe et al., "Short Bowel Syndrome and Intestinal Failure: Consensus Definitions and Overview," *Clinical Gastroenterology and Hepatology* 4, no. 1 (2006): 6–10.
19. M. D. Sitrin, "Absorption of Water-Soluble Vitamins and Minerals," in *The Gastrointestinal System: Gastrointestinal, Nutritional and Hepatobiliary Physiology*, ed. P. S. Leung (New York: Springer, 2014).

20. R. Bowen, "Absorption of Water and Electrolytes," VIVO Pathophysiology, http://www.vivo.colostate.edu /hbooks/pathphys/digestion/smallgut/absorb_water.html.
21. R. J. Maughan and J. B. Leiper, "Limitations to Fluid Replacement During Exercise," *Canadian Journal of Applied Physiology* 24, no. 2 (1999): 173–187.
22. E. B. Chang and P. S. Leung, "Gastrointestinal Motility," in *The Gastrointestinal System: Gastrointestinal, Nutritional and Hepatobiliary Physiology*, ed. P. S. Leung (New York: Springer, 2014).
23. S. M. K. H. Asl et al., "Determination of the Mean Daily Stool Weight, Frequency of Defecation and Bowel Transit Time: Assessment of 1000 Healthy Subjects," *Archives of Iranian Medicine* 3 (2000): 101–105.
24. J. H. Cummings et al., "Fecal Weight, Colon Cancer Risk, and Dietary Intake of Nonstarch Polysaccharides (Dietary Fiber)," *Gastroenterology* 103, no. 6 (1992): 1783–1789.
25. G. I. Sandle, "Salt and Water Absorption in the Human Colon: A Modern Appraisal," *Gut* 43, no. 2 (1998): 294–299.
26. R. Sender, S. Fuchs, and R. Milo, "Revised Estimates for the Number of Human and Bacteria Cells in the Body," *PLoS Biology* 14, no. 8 (2016): e1002533, https://doi.org/10.1371/journal.pbio.1002533.
27. G. T. Macfarlane and S. Macfarlane, "Bacteria, Colonic Fermentation, and Gastrointestinal Health," *Journal of AOAC International* 95, no. 1 (2012): 50–60.
28. D. Ríos-Covián et al., "Intestinal Short Chain Fatty Acids and Their Link with Diet and Human Health," *Frontiers in Microbiology* 7 (2016): 185, https://doi.org/10.3389/fmicb.2016.00185.
29. M. W. Bourassa et al., "Butyrate, Neuroepigenetics and the Gut Microbiome: Can a High Fiber Diet Improve Brain Health?" *Neuroscience Letters* 625 (2016): 56–63.
30. C. M. Mitchell et al., "Does Exercise Alter Gut Microbial Composition? A Systematic Review," *Medicine and Science in Sports and Exercise* 51, no. 1 (2019): 160–167.
31. *Encyclopedia Britannica*, s.v. "anal canal," July 20, 1998, https://www.britannica.com/science/anal-canal.
32. J. Fantozzi, "Foods You Eat Every Day Like Chocolate, Coffee, and Beer All Contain Thousands of Insect Bits," *Business Insider*, June 21, 2017, https://www.businessinsider.com/foods-full-of-insects-bugs-2017-6.
33. E. A. Mayer, "Gut Feelings: The Emerging Biology of Gut–Brain Communication," *Nature Reviews Neuroscience* 12, no. 8 (2011): 453–466.
34. M. B. Hansen, "The Enteric Nervous System I: Organisation and Classification," *Pharmacology and Toxicology* 92, no. 3 (2003): 105–113.
35. G. Roth and U. Dicke, "Evolution of the Brain and Intelligence," *Trends in Cognitive Sciences* 9, no. 5 (2005): 250–257.
36. M. Rao and M. D. Gershon, "The Bowel and Beyond: The Enteric Nervous System in Neurological Disorders," *Nature Reviews Gastroenterology and Hepatology* 13, no. 9 (2016): 517–528.
37. W. M. Bayliss and E. H. Starling, "The Movements and Innervation of the Small Intestine," *Journal of Physiology* 24, no. 2 (1899): 99–143.
38. A. J. Page, "Vagal Afferent Dysfunction in Obesity: Cause or Effect?" *Journal of Physiology* 594, no. 1 (2016): 5–6.
39. M. Klarer et al., "Gut Vagal Afferents Differentially Modulate Innate Anxiety and Learned Fear," *Journal of Neuroscience* 34, no. 21 (2014): 7067–7076.
40. L. Van Oudenhove et al., "Fatty Acid–Induced Gut-Brain Signaling Attenuates Neural and Behavioral Effects of Sad Emotion in Humans," *Journal of Clinical Investigation* 121, no. 8 (2011): 3094–3099.

Chapter 2

1. J. Aronson, "Nauseated/nauseous," *BMJ* 332, no. 7552 (2006): 1271.
2. M. D. Hoffman and K. Fogard, "Factors Related to Successful Completion of a 161-km Ultramarathon," *International Journal of Sports Physiology and Performance* 6, no. 1 (2011): 25–37.
3. N. J. Rehrer et al., "Fluid Intake and Gastrointestinal Problems in Runners Competing in a 25-km Race and a Marathon," *International Journal of Sports Medicine* 10, no. S1 (1989): S22–S25.
4. E. B. Keeffe et al., "Gastrointestinal Symptoms of Marathon Runners," *Western Journal of Medicine* 141, no. 4 (1984): 481–484.
5. P. B. Wilson, G. S. Rhodes, and S. J. Ingraham, "Saccharide Composition of Carbohydrates Consumed During an Ultra-endurance Triathlon," *Journal of the American College of Nutrition* 34, no. 6 (2015): 497–506.
6. R. Bowen, "Physiology of Vomiting," VIVO Pathophysiology, http://www.vivo.colostate.edu/hbooks /pathphys/digestion/stomach/vomiting.html.

7. M. Wada, M. Seo, and K. Abe, "Effect of Muscular Exercise upon the Epinephrine Secretion from the Suprarenal Gland," *Tohoku Journal of Experimental Medicine* 27, no. 1 (1935): 65–86.
8. E. W. Banister and J. Griffiths, "Blood Levels of Adrenergic Amines During Exercise," *Journal of Applied Physiology* 33, no. 5 (1972): 674–676.
9. E. Chong, K. J. Guelfi, and P. A. Fournier, "Effect of a Carbohydrate Mouth Rinse on Maximal Sprint Performance in Competitive Male Cyclists," *Journal of Science and Medicine in Sport* 14, no. 2 (2011): 162–167.
10. "Did You Know? Wayde van Niekerk," *Spikes*, World Athletics, May 4, 2016, https://spikes.iaaf.org/post/did-you-know-wayde-van-niekerk.
11. N. Lancefield, "Breaking World Record Has Mo Farah Sick to the Stomach," *Belfast Telegraph*, February 23, 2015, https://www.belfasttelegraph.co.uk/sport/othersports/breaking-world-record-has-mo-farah-sick-to-the-stomach-31012887.html.
12. J. McDermott, "Jim Ryun's Mile-High Mission," *Life Magazine*, October 11, 1968.
13. L. Carpenter, "Rio 2016: USA's Katie Ledecky Fights Off Exhaustion and Vomit for Second Gold," *Guardian*, August 9, 2016, https://www.theguardian.com/sport/2016/aug/09/rio-2016-katie-ledecky-swimming-gold-200m-freestyle.
14. J. Drayton, "'This Is What It Takes to Be No 1!' Bolt Posts Video of Himself Throwing Up After Training," *Mail Online*, January 3, 2014, https://www.dailymail.co.uk/sport/othersports/article-2533208/Usain-Bolt-posts-video-throwing-training.html.
15. G. H. Kamimori et al., "Catecholamine Levels in Hypoxia-Induced Acute Mountain Sickness," *Aviation, Space, and Environmental Medicine* 80, no. 4 (2009): 376–380.
16. A. M. Luks, E. R. Swenson, and P. Bärtsch, "Acute High-Altitude Sickness," *European Respiratory Review* 26, no. 143 (2017): 160096. https://doi.org/10.1183/16000617.0096-2016.
17. F. H. Maniyar et al., "The Origin of Nausea in Migraine–A PET Study," *Journal of Headache and Pain* 15, no. 1 (2014): 84, https://doi.org/10.1186/1129-2377-15-84.
18. J. Acosta, *The Natural and Moral History of the Indies*, ed. C. Markham, tran. E. Grimston (London: Hakluyt Society, 1880).
19. L. Bergeron et al., "Spinal Procaine With and Without Epinephrine and Its Relation to Transient Radicular Irritation," *Canadian Journal of Anesthesia* 46, no. 9 (1999): 846–849.
20. D. C. Campbell et al., "Addition of Epinephrine to Intrathecal Bupivacaine and Sufentanil for Ambulatory Labor Analgesia," *Anesthesiology: Journal of the American Society of Anesthesiologists* 86, no. 3 (1997): 525–531.
21. H. Heilborn et al., "Comparison of Subcutaneous Injection and High-Dose Inhalation of Epinephrine—Implications for Self-Treatment to Prevent Anaphylaxis," *Journal of Allergy and Clinical Immunology* 78, no. 6 (1986): 1174–1179.
22. K. S. King et al., "Exercise-Induced Nausea and Vomiting: Another Sign and Symptom of Pheochromocytoma and Paraganglioma," *Endocrine* 37, no. 3 (2010): 403–407.
23. J. M. Davis et al., "Effects of Ingesting 6% and 12% Glucose/Electrolyte Beverages During Prolonged Intermittent Cycling in the Heat," *European Journal of Applied Physiology and Occupational Physiology* 57, no. 5 (1988): 563–569.
24. C. Feinle, D. Grundy, and M. Fried, "Modulation of Gastric Distension-Induced Sensations by Small Intestinal Receptors," *American Journal of Physiology-Gastrointestinal and Liver Physiology* 280, no. 1 (2001): G51–G57.
25. G. P. Smith, "The Therapeutic Potential of Cholecystokinin," *International Journal of Obesity* 8 (1984): 35–38.
26. C. Feinle et al., "Fat Digestion Modulates Gastrointestinal Sensations Induced by Gastric Distention and Duodenal Lipid in Humans," *Gastroenterology* 120, no. 5 (2001): 1100–1107.
27. S. Himeno et al., "Plasma Cholecystokinin Responses After Ingestion of Liquid Meal and Intraduodenal Infusion of Fat, Amino Acids, or Hydrochloric Acid in Man: Analysis with Region Specific Radioimmunoassay," *American Journal of Gastroenterology* 78, no. 11 (1983): 703–707.
28. N. J. Rehrer et al., "Effect of Exercise on Portal Vein Blood Flow in Man," *Medicine and Science in Sports and Exercise* 33, no. 9 (2001): 1533–1537.
29. M. A. van Nieuwenhoven et al., "Effect of Dehydration on Gastrointestinal Function at Rest and During Exercise in Humans," *European Journal of Applied Physiology* 83, no. 6 (2000): 578–584.
30. A. Richardson, P. Watt, and N. Maxwell, "The Effect of Hypohydration Severity on the Physiological, Psychological and Renal Hormonal Responses to Hypoxic Exercise," *European Journal of Applied Physiology* 106, no. 1 (2009): 123–130.

31. N. J. Rehrer et al., "Effects of Dehydration on Gastric Emptying and Gastrointestinal Distress While Running," *Medicine and Science in Sports and Exercise* 22, no. 6 (1990): 790–795.
32. R. Snipe et al., "The Impact of Exertional-Heat Stress on Gastrointestinal Integrity, Gastrointestinal Symptoms, Systemic Endotoxin and Cytokine Profile," *European Journal of Applied Physiology* 118, no. 2 (2018): 389–400.
33. S. J. Montain et al., "Aldosterone and Vasopressin Responses in the Heat: Hydration Level and Exercise Intensity Effects," *Medicine and Science in Sports and Exercise* 29, no. 5 (1997): 661–668.
34. S. D. Caras et al., "The Effect of Intravenous Vasopressin on Gastric Myoelectrical Activity in Human Subjects," *Neurogastroenterology and Motility* 9, no. 3 (1997): 151–156.
35. M. S. Kim et al., "Role of Plasma Vasopressin as a Mediator of Nausea and Gastric Slow Wave Dysrhythmias in Motion Sickness," *American Journal of Physiology-Gastrointestinal and Liver Physiology* 272, no. 4 (1997): G853–G862.
36. K. J. Stuempfle et al., "Nausea Is Associated with Endotoxemia During a 161-km Ultramarathon," *Journal of Sports Sciences* 34, no. 17 (2016): 1662–1668.
37. J. G. Brock-Utne et al., "Endotoxaemia in Exhausted Runners After a Long-Distance Race," *South African Medical Journal* 73, no. 9 (1988): 533–536.
38. K. J. Van Zee et al., "Influence of IL-1 Receptor Blockade on the Human Response to Endotoxemia," *Journal of Immunology* 154, no. 3 (1995): 1499–1507.
39. A. Januszkiewicz et al., "Response of In Vivo Protein Synthesis in T Lymphocytes and Leucocytes to an Endotoxin Challenge in Healthy Volunteers," *Clinical and Experimental Immunology* 130, no. 2 (2002): 263–270.
40. A. Wegner et al., "Inflammation-Induced Pain Sensitization in Men and Women: Does Sex Matter in Experimental Endotoxemia?" *Pain* 156, no. 10 (2015): 1954–1964.
41. S. T. O'Dwyer et al., "A Single Dose of Endotoxin Increases Intestinal Permeability in Healthy Humans," *Archives of Surgery* 123, no. 12 (1988): 1459–1464.
42. R. Dantzer et al., "From Inflammation to Sickness and Depression: When the Immune System Subjugates the Brain," *Nature Reviews Neuroscience* 9, no. 1 (2008): 46–56.
43. M. Blick et al., "Phase I Study of Recombinant Tumor Necrosis Factor in Cancer Patients," *Cancer Research* 47, no. 11 (1987): 2986–2989.
44. W. G. Schucany, "Exercise-Associated Hyponatremia," *Baylor University Medical Center Proceedings* 20, no. 4 (2007): 398–401.
45. C. Almond et al., "Hyponatremia Among Runners in the Boston Marathon," *New England Journal of Medicine* 352, no. 15 (2005): 1550–1556.
46. E. F. Coyle et al., "Carbohydrate Feeding During Prolonged Strenuous Exercise Can Delay Fatigue," *Journal of Applied Physiology* 55, no. 1 (1983): 230–235.
47. P. Felig et al., "Hypoglycemia During Prolonged Exercise in Normal Men," *New England Journal of Medicine* 306, no. 15 (1982): 895–900.
48. S. M. Chernish and D. D. Maglinte, "Glucagon: Common Untoward Reactions—Review and Recommendations," *Radiology* 177, no. 1 (1990): 145–146.
49. D. Robertson et al., "Effects of Caffeine on Plasma Renin Activity, Catecholamines and Blood Pressure," *New England Journal of Medicine* 298, no. 4 (1978): 181–186.
50. J. M. Pequignot, L. Peyrin, and G. Peres, "Catecholamine-Fuel Interrelationships During Exercise in Fasting Men," *Journal of Applied Physiology* 48, no. 1 (1980): 109–113.
51. G. B. Kaplan et al., "Dose-Dependent Pharmacokinetics and Psychomotor Effects of Caffeine in Humans," *Journal of Clinical Pharmacology* 37, no. 8 (1997): 693–703.
52. D. G. Bell et al., "Effects of Caffeine, Ephedrine and Their Combination on Time to Exhaustion During High-Intensity Exercise," *European Journal of Applied Physiology and Occupational Physiology* 77, no. 5 (1998): 427–433.
53. D. G. Bell et al., "Reducing the Dose of Combined Caffeine and Ephedrine Preserves the Ergogenic Effect," *Aviation, Space, and Environmental Medicine* 71, no. 4 (2000): 415–419.
54. H. B. El-Serag et al., "Update on the Epidemiology of Gastro-Oesophageal Reflux Disease: A Systematic Review," *Gut* 63, no. 6 (2014): 871–880.
55. C. Riddoch and T. Trinick, "Gastrointestinal Disturbances in Marathon Runners," *British Journal of Sports Medicine* 22, no. 2 (1988): 71–74.
56. S. N. Sullivan, "Exercise-Associated Symptoms in Triathletes," *The Physician and Sportsmedicine* 15, no. 9 (1987): 105–108.

57. D. S. M. Ten Haaf et al., "Nutritional Indicators for Gastrointestinal Symptoms in Female Runners: The 'Marikenloop Study,'" *BMJ Open* 4, no. 8 (2014): e005780, https://doi.org/10.1136/bmjopen-2014-005780.
58. P. B. Wilson, "Dietary and Non-dietary Correlates of Gastrointestinal Distress During the Cycle and Run of a Triathlon," *European Journal of Sport Science* 16, no. 4 (2016): 448–454.
59. G. E. Boeckxstaens, "The Lower Oesophageal Sphincter," *Neurogastroenterology and Motility* 17 (2005): 13–21.
60. J. B. Wyman et al., "Control of Belching by the Lower Oesophageal Sphincter," *Gut* 31, no. 6 (1990): 639–646.
61. H. I. Kim et al., "Specific Movement of Esophagus During Transient Lower Esophageal Sphincter Relaxation in Gastroesophageal Reflux Disease," *Journal of Neurogastroenterology and Motility* 19, no. 3 (2013): 332–337.
62. E. E. Soffer et al., "Effect of Graded Exercise on Esophageal Motility and Gastroesophageal Reflux in Trained Athletes," *Digestive Diseases and Sciences* 38, no. 2 (1993): 220–224.
63. E. E. Soffer et al., "Effect of Graded Exercise on Esophageal Motility and Gastroesophageal Reflux in Nontrained Subjects," *Digestive Diseases and Sciences* 39, no. 1 (1994): 193–198.
64. E. P. de Oliveira and R. C. Burini, "The Impact of Physical Exercise on the Gastrointestinal Tract," *Current Opinion in Clinical Nutrition and Metabolic Care* 12, no. 5 (2009): 533–538.
65. C. S. Clark et al., "Gastroesophageal Reflux Induced by Exercise in Healthy Volunteers," *JAMA* 261, no. 24 (1989): 3599–3601.
66. K. L. Collings et al., "Esophageal Reflux in Conditioned Runners, Cyclists, and Weightlifters," *Medicine and Science in Sports and Exercise* 35, no. 5 (2003): 730–735.
67. E. A. Harman et al., "Intra-abdominal and Intra-thoracic Pressures During Lifting and Jumping," *Medicine and Science in Sports and Exercise* 20, no. 2 (1988): 195–201.
68. K. Iwakiri et al., "Relationship Between Postprandial Esophageal Acid Exposure and Meal Volume and Fat Content," *Digestive Diseases and Sciences* 41, no. 5 (1996): 926–930.
69. T. V. K. Herregods, A. J. Bredenoord, and A. J. Smout, "Pathophysiology of Gastroesophageal Reflux Disease: New Understanding in a New Era," *Neurogastroenterology and Motility* 27, no. 9 (2015): 1202–1213.
70. D. P. Morton, L. P. Aragón-Vargas, and R. Callister, "Effect of Ingested Fluid Composition on Exercise-Related Transient Abdominal Pain," *International Journal of Sport Nutrition and Exercise Metabolism* 14, no. 2 (2004): 197–208.
71. S. Sethi and J. E. Richter, "Diet and Gastroesophageal Reflux Disease: Role in Pathogenesis and Management," *Current Opinion in Gastroenterology* 33, no. 2 (2017): 107–111.
72. C. Newberry and K. Lynch, "Can We Use Diet to Effectively Treat Esophageal Disease? A Review of the Current Literature," *Current Gastroenterology Reports* 19, no. 8 (2017): 38, https://doi.org/10.1007/s11894-017-0578-5.
73. H. P. Peters et al., "The Effect of Omeprazole on Gastro-Oesophageal Reflux and Symptoms During Strenuous Exercise," *Alimentary Pharmacology and Therapeutics* 13, no. 8 (1999): 1015–1022.
74. B. B. Kraus, J. W. Sinclair, and D. O. Castell, "Gastroesophageal Reflux in Runners: Characteristics and Treatment," *Annals of Internal Medicine* 112, no. 6 (1990): 429–433.
75. C. H. Jansson et al., "Severe Gastro-Oesophageal Reflux Symptoms in Relation to Anxiety, Depression and Coping in a Population-Based Study," *Alimentary Pharmacology and Therapeutics* 26, no. 5 (2007): 683–691.
76. L. A. Bradley et al., "The Relationship Between Stress and Symptoms of Gastroesophageal Reflux: The Influence of Psychological Factors," *American Journal of Gastroenterology* 88, no. 1 (1993): 11–19.
77. J. McDonald-Haile et al., "Relaxation Training Reduces Symptom Reports and Acid Exposure in Patients with Gastroesophageal Reflux Disease," *Gastroenterology* 107, no. 1 (1994): 61–69.
78. A. J. Eherer et al., "Positive Effect of Abdominal Breathing Exercise on Gastroesophageal Reflux Disease: A Randomized, Controlled Study," *American Journal of Gastroenterology* 107, no. 3 (2012): 372–378.
79. M. S. Spetter et al., "The Sum of Its Parts—Effects of Gastric Distention, Nutrient Content and Sensory Stimulation on Brain Activation," *PLoS One* 9, no. 3 (2014): e90872, https://doi.org/10.1371/journal.pone.0090872.
80. B. J. Rolls et al., "Volume of Food Consumed Affects Satiety in Men," *American Journal of Clinical Nutrition* 67, no. 6 (1998): 1170–1177.
81. F. Azpiroz and J. R. Malagelada, "Abdominal Bloating," *Gastroenterology* 129, no. 3 (2005): 1060–1078.
82. P. Alonso-Coello et al., "Fiber for the Treatment of Hemorrhoids Complications: A Systematic Review and Meta-Analysis," *American Journal of Gastroenterology* 101, no. 1 (2006): 181–188.
83. R. Meier et al., "Influence of Age, Gender, Hormonal Status and Smoking Habits on Colonic Transit Time," *Neurogastroenterology and Motility* 7, no. 4 (1995): 235–238.

84. R. S. Sandler et al., "Abdominal Pain, Bloating, and Diarrhea in the United States," *Digestive Diseases and Sciences* 45, no. 6 (2000): 1166–1171.

85. A. J. Ryan, A. E. Navarre, and C. V. Gisolfi, "Consumption of Carbonated and Noncarbonated Sports Drinks During Prolonged Treadmill Exercise in the Heat," *International Journal of Sport Nutrition* 1, no. 3 (1991): 225–239.

86. J. J. Zachwieja et al., "The Effects of a Carbonated Carbohydrate Drink on Gastric Emptying, Gastrointestinal Distress, and Exercise Performance," *International Journal of Sport Nutrition* 2, no. 3 (1992): 239–250.

87. G. P. Lambert et al., "Effects of Carbonated and Noncarbonated Beverages at Specific Intervals During Treadmill Running in the Heat," *International Journal of Sport Nutrition* 3, no. 2 (1993): 177–193.

88. R. Cuomo et al., "Carbonated Beverages and Gastrointestinal System: Between Myth and Reality," *Nutrition, Metabolism and Cardiovascular Diseases* 19, no. 10 (2009): 683–689.

89. J. R. Malagelada, A. Accarino, and F. Azpiroz, "Bloating and Abdominal Distension: Old Misconceptions and Current Knowledge," *American Journal of Gastroenterology* 112, no. 8 (2017): 1221–1231.

90. B. McGann and C. McGann, *The Story of the Tour de France: How a Newspaper Promotion Became the Greatest Sporting Event in the World, Volume 1: 1903-1964* (Indianapolis: Dog Ear Publishing, 2006).

91. J. Cart, "Samuelson Hits Some Obstacles: Stomach Cramps, Collision Mark Return to Marathon," *Los Angeles Times*, November 7, 1988, http://articles.latimes.com/1988-11-07/sports/sp-213_1_stomach-cramps.

92. F. Bondy, "From Back of Pack, Kenyan Seizes Race," *New York Times*, April 20, 1993, https://www.nytimes.com/1993/04/20/sports/boston-marathon-from-back-of-pack-kenyan-seizes-race.html.

93. T. Odula, "Injured Mosop Out of Kenya's Olympic Marathon Team," *San Diego Tribune*, June 12, 2012, https://www.sandiegouniontribune.com/sdut-injured-mosop-out-of-kenyas-olympic-marathon-team-2012 jun12-story.html.

94. D. S. Rowlands et al., "Composite Versus Single Transportable Carbohydrate Solution Enhances Race and Laboratory Cycling Performance," *Applied Physiology, Nutrition, and Metabolism* 37, no. 3 (2012): 425–436.

95. M. C. E. Lomer, G. C. Parkes, and J. D. Sanderson, "Lactose Intolerance in Clinical Practice—Myths and Realities," *Alimentary Pharmacology and Therapeutics* 27, no. 2 (2008): 93–103.

96. W. J. Ravich, T. M. Bayless, and M. Thomas, "Fructose: Incomplete Intestinal Absorption in Humans," *Gastroenterology* 84, no. 1 (1983): 26–29.

97. W. L. Straus et al., "Do NSAIDs Cause Dyspepsia? A Meta-Analysis Evaluating Alternative Dyspepsia Definitions," *American Journal of Gastroenterology* 97, no. 8 (2002): 1951–1958.

98. M. Küster et al., "Consumption of Analgesics Before a Marathon and the Incidence of Cardiovascular, Gastrointestinal and Renal Problems: A Cohort Study," *BMJ Open* 3, no. 4 (2013): e002090, https://doi.org/10.1136/bmjopen-2012-002090.

99. D. Morton and R. Callister, "Characteristics and Etiology of Exercise-Related Transient Abdominal Pain," *Medicine and Science in Sports and Exercise* 32, no. 2 (2000): 432–438.

100. D. Morton and R. Callister, "Exercise-Related Transient Abdominal Pain (ETAP)," *Sports Medicine* 45, no. 1 (2015): 23–35.

101. R. Goldstein, "Johnny Miles, Upset Winner of the Boston Marathon, Dies at 97," *New York Times*, June 22, 2003, https://www.nytimes.com/2003/06/22/sports/johnny-miles-upset-winner-of-the-boston-marathon-dies-at -97.html.

102. C. V. Almario et al., "Old Farts—Fact or Fiction? Results from a Population-Based Survey of 16,000 Americans Examining the Association Between Age and Flatus," *Clinical Gastroenterology and Hepatology* 15, no. 8 (2017): 1308–1310.

103. G. Dunea, "The Gas We Pass," *BMJ* 329, no. 7471 (2004): 925.

104. C. D. Spivak, "Aerophagia and Flatulence," *Medical Record (1866-1922)* 67, no. 17 (1905): 649.

105. R. Dainese et al., "Effects of Physical Activity on Intestinal Gas Transit and Evacuation in Healthy Subjects," *American Journal of Medicine* 116, no. 8 (2004): 536–539.

106. A. Villoria et al., "Physical Activity and Intestinal Gas Clearance in Patients with Bloating," *American Journal of Gastroenterology* 101, no. 11 (2006): 2552–2557.

107. S. Kurbel, B. Kurbel, and A. Včev, "Intestinal Gases and Flatulence: Possible Causes of Occurrence," *Medical Hypotheses* 67, no. 2 (2006): 235–239.

108. J. Tomlin, C. Lowis, and N. W. Read, "Investigation of Normal Flatus Production in Healthy Volunteers," *Gut* 32, no. 6 (1991): 665–669.

109. S. Christodoulides et al., "Systematic Review with Meta-Analysis: Effect of Fibre Supplementation on Chronic Idiopathic Constipation in Adults," *Alimentary Pharmacology and Therapeutics* 44, no. 2 (2016): 103–116.

110. B. Pfeiffer et al., "Nutritional Intake and Gastrointestinal Problems During Competitive Endurance Events," *Medicine and Science in Sports and Exercise* 44, no. 2 (2012): 344–351.
111. Y. A. McKenzie et al., "British Dietetic Association Systematic Review of Systematic Reviews and Evidence-Based Practice Guidelines for the Use of Probiotics in the Management of Irritable Bowel Syndrome in Adults (2016 Update)," *Journal of Human Nutrition and Dietetics* 29, no. 5 (2016): 576–592.
112. M. Ortiz-Lucas et al., "Effect of Probiotic Species on Irritable Bowel Syndrome Symptoms: A Bring Up To Date Meta-Analysis," *Revista Espanola de Enfermedades Digestivas* 105, no. 1 (2013): 19–36.
113. N. P. West et al., "Lactobacillus Fermentum (PCC®) Supplementation and Gastrointestinal and Respiratory-Tract Illness Symptoms: A Randomised Control Trial in Athletes," *Nutrition Journal* 10 (2011): 30, https://doi.org/10.1186/1475-2891-10-30.
114. S. Doron and D. R. Snydman, "Risk and Safety of Probiotics," *Clinical Infectious Diseases* 60, no. S2 (2015): S129–S134.
115. M. D. Levitt et al., "Evaluation of an Extremely Flatulent Patient: Case Report and Proposed Diagnostic and Therapeutic Approach," *American Journal of Gastroenterology* 93, no. 11 (1998): 2276–2281.
116. F. L. Suarez, J. Springfield, and M. D. Levitt, "Identification of Gases Responsible for the Odour of Human Flatus and Evaluation of a Device Purported to Reduce This Odour," *Gut* 43, no. 1 (1998): 100–104.
117. F. Azpiroz and J. Serra, "Treatment of Excessive Intestinal Gas," *Current Treatment Options in Gastroenterology* 7, no. 4 (2004): 299–305.
118. D. Fleming, "Tao of Poo," *ESPN the Magazine*, April 10, 2013, http://www.espn.com/espn/news/story?page=Mag15taoofpoo.
119. B. P. Abraham and J. H. Sellin, "Drug-Induced Diarrhea," in *Diarrhea*, ed. S. Guandalini and H. Vaziri (Totowa, NJ: Humana Press, 2010).
120. R. L. Scharff, "Economic Burden from Health Losses Due to Foodborne Illness in the United States," *Journal of Food Protection* 75, no. 1 (2012): 123–131.
121. M. S. Riddle et al., "Guidelines for the Prevention and Treatment of Travelers' Diarrhea: A Graded Expert Panel Report," *Journal of Travel Medicine* 24, no. S1 (2017): S63–S80.
122. T. T. Haug, A. Mykletun, and A. A. Dahl, "Are Anxiety and Depression Related to Gastrointestinal Symptoms in the General Population?" *Scandinavian Journal of Gastroenterology* 37, no. 3 (2002): 294–298.
123. P. B. Wilson, "Perceived Life Stress and Anxiety Correlate with Chronic Gastrointestinal Symptoms in Runners," *Journal of Sports Sciences* 36, no. 15 (2018): 1713–1719.
124. W. J. Snape et al., "The Gastrocolic Response: Evidence for a Neural Mechanism," *Gastroenterology* 77, no. 6 (1979): 1235–1240.
125. H. F. Hammer et al., "Carbohydrate Malabsorption. Its Measurement and its Contribution to Diarrhea," *Journal of Clinical Investigation* 86, no. 6 (1990): 1936–1944.
126. L. S. Stephenson and M. C. Latham, "Lactose Intolerance and Milk Consumption: The Relation of Tolerance to Symptoms," *American Journal of Clinical Nutrition* 27, no. 3 (1974): 296–303.
127. Y. Deng et al., "Lactose Intolerance in Adults: Biological Mechanism and Dietary Management," *Nutrients* 7, no. 9 (2015): 8020–8035.
128. P. M. Christensen et al., "Caffeine and Bicarbonate for Speed. A Meta-Analysis of Legal Supplements Potential for Improving Intense Endurance Exercise Performance," *Frontiers in Physiology* 8 (2017): 240, https://doi.org/10.3389/fphys.2017.00240.
129. A. Hutchinson, "Does Baking Soda Boost Endurance? It's a Commonly Used Performance Enhancer, but It Has Some Limitations," *Runner's World*, August 22, 2017, https://www.runnersworld.com/sweat-science/does-baking-soda-boost-endurance.
130. P. D. Chilibeck et al., "Effects of Creatine and Resistance Training on Bone Health in Postmenopausal Women," *Medicine and Science in Sports and Exercise* 47, no. 8 (2015): 1587–1595.
131. K. Clarke et al., "Kinetics, Safety and Tolerability of (R)-3-Hydroxybutyl (R)-3-Hydroxybutyrate in Healthy Adult Subjects," *Regulatory Toxicology and Pharmacology* 63, no. 3 (2012): 401–408.
132. J. Y. Chang et al., "Impact of Functional Gastrointestinal Disorders on Survival in the Community," *American Journal of Gastroenterology* 105, no. 4 (2010): 822–832.
133. T. Sommers et al., "Emergency Department Burden of Constipation in the United States from 2006 to 2011," *American Journal of Gastroenterology* 110, no. 4 (2015): 572–579.
134. A. G. Klauser et al., "Behavioral Modification of Colonic Function," *Digestive Diseases and Sciences* 35, no. 10 (1990): 1271–1275.
135. H. C. Tjeerdsma, A. J. Smout, and L. M. Akkermans, "Voluntary Suppression of Defecation Delays Gastric Emptying," *Digestive Diseases and Sciences* 38, no. 5 (1993): 832–836.

136. J. E. Kellow, R. C. Gill, and D. L. Wingate, "Modulation of Human Upper Gastrointestinal Motility by Rectal Distension," *Gut* 28, no. 7 (1987): 864–868.

137. K. Krogh, G. Chiarioni, and W. Whitehead, "Management of Chronic Constipation in Adults," *United European Gastroenterology Journal* 5, no. 4 (2017): 465–472.

138. A. C. Ford et al., "American College of Gastroenterology Monograph on the Management of Irritable Bowel Syndrome and Chronic Idiopathic Constipation," *American Journal of Gastroenterology* 109, no. S1 (2014): S2–S26.

139. R. W. F. ter Steege and J. J. Kolkman, "The Pathophysiology and Management of Gastrointestinal Symptoms During Physical Exercise, and the Role of Splanchnic Blood Flow," *Alimentary Pharmacology and Therapeutics* 35, no. 5 (2012): 516–528.

140. S. M. Simons and R. G. Kennedy, "Gastrointestinal Problems in Runners," *Current Sports Medicine Reports* 3, no. 2 (2004): 112–116.

141. M. E. McCabe et al., "Gastrointestinal Blood Loss Associated with Running a Marathon," *Digestive Diseases and Sciences* 31, no. 11 (1986): 1229–1232.

142. F. A. Halvorsen, J. Lyng, and S. Ritland, "Gastrointestinal Bleeding in Marathon Runners," *Scandinavian Journal of Gastroenterology* 21, no. 4 (1986): 493–497.

143. R. S. Baska et al., "Gastrointestinal Bleeding During an Ultramarathon," *Digestive Diseases and Sciences* 35, no. 2 (1990): 276–279.

144. G. W. Ho, "Lower Gastrointestinal Distress in Endurance Athletes," *Current Sports Medicine Reports* 8, no. 2 (2009): 85–91.

145. J. D. Adams et al., "Gastrointestinal Bleeding Following a 161-km Cycling Race in the Heat: A Pilot Study," *Asian Journal of Sports Medicine* 9, no. 1 (2018): e60900, https://doi.org/10.5812/asjsm.60900.

146. E. P. de Oliveira, R. C. Burini, and A. Jeukendrup, "Gastrointestinal Complaints During Exercise: Prevalence, Etiology, and Nutritional Recommendations," *Sports Medicine* 44, no. 1 (2014): 79–85.

147. A. M. Porter, "Marathon Running and the Caecal Slap Syndrome," *British Journal of Sports Medicine* 16, no. 3 (1982): 178.

148. I. Alaunyte, V. Stojceska, and A. Plunkett, "Iron and the Female Athlete: A Review of Dietary Treatment Methods for Improving Iron Status and Exercise Performance," *Journal of the International Society of Sports Nutrition* 12 (2015): 38, https://doi.org/10.1186/s12970-015-0099-2.

149. B. T. Cooper et al., "Erosive Gastritis and Gastrointestinal Bleeding in a Female Runner: Prevention of the Bleeding and Healing of the Gastritis with H2-Receptor Antagonists," *Gastroenterology* 92, no. 6 (1987): 2019–2023.

150. W. Lucas and P. C. Schroy III, "Reversible Ischemic Colitis in a High Endurance Athlete," *American Journal of Gastroenterology* 93, no. 11 (1998): 2231–2234.

151. M. Thalmann et al., "Proton Pump Inhibition Prevents Gastrointestinal Bleeding in Ultramarathon Runners: A Randomised, Double Blinded, Placebo Controlled Study," *British Journal of Sports Medicine* 40, no. 4 (2006): 359–362.

152. N. J. Rehrer and G. A. Meijer, "Biomechanical Vibration of the Abdominal Region During Running and Bicycling," *Journal of Sports Medicine and Physical Fitness* 31, no. 2 (1991): 231–234.

153. R. M. McAllister, "Adaptations in Control of Blood Flow with Training: Splanchnic and Renal Blood Flows," *Medicine and Science in Sports and Exercise* 30, no. 3 (1998): 375–381.

154. R. D. Smetanka et al., "Intestinal Permeability in Runners in the 1996 Chicago Marathon," *International Journal of Sport Nutrition* 9, no. 4 (1999): 426–433.

155. R. W. F. ter Steege, J. Van Der Palen, and J. J. Kolkman, "Prevalence of Gastrointestinal Complaints in Runners Competing in a Long-Distance Run: An Internet-Based Observational Study in 1281 Subjects," *Scandinavian Journal of Gastroenterology* 43, no. 12 (2008): 1477–1482.

156. G. Tibblin et al., "Symptoms by Age and Sex: The Population Studies of Men and Women in Gothenburg, Sweden," *Scandinavian Journal of Primary Health Care* 8, no. 1 (1990): 9–17.

157. N. J. Talley et al., "Onset and Disappearance of Gastrointestinal Symptoms and Functional Gastrointestinal Disorders," *American Journal of Epidemiology* 136, no. 2 (1992): 165–177.

158. K. van Wijck et al., "Physiology and Pathophysiology of Splanchnic Hypoperfusion and Intestinal Injury During Exercise: Strategies for Evaluation and Prevention," *American Journal of Physiology-Gastrointestinal and Liver Physiology* 303, no. 2 (2012): G155–G168.

159. P. Bytzer et al., "Low Socioeconomic Class Is a Risk Factor for Upper and Lower Gastrointestinal Symptoms: A Population Based Study in 15 000 Australian Adults," *Gut* 49, no. 1 (2001): 66–72.
160. A. C. Ford et al., "Global Prevalence of, and Risk Factors for, Uninvestigated Dyspepsia: A Meta-Analysis," *Gut* 64, no. 7 (2015): 1049–1057.
161. A. J. Barsky, H. M. Peekna, and J. F. Borus, "Somatic Symptom Reporting in Women and Men," *Journal of General Internal Medicine* 16, no. 4 (2001): 266–275.
162. B. K. Diduch, "Gastrointestinal Conditions in the Female Athlete," *Clinics in Sports Medicine* 36, no. 4 (2017): 655–669.
163. B. Pfeiffer et al., "The Effect of Carbohydrate Gels on Gastrointestinal Tolerance During a 16-km Run," *International Journal of Sport Nutrition and Exercise Metabolism* 19, no. 5 (2009): 485–503.
164. P. B. F. Mensink et al., "Gastric Exercise Tonometry: The Key Investigation in Patients with Suspected Celiac Artery Compression Syndrome," *Journal of Vascular Surgery* 44, no. 2 (2006): 277–281.
165. B. V. Vaughn, S. Rotolo, and H. L. Roth, "Circadian Rhythm and Sleep Influences on Digestive Physiology and Disorders," *ChronoPhysiology Therapy* 4 (2014): 67–77.
166. A. Knutsson and H. Bøggild, "Gastrointestinal Disorders Among Shift Workers," *Scandinavian Journal of Work, Environment and Health* (2010): 85–95.
167. W. A. Hoogerwerf, "Role of Clock Genes in Gastrointestinal Motility," *American Journal of Physiology-Gastrointestinal and Liver Physiology* 299, no. 3 (2010): G549–G555.
168. R. Schey et al., "Sleep Deprivation Is Hyperalgesic in Patients with Gastroesophageal Reflux Disease," *Gastroenterology* 133, no. 6 (2007): 1787–1795.
169. M. Haack, E. Sanchez, and J. M. Mullington, "Elevated Inflammatory Markers in Response to Prolonged Sleep Restriction Are Associated with Increased Pain Experience in Healthy Volunteers," *Sleep* 30, no. 9 (2007): 1145–1152.

Chapter 3

1. S. Howell and R. Kones, "'Calories in, Calories out' and Macronutrient Intake: The Hope, Hype, and Science of Calories," *American Journal of Physiology-Endocrinology and Metabolism* 313, no. 5 (2017): E608–E612.
2. W. H. Saris et al., "Study on Food Intake and Energy Expenditure During Extreme Sustained Exercise: The Tour de France," *International Journal of Sports Medicine* 10, no. S1 (1989): S26–S31.
3. G. Plasqui et al., "Energy Expenditure During Extreme Endurance Exercise: The Giro d'Italia," *Medicine and Science in Sports and Exercise* 51, no. 3 (2019): 568–574.
4. J. K. Enqvist et al., "Energy Turnover During 24 Hours and 6 Days of Adventure Racing," *Journal of Sports Sciences* 28, no. 9 (2010): 947–955.
5. A. Drewnowski and S. E. Specter, "Poverty and Obesity: The Role of Energy Density and Energy Costs," *American Journal of Clinical Nutrition* 79, no. 1 (2004): 6–16.
6. P. M. Garcia-Roves et al., "Macronutrients Intake of Top Level Cyclists During Continuous Competition-Change in the Feeding Pattern," *International Journal of Sports Medicine* 19, no. 01 (1998): 61–67.
7. B. Corvilain et al., "Effect of Short-Term Starvation on Gastric Emptying in Humans: Relationship to Oral Glucose Tolerance," *American Journal of Physiology-Gastrointestinal and Liver Physiology* 269, no. 4 (1995): G512–G517.
8. E. S. Rome and S. Ammerman, "Medical Complications of Eating Disorders: An Update," *Journal of Adolescent Health* 33, no. 6 (2003): 418–426.
9. N. Kamal et al., "Delayed Gastrointestinal Transit Times in Anorexia Nervosa and Bulimia Nervosa," *Gastroenterology* 101, no. 5 (1991): 1320–1324.
10. A. B. Chun et al., "Colonic and Anorectal Function in Constipated Patients with Anorexia Nervosa," *American Journal of Gastroenterology* 92, no. 10 (1997): 1879–1883.
11. E. Joy, A. Kussman, and A. Nattiv, "2016 Update on Eating Disorders in Athletes: A Comprehensive Narrative Review with a Focus on Clinical Assessment and Management," *British Journal of Sports Medicine* 50, no. 3 (2016): 154–162.
12. H. Murakami et al., "Accuracy of Wearable Devices for Estimating Total Energy Expenditure: Comparison with Metabolic Chamber and Doubly Labeled Water Method," *JAMA Internal Medicine* 176, no. 5 (2016): 702–703.

Chapter 4

1. D. T. Thomas, K. A. Erdman, and L. M. Burke, "American College of Sports Medicine Joint Position Statement: Nutrition and Athletic Performance," *Medicine and Science in Sports and Exercise* 48, no. 3 (2016): 543–568.
2. M. C. Venables, J. Achten, and A. E. Jeukendrup, "Determinants of Fat Oxidation During Exercise in Healthy Men and Women: A Cross-Sectional Study," *Journal of Applied Physiology* 98, no. 1 (2005): 160–167.
3. T. Purdom et al., "Understanding the Factors That Effect Maximal Fat Oxidation," *Journal of the International Society of Sports Nutrition* 15 (2018): 3, https://doi.org/10.1186/s12970-018-0207-1.
4. J. Jeppesen and B. Kiens, "Regulation and Limitations to Fatty Acid Oxidation During Exercise," *Journal of Physiology* 590, no. 5 (2012): 1059–1068.
5. T. Fordyce, "Chris Froome: Team Sky's Unprecedented Release of Data Reveals How British Rider Won Giro d'Italia," *BBC Sport*, July 4, 2018, https://www.bbc.com/sport/cycling/44694122.
6. J. J. Wan et al., "Muscle Fatigue: General Understanding and Treatment," *Experimental and Molecular Medicine* 49, no. 10 (2017): e384, https://doi.org/10.1038/emm.2017.194.
7. D. J. Peart, "Quantifying the Effect of Carbohydrate Mouth Rinsing on Exercise Performance," *Journal of Strength and Conditioning Research* 31, no. 6 (2017): 1737–1743.
8. A. E. Jeukendrup and E. S. Chambers, "Oral Carbohydrate Sensing and Exercise Performance," *Current Opinion in Clinical Nutrition and Metabolic Care* 13, no. 4 (2010): 447–451.
9. E. S. Chambers, M. W. Bridge, and D. A. Jones, "Carbohydrate Sensing in the Human Mouth: Effects on Exercise Performance and Brain Activity," *Journal of Physiology* 587, no. 8 (2009): 1779–1794.
10. A. E. Jeukendrup, "Training the Gut for Athletes," *Sports Medicine* 47, no. 1 (2017): 101–110.
11. P. B. Wilson, "Multiple Transportable Carbohydrates During Exercise: Current Limitations and Directions for Future Research," *Journal of Strength and Conditioning Research* 29, no. 7 (2015): 2056–2070.
12. P. B. Wilson and S. J. Ingraham, "Glucose-Fructose Likely Improves Gastrointestinal Comfort and Endurance Running Performance Relative to Glucose-Only," *Scandinavian Journal of Medicine and Science in Sports* 25, no. 6 (2015): e613–e620.
13. M. Kelly, "Kipchoge's Berlin Nutrition Plan," *Canadian Running*, September 21, 2018, https://runningmagazine.ca/health-nutrition/kipchoges-berlin-nutrition-plan/.
14. G. E. Vist and R. J. Maughan, "The Effect of Osmolality and Carbohydrate Content on the Rate of Gastric Emptying of Liquids in Man," *Journal of Physiology* 486, no. 2 (1995): 523–531.
15. B. Pfeiffer et al., "Oxidation of Solid Versus Liquid CHO Sources During Exercise," *Medicine and Science in Sports and Exercise* 42, no. 11 (2010): 2030–2037.
16. M. Sareban et al., "Carbohydrate Intake in Form of Gel Is Associated with Increased Gastrointestinal Distress but Not with Performance Differences Compared with Liquid Carbohydrate Ingestion During Simulated Long-Distance Triathlon," *International Journal of Sport Nutrition and Exercise Metabolism* 26, no. 2 (2016): 114–122.
17. M. Guillochon and D. S. Rowlands, "Solid, Gel, and Liquid Carbohydrate Format Effects on Gut Comfort and Performance," *International Journal of Sport Nutrition and Exercise Metabolism* 27, no. 3 (2017): 247–254.
18. P. Pera et al., "Influence of Mastication on Gastric Emptying," *Journal of Dental Research* 81, no. 3 (2002): 179–181.
19. S. Holt et al., "Gastric Emptying of Solids in Man," *Gut* 23, no. 4 (1982): 292–296.
20. J. R. Malagelada, V. L. W. Go, and W. H. J. Summerskill, "Different Gastric, Pancreatic, and Biliary Responses to Solid-Liquid or Homogenized Meals," *Digestive Diseases and Sciences* 24, no. 2 (1979): 101–110.
21. S. Sutehall et al., "The Addition of a Sodium Alginate-Pectin Hydrogel to a Carbohydrate Beverage Significantly Enhances Gastric Emptying in Humans," (presentation, American College of Sports Medicine Conference, Orlando, FL, May 28, 2019), https://www.abstractsonline.com/pp8/#!/5776/presentation/8470.
22. A. McCubbin et al., "Hydrogel Carbohydrate-Electrolyte Beverage Does Not Improve Glucose Availability, Substrate Oxidation, Gastrointestinal Symptoms or Exercise Performance, Compared with a Concentration and Nutrient-Matched Placebo," *International Journal of Sport Nutrition and Exercise Metabolism* (2019): 1–9, https://doi.org/10.1123/ijsnem.2019-0090.
23. C. L. Lim and K. Suzuki, "Systemic Inflammation Mediates the Effects of Endotoxemia in the Mechanisms of Heat Stroke," *Biology and Medicine* 9, no. 376 (2017), https://doi.org/10.4172/0974-8369.1000376.

24. G. P. Lambert et al., "Fluid Restriction During Running Increases GI Permeability," *International Journal of Sports Medicine* 29, no. 3 (2008): 194–198.

25. R. M. J. Snipe et al., "Carbohydrate and Protein Intake During Exertional Heat Stress Ameliorates Intestinal Epithelial Injury and Small Intestine Permeability," *Applied Physiology, Nutrition, and Metabolism* 42, no. 12 (2017): 1283–1292.

26. G. P. Lambert et al., "Gastrointestinal Permeability During Exercise: Effects of Aspirin and Energy-Containing Beverages," *Journal of Applied Physiology* 90, no. 6 (2001): 2075–2080.

27. M. I. Qamar and A. E. Read, "Effects of Ingestion of Carbohydrate, Fat, Protein, and Water on the Mesenteric Blood Flow in Man," *Scandinavian Journal of Gastroenterology* 23, no. 1 (1988): 26–30.

28. H. M. Staudacher and K. Whelan, "The Low FODMAP Diet: Recent Advances in Understanding Its Mechanisms and Efficacy in IBS," *Gut* 66, no. 8 (2017): 1517–1527.

29. M. Wiffin et al., "Effect of a Short-Term Low Fermentable Oligosaccharide, Disaccharide, Monosaccharide and Polyol (FODMAP) Diet on Exercise-Related Gastrointestinal Symptoms," *Journal of the International Society of Sports Nutrition* 16 (2019): 1, doi:10.1186/s12970-019-0268-9.

30. D. Lis et al., "Low FODMAP: A Preliminary Strategy to Reduce Gastrointestinal Distress in Athletes," *Medicine and Science in Sports and Exercise* 50, no. 1 (2018): 116–123.

31. S. K. Gaskell et al., "Impact of 24-hour High and Low Fermentable Oligo- Di- Mono- Saccharide Polyol Diets on Markers of Exercise-Induced Gastrointestinal Syndrome in Response to Exertional-Heat Stress," *Applied Physiology, Nutrition, and Metabolism* (2019): https://doi.org/10.1139/apnm-2019-0187.

32. E. P. Halmos et al., "Diets That Differ in Their FODMAP Content Alter the Colonic Luminal Microenvironment," *Gut* 64, no. 1 (2015): 93–100.

33. W. J. Dahl and M. L. Stewart, "Position of the Academy of Nutrition and Dietetics: Health Implications of Dietary Fiber," *Journal of the Academy of Nutrition and Dietetics* 115, no. 11 (2015): 1861–1870.

34. K. N. Grooms et al., "Dietary Fiber Intake and Cardiometabolic Risks Among US Adults, NHANES 1999–2010," *American Journal of Medicine* 126, no. 12 (2013): 1059–1067.

35. J. L. Slavin, "Dietary Fiber and Body Weight," *Nutrition* 21, no. 3 (2005): 411–418.

36. J. P. Kirwan, D. O'Gorman, and W. J. Evans, "A Moderate Glycemic Meal Before Endurance Exercise Can Enhance Performance," *Journal of Applied Physiology* 84, no. 1 (1998): 53–59.

37. D. E. Thomas, J. R. Brotherhood, and J. C. Brand, "Carbohydrate Feeding Before Exercise: Effect of Glycemic Index," *International Journal of Sports Medicine* 12, no. 2 (1991): 180–186.

38. C. L. Wu and C. Williams, "A Low Glycemic Index Meal Before Exercise Improves Endurance Running Capacity in Men," *International Journal of Sport Nutrition and Exercise Metabolism* 16, no. 5 (2006): 510–527.

39. B. Glace, C. Murphy, and M. McHugh, "Food and Fluid Intake and Disturbances in Gastrointestinal and Mental Function During an Ultramarathon," *International Journal of Sport Nutrition and Exercise Metabolism* 12, no. 4 (2002): 414–427.

40. B. Pfeiffer et al., "Nutritional Intake and Gastrointestinal Problems During Competitive Endurance Events," *Medicine and Science in Sports and Exercise* 44, no. 2 (2012): 344–351.

41. J. de Vries et al., "Effects of Cereal, Fruit and Vegetable Fibers on Human Fecal Weight and Transit Time: A Comprehensive Review of Intervention Trials," *Nutrients* 8, no. 3 (2016): 130, https://doi.org/10.3390/nu8030130.

42. S. Christodoulides et al., "Systematic Review with Meta-Analysis: Effect of Fibre Supplementation on Chronic Idiopathic Constipation in Adults," *Alimentary Pharmacology and Therapeutics* 44, no. 2 (2016): 103–116.

43. P. Alonso-Coello et al., "Fiber for the Treatment of Hemorrhoids Complications: A Systematic Review and Meta-Analysis," *American Journal of Gastroenterology* 101, no. 1 (2006): 181–188.

44. C. Bonithon-Kopp et al., "Calcium and Fibre Supplementation in Prevention of Colorectal Adenoma Recurrence: A Randomised Intervention Trial," *The Lancet* 356, no. 9238 (2000): 1300–1306.

45. D. S. Alberts et al., "Lack of Effect of a High-Fiber Cereal Supplement on the Recurrence of Colorectal Adenomas," *New England Journal of Medicine* 342, no. 16 (2000): 1156–1162.

46. A. Schatzkin et al., "Lack of Effect of a Low-Fat, High-Fiber Diet on the Recurrence of Colorectal Adenomas," *New England Journal of Medicine* 342, no. 16 (2000): 1149–1155.

47. C. Hillemeier, "An Overview of the Effects of Dietary Fiber on Gastrointestinal Transit," *Pediatrics* 96, no. 5 (1995): 997–999.

Chapter 5

1. E. Cohen et al., "Statistical Review of US Macronutrient Consumption Data, 1965–2011: Americans Have Been Following Dietary Guidelines, Coincident with the Rise in Obesity," *Nutrition* 31, no. 5 (2015): 727–732.

2. B. Glace, C. Murphy, and M. McHugh, "Food and Fluid Intake and Disturbances in Gastrointestinal and Mental Function During an Ultramarathon," *International Journal of Sport Nutrition and Exercise Metabolism* 12, no. 4 (2002): 414–427.

3. N. J. Rehrer et al., "Gastrointestinal Complaints in Relation to Dietary Intake in Triathletes," *International Journal of Sport Nutrition* 2, no. 1 (1992): 48–59.

4. P. Satabin et al., "Metabolic and Hormonal Responses to Lipid and Carbohydrate Diets During Exercise in Man," *Medicine and Science in Sports and Exercise* 19, no. 3 (1987): 218–223.

5. A. E. Jeukendrup and S. Aldred, "Fat Supplementation, Health, and Endurance Performance," *Nutrition* 20, no. 7–8 (2004): 678–688.

6. D. S. Rowlands and W. G. Hopkins, "Effect of High-Fat, High-Carbohydrate, and High-Protein Meals on Metabolism and Performance During Endurance Cycling," *International Journal of Sport Nutrition and Exercise Metabolism* 12, no. 3 (2002): 318–335.

7. G. Okano et al., "Effect of 4h Preexercise High Carbohydrate and High Fat Meal Ingestion on Endurance Performance and Metabolism," *International Journal of Sports Medicine* 17, no. 7 (1996): 530–534.

8. H. A. Whitley et al., "Metabolic and Performance Responses During Endurance Exercise After High-Fat and High-Carbohydrate Meals," *Journal of Applied Physiology* 85, no. 2 (1998): 418–424.

9. M. B. Sidery, I. A. Macdonald, and P. E. Blackshaw, "Superior Mesenteric Artery Blood Flow and Gastric Emptying in Humans and the Differential Effects of High Fat and High Carbohydrate Meals," *Gut* 35, no. 2 (1994): 186–190.

10. L. M. Burke, "Re-examining High-Fat Diets for Sports Performance: Did We Call the 'Nail in the Coffin' Too Soon?" *Sports Medicine* 45, no. 1 (2015): 33–49.

11. L. M. Burke et al., "Low Carbohydrate, High Fat Diet Impairs Exercise Economy and Negates the Performance Benefit from Intensified Training in Elite Race Walkers," *Journal of Physiology* 595, no. 9 (2017): 2785–2807.

12. G. D. Brinkworth et al., "Comparative Effects of Very Low-Carbohydrate, High-Fat and High-Carbohydrate, Low-Fat Weight-Loss Diets on Bowel Habit and Faecal Short-Chain Fatty Acids and Bacterial Populations," *British Journal of Nutrition* 101, no. 10 (2009): 1493–1502.

13. D. Aune et al., "Fruit and Vegetable Intake and the Risk of Cardiovascular Disease, Total Cancer and All-Cause Mortality—A Systematic Review and Dose-Response Meta-Analysis of Prospective Studies," *International Journal of Epidemiology* 46, no. 3 (2017): 1029–1056.

14. J. N. Hunt and M. T. Knox, "A Relation Between the Chain Length of Fatty Acids and the Slowing of Gastric Emptying," *Journal of Physiology* 194, no. 2 (1968): 327–336.

15. T. J. Little, M. Horowitz, and C. Feinle-Bisset, "Modulation by High-Fat Diets of Gastrointestinal Function and Hormones Associated with the Regulation of Energy Intake: Implications for the Pathophysiology of Obesity," *American Journal of Clinical Nutrition* 86, no. 3 (2007): 531–541.

16. J. L. Ivy et al., "Contribution of Medium and Long Chain Triglyceride Intake to Energy Metabolism During Prolonged Exercise," *International Journal of Sports Medicine* 1, no. 1 (1980): 15–20.

17. J. H. Goedecke et al., "The Effects of Medium-Chain Triacylglycerol and Carbohydrate Ingestion on Ultra-Endurance Exercise Performance," *International Journal of Sport Nutrition and Exercise Metabolism* 15, no. 1 (2005): 15–27.

18. R. H. Eckel et al., "Dietary Substitution of Medium-Chain Triglycerides Improves Insulin-Mediated Glucose Metabolism in NIDDM Subjects," *Diabetes* 41, no. 5 (1992): 641–647.

19. T. J. Yost and R. H. Eckel, "Hypocaloric Feeding in Obese Women: Metabolic Effects of Medium-Chain Triglyceride Substitution," *American Journal of Clinical Nutrition* 49, no. 2 (1989): 326–330.

20. T. Ohnuma et al., "Benefits of Use, and Tolerance of, Medium-Chain Triglyceride Medical Food in the Management of Japanese Patients with Alzheimer's Disease: A Prospective, Open-Label Pilot Study," *Clinical Interventions in Aging* 11 (2016): 29–36.

Chapter 6

1. D. T. Thomas, K. A. Erdman, and L. M. Burke, "American College of Sports Medicine Joint Position Statement. Nutrition and Athletic Performance," *Medicine and Science in Sports and Exercise* 48, no. 3 (2016): 543–568.
2. H. L. Gentle et al., "A Randomised Trial of Pre-exercise Meal Composition on Performance and Muscle Damage in Well-Trained Basketball Players," *Journal of the International Society of Sports Nutrition* 11 (2014): 33, https://doi.org/10.1186/1550-2783-11-33.
3. E. C. Haakonssen et al., "Dairy-Based Preexercise Meal Does Not Affect Gut Comfort or Time-Trial Performance in Female Cyclists," *International Journal of Sport Nutrition and Exercise Metabolism* 24, no. 5 (2014): 553–558.
4. H. J. Leidy et al., "The Role of Protein in Weight Loss and Maintenance," *American Journal of Clinical Nutrition* 101, no. 6 (2015): 1320S–1329S.
5. Pera et al., "Influence of Mastication on Gastric Emptying," *Journal of Dental Research* 81, no. 3 (2002): 179–181.
6. K. J. Carpenter, "A Short History of Nutritional Science: Part 1 (1785–1885)," *Journal of Nutrition* 133, no. 3 (2003): 638–645.
7. K. J. Carpenter, "The History of Enthusiasm for Protein," *Journal of Nutrition* 116, no. 7 (1986): 1364–1370.
8. G. A. Brooks, "Amino Acid and Protein Metabolism During Exercise and Recovery," *Medicine and Science in Sports and Exercise* 19, no. S5 (1987): S150–S156.
9. T. M. McLellan, S. M. Pasiakos, and H. R. Lieberman, "Effects of Protein in Combination with Carbohydrate Supplements on Acute or Repeat Endurance Exercise Performance: A Systematic Review," *Sports Medicine* 44, no. 4 (2014): 535–550.
10. V. L. Fulgoni 3rd., "Current Protein Intake in America: Analysis of the National Health and Nutrition Examination Survey, 2003–2004," *American Journal of Clinical Nutrition* 87, no. 5 (2008): 1554S–1557S.
11. S. M. Phillips, S. Chevalier, and H. J. Leidy, "Protein 'Requirements' Beyond the RDA: Implications for Optimizing Health," *Applied Physiology, Nutrition, and Metabolism* 41, no. 5 (2016): 565–572.
12. S. Mettler, N. Mitchell, and K. D. Tipton, "Increased Protein Intake Reduces Lean Body Mass Loss During Weight Loss in Athletes," *Medicine and Science in Sports and Exercise* 42, no. 2 (2010): 326–337.
13. W. R. Russell et al., "High-Protein, Reduced-Carbohydrate Weight-Loss Diets Promote Metabolite Profiles Likely to Be Detrimental to Colonic Health," *American Journal of Clinical Nutrition* 93, no. 5 (2011): 1062–1072.
14. L. J. Appel et al., "Effects of Protein, Monounsaturated Fat, and Carbohydrate Intake on Blood Pressure and Serum Lipids: Results of the Omniheart Randomized Trial," *JAMA* 294, no. 19 (2005): 2455–2464.
15. W. S. Yancy et al., "A Low-Carbohydrate, Ketogenic Diet Versus a Low-Fat Diet to Treat Obesity and Hyperlipidemia: A Randomized, Controlled Trial," *Annals of Internal Medicine* 140, no. 10 (2004): 769–777.
16. J. J. Knapik et al., "Prevalence of Dietary Supplement Use by Athletes: Systematic Review and Meta-Analysis," *Sports Medicine* 46, no. 1 (2016): 103–123.
17. T. He and M. L. F. Giuseppin, "Slow and Fast Dietary Proteins Differentially Modulate Postprandial Metabolism," *International Journal of Food Sciences and Nutrition* 65, no. 3 (2014): 386–390.
18. J. R. Brooks et al., "Safety and Performance Benefits of Arginine Supplements for Military Personnel: A Systematic Review," *Nutrition Reviews* 74, no. 11 (2016): 708–721.
19. G. K. Grimble, "Adverse Gastrointestinal Effects of Arginine and Related Amino Acids," *Journal of Nutrition* 137, no. 6 (2007): 1693S–1701S.
20. R. R. Wolfe, "Branched-Chain Amino Acids and Muscle Protein Synthesis in Humans: Myth or Reality?" *Journal of the International Society of Sports Nutrition* 14, (2017): 30, https://doi.org/10.1186/s12970-017-0184-9.
21. L. Chen et al., "Efficacy and Safety of Oral Branched-Chain Amino Acid Supplementation in Patients Undergoing Interventions for Hepatocellular Carcinoma: A Meta-Analysis," *Nutrition Journal* 14, no. 1 (2015): 67, https://doi.org/10.1186/s12937-015-0056-6.
22. L. L. Gluud et al., "Oral Branched-Chain Amino Acids Have a Beneficial Effect on Manifestations of Hepatic Encephalopathy in a Systematic Review with Meta-Analyses of Randomized Controlled Trials," *Journal of Nutrition* 143, no. 8 (2013): 1263–1268.

Chapter 7

1. M. N. Sawka, S. N. Cheuvront, and R. Carter, "Human Water Needs," *Nutrition Reviews* 63, no. S1 (2005): S30–S39.
2. V. A. Convertino, "Blood Volume: Its Adaptation to Endurance Training," *Medicine and Science in Sports and Exercise* 23, no. 12 (1991): 1338–1348.
3. M. N. Sawka et al., "Thermoregulatory and Blood Responses During Exercise at Graded Hypohydration Levels," *Journal of Applied Physiology* 59, no. 5 (1985): 1394–1401.
4. P. D. Neufer, A. J. Young, and M. N. Sawka, "Gastric Emptying During Exercise: Effects of Heat Stress and Hypohydration," *European Journal of Applied Physiology and Occupational Physiology* 58, no. 4 (1989): 433–439.
5. V. A. Convertino et al., "American College of Sports Medicine Position Stand. Exercise and Fluid Replacement," *Medicine and Science in Sports and Exercise* 28, no. 1 (1996): i–vii.
6. D. J. Casa et al., "National Athletic Trainers' Association Position Statement: Fluid Replacement for Athletes," *Journal of Athletic Training* 35, no. 2 (2000): 212–224.
7. M. N. Sawka et al., "American College of Sports Medicine Position Stand. Exercise and Fluid Replacement," *Medicine and Science in Sports and Exercise* 39, no. 2 (2007): 377–390.
8. T. Hew-Butler, J. G. Verbalis, and T. D. Noakes, "Updated Fluid Recommendation: Position Statement from the International Marathon Medical Directors Association (IMMDA)," *Clinical Journal of Sport Medicine* 16, no. 4 (2006): 283–292.
9. E. D. Goulet, "Effect of Exercise-Induced Dehydration on Time-Trial Exercise Performance: A Meta-Analysis," *British Journal of Sports Medicine* 45, no. 14 (2011): 1149–1156.
10. E. D. Goulet, "Effect of Exercise-Induced Dehydration on Endurance Performance: Evaluating the Impact of Exercise Protocols on Outcomes Using a Meta-Analytic Procedure," *British Journal of Sports Medicine* 47, no. 11 (2013): 679–686.
11. E. D. Goulet and M. D. Hoffman, "Impact of Ad Libitum Versus Programmed Drinking on Endurance Performance: A Systematic Review with Meta-Analysis," *Sports Medicine* 49, no. 12 (2019): 221–232
12. J. B. Mitchell and K. W. Voss, "The Influence of Volume on Gastric Emptying and Fluid Balance During Prolonged Exercise," *Medicine and Science in Sports and Exercise* 23, no. 3 (1991): 314–319.
13. T. A. Robinson et al., "Water Ingestion Does Not Improve 1-h Cycling Performance in Moderate Ambient Temperatures," *European Journal of Applied Physiology and Occupational Physiology* 71, no. 2–3 (1995): 153–160.
14. H. N. Daries, T. D. Noakes, and S. C. Dennis, "Effect of Fluid Intake Volume on 2-h Running Performances in a 25 Degrees C Environment," *Medicine and Science in Sports and Exercise* 32, no. 10 (2000): 1783–1789.
15. T. Dion et al., "Half-Marathon Running Performance Is Not Improved by a Rate of Fluid Intake Above That Dictated by Thirst Sensation in Trained Distance Runners," *European Journal of Applied Physiology* 113, no. 12 (2013): 3011–3020.
16. I. Rollo et al., "The Effect of Carbohydrate-Electrolyte Beverage Drinking Strategy on 10-Mile Running Performance," *International Journal of Sport Nutrition and Exercise Metabolism* 22, no. 5 (2012): 338–346.
17. D. L. Costill and B. Saltin, "Factors Limiting Gastric Emptying During Rest and Exercise," *Journal of Applied Physiology* 37, no. 5 (1974): 679–683.
18. J. J. Holland et al., "The Influence of Drinking Fluid on Endurance Cycling Performance: A Meta-Analysis," *Sports Medicine* 47, no. 11 (2017): 2269–2284.
19. E. D. Goulet et al., "A Meta-Analysis of the Effects of Glycerol-Induced Hyperhydration on Fluid Retention and Endurance Performance," *International Journal of Sport Nutrition and Exercise Metabolism* 17, no. 4 (2007): 391–410.
20. K. Koehler, M. Thevis, and W. Schaenzer, "Meta-Analysis: Effects of Glycerol Administration on Plasma Volume, Haemoglobin, and Haematocrit," *Drug Testing and Analysis* 5, no. 11–12 (2013): 896–899.
21. S. P. van Rosendal et al., "Guidelines for Glycerol Use in Hyperhydration and Rehydration Associated with Exercise," *Sports Medicine* 40, no. 2 (2010): 113–139.
22. S. T. Sims et al., "Sodium Loading Aids Fluid Balance and Reduces Physiological Strain of Trained Men Exercising in the Heat," *Medicine and Science in Sports and Exercise* 39, no. 1 (2007): 123–130.
23. S. T. Sims et al., "Preexercise Sodium Loading Aids Fluid Balance and Endurance for Women Exercising in the Heat," *Journal of Applied Physiology* 103, no. 2 (2007): 534–541.
24. W. M. Sun et al., "Effect of Meal Temperature on Gastric Emptying of Liquids in Man," *Gut* 29, no. 3 (1988): 302–305.

25. J. K. Lee, S. M. Shirreffs, and R. J. Maughan, "Cold Drink Ingestion Improves Exercise Endurance Capacity in the Heat," *Medicine and Science in Sports and Exercise* 40, no. 9 (2008): 1637–1644.
26. X. Shi et al., "Gastric Emptying of Cold Beverages in Humans: Effect of Transportable Carbohydrates," *International Journal of Sport Nutrition and Exercise Metabolism* 10, no. 4 (2000): 394–403.
27. T. D. Noakes, N. J. Rehrer, and R. J. Maughan, "The Importance of Volume in Regulating Gastric Emptying," *Medicine and Science in Sports and Exercise* 23, no. 3 (1991): 307–313.

Chapter 8

1. I. J. Brown et al., "Salt Intakes Around the World: Implications for Public Health," *International Journal of Epidemiology* 38, no. 3 (2009): 791–813.
2. D. Mozaffarian et al., "Global Sodium Consumption and Death from Cardiovascular Causes," *New England Journal of Medicine* 371, no. 7 (2014): 624–634.
3. M. D. Hoffman and K. J. Stuempfle, "Is Sodium Supplementation Necessary to Avoid Dehydration During Prolonged Exercise in the Heat?" *Journal of Strength and Conditioning Research* 30, no. 3 (2016): 615–620.
4. T. D. Hew-Butler et al., "Sodium Supplementation Is Not Required to Maintain Serum Sodium Concentrations During an Ironman Triathlon," *British Journal of Sports Medicine* 40, no. 3 (2006): 255–259.
5. S. D. Cosgrove and K. E. Black, "Sodium Supplementation Has No Effect on Endurance Performance During a Cycling Time-Trial in Cool Conditions: A Randomised Cross-Over Trial," *Journal of the International Society of Sports Nutrition* 10 (2013): 30, https://doi.org/10.1186/1550-2783-10-30.
6. E. L. Earhart et al., "Effects of Oral Sodium Supplementation on Indices of Thermoregulation in Trained, Endurance Athletes," *Journal of Sports Science and Medicine* 14, no. 1 (2015): 172–178.
7. J. C. Del Coso et al., "Effects of Oral Salt Supplementation on Physical Performance During a Half-Ironman: A Randomized Controlled Trial," *Scandinavian Journal of Medicine and Science in Sports* 26, no. 2 (2016): 156–164.
8. J. R. Stofan et al., "Sweat and Sodium Losses in NCAA Football Players: A Precursor to Heat Cramps?" *International Journal of Sport Nutrition and Exercise Metabolism* 15, no. 6 (2005): 641–652.
9. P. Smith, "How Pickle Juice Changed the World of Sports: Food Innovations from the Football Field," *Good*, February 11, 2011, https://www.good.is/articles/how-pickle-juice-changed-the-world-of-sports-food-innovations-from-the-football-field.
10. K. C. Miller, K. L. Knight, and R. B. Williams, "Athletic Trainers' Perceptions of Pickle Juice's Effects on Exercise Associated Muscle Cramps," *Athletic Therapy Today* 13, no. 5 (2008): 31–34.
11. K. C. Miller et al., "Reflex Inhibition of Electrically Induced Muscle Cramps in Hypohydrated Humans," *Medicine and Science in Sports and Exercise* 42, no. 5 (2010): 953–961.
12. D. Alvarez-Berdugo et al., "Localization and Expression of TRPV1 And TRPA1 in the Human Oropharynx and Larynx," *Neurogastroenterology and Motility* 28, no. 1 (2016): 91–100.
13. M. Behringer et al., "Effects of TRPV1 and TRPA1 Activators on the Cramp Threshold Frequency: A Randomized, Double-Blind Placebo-Controlled Trial," *European Journal of Applied Physiology* 117, no. 8 (2017): 1641–1647.
14. D. H. Craighead et al., "Ingestion of Transient Receptor Potential Channel Agonists Attenuates Exercise-Induced Muscle Cramps," *Muscle and Nerve* 56, no. 3 (2017): 379–385.
15. J. N. Hunt and J. D. Pathak, "The Osmotic Effects of Some Simple Molecules and Ions on Gastric Emptying," *Journal of Physiology* 154, no. 2 (1960): 254–269.

Chapter 9

1. S. J. Colcombe et al., "Aerobic Exercise Training Increases Brain Volume in Aging Humans," *Journals of Gerontology Series A: Biological Sciences and Medical Sciences* 61, no. 11 (2006): 1166–1170.
2. K. I. Erickson et al., "Exercise Training Increases Size of Hippocampus and Improves Memory," *Proceedings of the National Academy of Sciences* 108, no. 7 (2011): 3017–3022.
3. R. Donaghey, "Kobayashi Taught Me to Be a Champion Hot Dog Eater," *Munchies*, July 3, 2015, https://munchies.vice.com/en_us/article/pgxvmy/kobayashi-taught-me-to-be-a-champion-hot-dog-eater.
4. M. J. Joyner and D. P. Casey, "Regulation of Increased Blood Flow (Hyperemia) to Muscles During Exercise: A Hierarchy of Competing Physiological Needs," *Physiological Reviews* 95, no. 2 (2015): 549–601.
5. N. J. Rehrer et al., "Effects of Dehydration on Gastric Emptying and Gastrointestinal Distress While Running," *Medicine and Science in Sports and Exercise* 22, no. 6 (1990): 790–795.

6. P. D. Neufer, A. J. Young, and M. N. Sawka, "Gastric Emptying During Exercise: Effects of Heat Stress and Hypohydration," *European Journal of Applied Physiology and Occupational Physiology* 58, no. 4 (1989): 433–439.

7. R. M. McAllister, "Adaptations in Control of Blood Flow with Training: Splanchnic and Renal Blood Flows," *Medicine and Science in Sports and Exercise* 30, no. 3 (1998): 375–381.

8. D. S. M. ten Haaf et al., "Nutritional Indicators for Gastrointestinal Symptoms in Female Runners: The 'Marikenloop Study,'" *BMJ Open* 4, no. 8 (2014): e005780, https://doi.org/10.1136/bmjopen-2014-005780.

9. R. W. ter Steege, J. Van Der Palen, and J. J. Kolkman, "Prevalence of Gastrointestinal Complaints in Runners Competing in a Long-Distance Run: An Internet-Based Observational Study in 1281 Subjects," *Scandinavian Journal of Gastroenterology* 43, no. 12 (2008): 1477–1482.

10. A. E. Jeukendrup, "Training the Gut for Athletes," *Sports Medicine* 47, no. S1 (2017): 101–110.

11. G. R. Cox et al., "Daily Training with High Carbohydrate Availability Increases Exogenous Carbohydrate Oxidation During Endurance Cycling," *Journal of Applied Physiology* 109, no. 1 (2010): 126–134.

12. R. J. S. Costa et al., "Gut-Training: The Impact of Two Weeks Repetitive Gut-Challenge During Exercise on Gastrointestinal Status, Glucose Availability, Fuel Kinetics, and Running Performance," *Applied Physiology, Nutrition, and Metabolism* 42, no. 5 (2017): 547–557.

13. K. M. Cunningham, M. Horowitz, and N. W. Read, "The Effect of Short-Term Dietary Supplementation with Glucose on Gastric Emptying in Humans," *British Journal of Nutrition* 65, no. 1 (1991): 15–19.

14. M. Horowitz et al., "The Effect of Short-Term Dietary Supplementation with Glucose on Gastric Emptying of Glucose and Fructose and Oral Glucose Tolerance in Normal Subjects," *Diabetologia* 39, no. 4 (1996): 481–486.

15. A. M. Yau et al., "Short-Term Dietary Supplementation with Fructose Accelerates Gastric Emptying of a Fructose but Not a Glucose Solution," *Nutrition* 30, no. 11–12 (2014): 1344–1348.

16. B. Corvilain et al., "Effect of Short-Term Starvation on Gastric Emptying in Humans: Relationship to Oral Glucose Tolerance," *American Journal of Physiology-Gastrointestinal and Liver Physiology* 269, no. 4 (1995): G512–G517.

17. P. H. Robinson, M. Clarke, and J. Barrett, "Determinants of Delayed Gastric Emptying in Anorexia Nervosa and Bulimia Nervosa," *Gut* 29, no. 4 (1988): 458–464.

18. M. Mountjoy et al., "The IOC Consensus Statement: Beyond the Female Athlete Triad—Relative Energy Deficiency in Sport (RED-S)," *British Journal of Sports Medicine* 48, no. 7 (2014): 491–497.

19. J. S. Volek, T. Noakes, and S. D. Phinney, "Rethinking Fat as a Fuel for Endurance Exercise," *European Journal of Sport Science* 15, no. 1 (2015): 13–20.

20. K. E. Castiglione, N. W. Read, and S. J. French, "Adaptation to High-Fat Diet Accelerates Emptying of Fat but Not Carbohydrate Test Meals in Humans," *American Journal of Physiology-Regulatory, Integrative and Comparative Physiology* 282, no. 2 (2002): R366–R371.

21. K. M. Cunningham et al., "Gastrointestinal Adaptation to Diets of Differing Fat Composition in Human Volunteers," *Gut* 32, no. 5 (1991): 483–486.

22. M. E. Clegg et al., "Gastrointestinal Transit, Post-Prandial Lipaemia and Satiety Following 3 Days High-Fat Diet in Men," *European Journal of Clinical Nutrition* 65, no. 2 (2011): 240–246.

23. M. E. Clegg and A. Shafat, "A High-Fat Diet Temporarily Accelerates Gastrointestinal Transit and Reduces Satiety in Men," *International Journal of Food Sciences and Nutrition* 62, no. 8 (2011): 857–864.

24. G. Shi et al., "Specific Adaptation of Gastric Emptying to Diets with Differing Protein Content in the Rat: Is Endogenous Cholecystokinin Implicated?" *Gut* 41, no. 5 (1997): 612–618.

25. V. Leray et al., "Adaptation to Low-Protein Diet Increases Inhibition of Gastric Emptying by CCK," *Peptides* 24, no. 12 (2003): 1929–1934.

26. D. T. Thomas, K. A. Erdman, and L. M. Burke, "American College of Sports Medicine Joint Position Statement. Nutrition and Athletic Performance," *Medicine and Science in Sports and Exercise* 48, no. 3 (2016): 543–568.

27. I. Rollo et al., "The Effect of Carbohydrate-Electrolyte Beverage Drinking Strategy on 10-Mile Running Performance," *International Journal of Sport Nutrition and Exercise Metabolism* 22, no. 5 (2012): 338–346.

28. T. Dion et al., "Half-Marathon Running Performance Is Not Improved by a Rate of Fluid Intake Above That Dictated by Thirst Sensation in Trained Distance Runners," *European Journal of Applied Physiology* 113, no. 12 (2013): 3011–3020.

29. G. P. Lambert et al., "Fluid Tolerance While Running: Effect of Repeated Trials," *International Journal of Sports Medicine* 29, no. 11 (2008): 878–882.

Chapter 10

1. E. D. Kantor et al., "Trends in Dietary Supplement Use Among US Adults from 1999-2012," *JAMA* 316, no. 14 (2016): 1464-1474.
2. P. A. Cohen, "Hazards of Hindsight—Monitoring the Safety of Nutritional Supplements," *New England Journal of Medicine* 370, no. 14 (2014): 1277-1280.
3. G. Skeie et al., "Use of Dietary Supplements in the European Prospective Investigation into Cancer and Nutrition Calibration Study," *European Journal of Clinical Nutrition* 63, no. S4 (2009): S226-S238.
4. S. M. Ock et al., "Dietary Supplement Use by South Korean Adults: Data from the National Complementary and Alternative Medicine Use Survey (NCAMUS) in 2006," *Nutrition Research and Practice* 4, no. 1 (2010): 69-74.
5. H. Yamashita, H. Tsukayama, and C. Sugishita, "Popularity of Complementary and Alternative Medicine in Japan: A Telephone Survey," *Complementary Therapies in Medicine* 10, no. 2 (2002): 84-93.
6. R. Bailey et al., "Why US Adults Use Dietary Supplements," *JAMA Internal Medicine* 173, no. 5 (2013): 355-361.
7. R. J. Maughan, "Quality Assurance Issues in the Use of Dietary Supplements, with Special Reference to Protein Supplements," *Journal of Nutrition* 143, no. 11 (2012): 1843S-1847S.
8. H. Geyer et al., "Analysis of Non-hormonal Nutritional Supplements for Anabolic-Androgenic Steroids-Results of an International Study," *International Journal of Sports Medicine* 25, no. 2 (2004): 124-129.
9. N. Zaccardi, "US Swimmer's Suspension Reduced from Two Years to Six Months," *NBC Sports*, September 3, 2018, https://olympics.nbcsports.com/2018/09/03/madisyn-cox-suspension-swimming/.
10. L. Carroll, "Many Multivitamins Don't Have Nutrients Claimed in Label," *NBC News*, June 20, 2011, http://www.nbcnews.com/id/43429680/ns/health-diet_and_nutrition/?ocid=twitter#.Wi1E-mfwm1A.
11. S. G. Newmaster et al., "DNA Barcoding Detects Contamination and Substitution in North American Herbal Products," *BMC Medicine* 11 (2013): 222, https://doi.org/10.1186/1741-7015-11-222.
12. A. O'Connor, "Herbal Supplements Are Often Not What They Seem," *New York Times*, November 3, 2013, http://www.nytimes.com/2013/11/05/science/herbal-supplements-are-often-not-what-they-seem.html.
13. A. O'Connor, "New York Attorney General Targets Supplements at Major Retailers," *New York Times*, February 3, 2015, https://well.blogs.nytimes.com/2015/02/03/new-york-attorney-general-targets-supplements-at-major-retailers/.
14. P. M. Ridker, "Fish Consumption, Fish Oils, and Cardiovascular Events: Still Waiting for Definitive Evidence," *American Journal of Clinical Nutrition* 104, no. 4 (2016): 951-952.
15. B. B. Albert et al., "Fish Oil Supplements in New Zealand Are Highly Oxidised and Do Not Meet Label Content of N-3 PUFA," *Scientific Reports* 5 (2015): 7928, https://doi.org/10.1038/srep07928.
16. B. L. Halvorsen and R. Blomhoff, "Determination of Lipid Oxidation Products in Vegetable Oils and Marine Omega-3 Supplements," *Food and Nutrition Research* 55, no. 1 (2011): 5792, https://doi.org/10.3402/fnr.v55i0.5792.
17. A. C. Kleiner, D. P. Cladis, and C. R. Santerre, "A Comparison of Actual Versus Stated Label Amounts of EPA and DHA in Commercial Omega-3 Dietary Supplements in the United States," *Journal of the Science of Food and Agriculture* 95, no. 6 (2015): 1260-1267.
18. A. I. Geller et al., "Emergency Department Visits for Adverse Events Related to Dietary Supplements," *New England Journal of Medicine* 373, no. 16 (2015): 1531-1540.
19. "Beware of Fraudulent Dietary Supplements," FDA, https://www.fda.gov/ForConsumers/ConsumerUpdates/ucm246744.htm.
20. D. Connolly, "Steve Bechler's Death Five Years Later," *The Baltimore Sun*, February 17, 2008, http://articles.baltimoresun.com/2008-02-17/sports/0802160233_1_steve-bechler-hailie-kiley.
21. P. A. Cohen et al., "Presence of Banned Drugs in Dietary Supplements Following FDA Recalls," *JAMA* 312, no. 16 (2014): 1691-1693.
22. A. R. Hoffmann et al., "The Microbiome: The Trillions of Microorganisms That Maintain Health and Cause Disease in Humans and Companion Animals," *Veterinary Pathology* 53, no. 1 (2016): 10-21.
23. C. Hill et al., "Expert Consensus Document: The International Scientific Association for Probiotics and Prebiotics Consensus Statement on the Scope and Appropriate Use of the Term Probiotic," *Nature Reviews Gastroenterology and Hepatology* 11, no. 8 (2014): 506-514.
24. G. T. Rijkers et al., "Guidance for Substantiating the Evidence for Beneficial Effects of Probiotics: Current Status and Recommendations for Future Research," *Journal of Nutrition* 140, no. 3 (2010): 671S-676S.
25. D. B. Pyne et al., "Probiotics Supplementation for Athletes-Clinical and Physiological Effects," *European Journal of Sport Science* 15, no. 1 (2015): 63-72.

26. R. Kekkonen et al., "The Effect of Probiotics on Respiratory Infections and Gastrointestinal Symptoms During Training in Marathon Runners," *International Journal of Sport Nutrition and Exercise Metabolism* 17, no. 4 (2007): 352–363.

27. J. N. Pugh et al., "Four Weeks of Probiotic Supplementation Reduces GI Symptoms During a Marathon Race," *European Journal of Applied Physiology* 119 (2019): 1491–1501, doi.org/10.1007/s00421-019-04136-3.

28. N. P. West et al., "Lactobacillus Fermentum (PCC®) Supplementation and Gastrointestinal and Respiratory-Tract Illness Symptoms: A Randomised Control Trial in Athletes," *Nutrition Journal* 10 (2011): 30, https://doi.org/10.1186/1475-2891-10-30.

29. C. N. Larsen et al., "Dose–Response Study of Probiotic Bacteria *Bifidobacterium Animalis* Subsp *Lactis* BB-12 and *Lactobacillus paracasei* Subsp *Paracasei* CRL-341 in Healthy Young Adults," *European Journal of Clinical Nutrition* 60, no. 11 (2006): 1284–1293.

30. K. R. Pandey, S. R. Naik, and B. V. Vakil, "Probiotics, Prebiotics and Synbiotics—a Review," *Journal of Food Science and Technology* 52, no. 12 (2015): 7577–7587.

31. M. Lamprecht et al., "Probiotic Supplementation Affects Markers of Intestinal Barrier, Oxidation, and Inflammation in Trained Men; A Randomized, Double-Blinded, Placebo-Controlled Trial," *Journal of the International Society of Sports Nutrition* 9 (2012): 45, https://doi.org/10.1186/1550-2783-9-45.

32. C. M. Shing et al., "Effects of Probiotics Supplementation on Gastrointestinal Permeability, Inflammation and Exercise Performance in the Heat," *European Journal of Applied Physiology* 114, no. 1 (2014): 93–103.

33. Q. Hao, B. R. Dong, and T. Wu, "Probiotics for Preventing Acute Upper Respiratory Tract Infections," *Cochrane Database of Systematic Reviews* no. 2 (2015): CD006895, https://doi.org/10.1002/14651858 .CD006895.pub3.

34. M. A. Ciorba, "A Gastroenterologist's Guide to Probiotics," *Clinical Gastroenterology and Hepatology* 10, no. 9 (2012): 960–968.

35. O. Ballard and A. L. Morrow, "Human Milk Composition: Nutrients and Bioactive Factors," *Pediatric Clinics of North America* 60, no. 1 (2013): 49–74.

36. A. W. Jones et al., "Bovine Colostrum Supplementation and Upper Respiratory Symptoms During Exercise Training: A Systematic Review and Meta-Analysis of Randomised Controlled Trials," *BMC Sports Science, Medicine and Rehabilitation* 8 (2016): 21, https://doi.org/10.1186/s13102-016-0047-8.

37. M. Rathe et al., "Clinical Applications of Bovine Colostrum Therapy: A Systematic Review," *Nutrition Reviews* 72, no. 4 (2014): 237–254.

38. T. Marchbank et al., "The Nutriceutical Bovine Colostrum Truncates the Increase in Gut Permeability Caused by Heavy Exercise in Athletes," *American Journal of Physiology-Gastrointestinal and Liver Physiology* 300, no. 3 (2010): G477–G484.

39. G. Davison et al., "Zinc Carnosine Works with Bovine Colostrum in Truncating Heavy Exercise–Induced Increase in Gut Permeability in Healthy Volunteers," *American Journal of Clinical Nutrition* 104, no. 2 (2016): 526–536.

40. M. Hałasa et al., "Oral Supplementation with Bovine Colostrum Decreases Intestinal Permeability and Stool Concentrations of Zonulin in Athletes," *Nutrients* 9, no. 4 (2017): 370, https://doi.org/10.3390 /nu9040370.

41. S. A. Morrison, S. S. Cheung, and J. D. Cotter, "Bovine Colostrum, Training Status, and Gastrointestinal Permeability During Exercise in the Heat: A Placebo-Controlled Double-Blind Study," *Applied Physiology, Nutrition, and Metabolism* 39, no. 9 (2014): 1070–1082.

42. Z. McKenna et al., "Bovine Colostrum Supplementation Does Not Affect Plasma I-FABP Concentrations Following Exercise in a Hot and Humid Environment," *European Journal of Applied Physiology* 117, no. 12 (2017): 2561–2567.

43. J. D. Buckley et al., "Bovine Colostrum Supplementation During Running Training Increases Intestinal Permeability," *Nutrients* 1, no. 2 (2009): 224–234.

44. L. Elfstrand et al., "Immunoglobulins, Growth Factors and Growth Hormone in Bovine Colostrum and the Effects of Processing," *International Dairy Journal* 12, no. 11 (2002): 879–887.

45. "Prohibited List," WADA, accessed December 17, 2017, https://www.wada-ama.org/en/questions-answers /prohibited-list.

46. R. Rao and G. Samak, "Role of Glutamine in Protection of Intestinal Epithelial Tight Junctions," *Journal of Epithelial Biology and Pharmacology* 5, no. S1-M7 (2012): 47–54.

47. D. E. Matthews, M. A. Marano, and R. G. Campbell, "Splanchnic Bed Utilization of Glutamine and Glutamic Acid in Humans," *American Journal of Physiology-Endocrinology and Metabolism* 264, no. 6 (1993): E848–E854.

48. M. Haisch, N. K. Fukagawa, and D. E. Matthews, "Oxidation of Glutamine by the Splanchnic Bed in Humans," *American Journal of Physiology-Endocrinology and Metabolism* 278, no. 4 (2000): E593–E602.

49. R. J. DeBerardinis and T. Cheng, "Q's Next: The Diverse Functions of Glutamine in Metabolism, Cell Biology and Cancer," *Oncogene* 29, no. 3 (2010): 313–324.

50. J. M. Williams et al., "Epithelial Cell Shedding and Barrier Function: A Matter of Life and Death at the Small Intestinal Villus Tip," *Veterinary Pathology* 52, no. 3 (2015): 445–455.

51. Q. H. Chen et al., "The Effect of Glutamine Therapy on Outcomes in Critically Ill Patients: A Meta-Analysis of Randomized Controlled Trials," *Critical Care* 18, no. 1 (2014): R8, https://doi.org/10.1186/cc13185.

52. N. P. Walsh et al., "Position Statement. Part Two: Maintaining Immune Health," *Exercise Immunology Review* 17 (2011): 64–103.

53. S. L. Bermon et al., "Consensus Statement Immunonutrition and Exercise," *Exercise Immunology Review* 23 (2017): 8–50.

54. J. N. Pugh et al., "Glutamine Supplementation Reduces Markers of Intestinal Permeability During Running in the Heat in a Dose-Dependent Manner," *European Journal of Applied Physiology* 117, no. 12 (2017): 2569–2577.

55. M. N. Zuhl et al., "Effects of Oral Glutamine Supplementation on Exercise-Induced Gastrointestinal Permeability and Tight Junction Protein Expression," *Journal of Applied Physiology* 116, no. 2 (2013): 183–191.

56. M. Zuhl et al., "The Effects of Acute Oral Glutamine Supplementation on Exercise-Induced Gastrointestinal Permeability and Heat Shock Protein Expression in Peripheral Blood Mononuclear Cells," *Cell Stress and Chaperones* 20, no. 1 (2015): 85–93.

57. R. C. Nava et al., "The Effect of Acute Glutamine Supplementation on Markers of Inflammation and Fatigue During Consecutive Days of Simulated Wildland Firefighting," *Journal of Occupational and Environmental Medicine* 61, no. 2 (2019): e33–e42.

58. G. P. Lambert et al., "Gastrointestinal Permeability During Exercise: Effects of Aspirin and Energy-Containing Beverages," *Journal of Applied Physiology* 90, no. 6 (2001): 2075–2080.

59. K. Van Wijck et al., "L-Citrulline Improves Splanchnic Perfusion and Reduces Gut Injury During Exercise," *Medicine and Science in Sports and Exercise* 46, no. 11 (2014): 2039–2046.

60. M. C. Szymanski et al., "Short-Term Dietary Curcumin Supplementation Reduces Gastrointestinal Barrier Damage and Physiological Strain Responses During Exertional Heat Stress," *Journal of Applied Physiology* 124, no. 2 (2017): 330–340.

61. A. M. Bode and Z. Dong, "The Amazing and Mighty Ginger," in *Herbal Medicine: Biomolecular and Clinical Aspects*, 2nd ed., ed. I. F. F. Benzie and S. Wachtel-Galor (Boca Raton, FL: CRC Press/Taylor and Francis, 2011), chap. 7.

62. B. H. Ali et al., "Some Phytochemical, Pharmacological and Toxicological Properties of Ginger (*Zingiber officinale* Roscoe): A Review of Recent Research," *Food and Chemical Toxicology* 46, no. 2 (2008): 409–420.

63. E. M. Bartels et al., "Efficacy and Safety of Ginger in Osteoarthritis Patients: A Meta-Analysis of Randomized Placebo-Controlled Trials," *Osteoarthritis and Cartilage* 23, no. 1 (2015): 13–21.

64. P. B. Wilson, "Ginger (*Zingiber officinale*) As an Analgesic and Ergogenic Aid in Sport: A Systemic Review," *Journal of Strength and Conditioning Research* 29, no. 10 (2015): 2980–2995.

65. W. Marx, N. Kiss, and L. Isenring, "Is Ginger Beneficial for Nausea and Vomiting? An Update of the Literature," *Current Opinion in Supportive and Palliative Care* 9, no. 2 (2015): 189–195.

66. M. D. Hoffman and K. Fogard, "Factors Related to Successful Completion of a 161-km Ultramarathon," *International Journal of Sports Physiology and Performance* 6, no. 1 (2011): 25–37.

67. M. N. Siddaraju and S. M. Dharmesh, "Inhibition of Gastric H+, K+-Atpase and Helicobacter Pylori Growth by Phenolic Antioxidants of *Zingiber officinale*," *Molecular Nutrition and Food Research* 51, no. 3 (2007): 324–332.

68. V. N. Drozdov et al., "Influence of a Specific Ginger Combination on Gastropathy Conditions in Patients with Osteoarthritis of the Knee or Hip," *Journal of Alternative and Complementary Medicine* 18, no. 6 (2012): 583–588.

69. L. L. Spriet, "Exercise and Sport Performance with Low Doses of Caffeine," *Sports Medicine* 44, no. 2 (2014): 175–184.

70. S. S. Rao et al., "Is Coffee a Colonic Stimulant?" *European Journal of Gastroenterology and Hepatology* 10, no. 2 (1998): 113–118.

71. M. Abo, "Effects of Caffeine on Gastrointestinal Myoelectric Activity and Colonic Spike Activity in Dogs," *Scandinavian Journal of Gastroenterology* 35, no. 4 (2000): 368–374.

72. P. B. Wilson, "Dietary and Non-dietary Correlates of Gastrointestinal Distress During the Cycle and Run of a Triathlon," *European Journal of Sport Science* 16, no. 4 (2016): 448–454.

73. P. M. Christensen et al., "Caffeine and Bicarbonate for Speed. A Meta-Analysis of Legal Supplements Potential for Improving Intense Endurance Exercise Performance," *Frontiers in Physiology* 8 (2017): 240, https://doi.org/10.3389/fphys.2017.00240.

74. S. L. Cameron, "Increased Blood Ph but Not Performance with Sodium Bicarbonate Supplementation in Elite Rugby Union Players," *International Journal of Sport Nutrition and Exercise Metabolism* 20, no. 4 (2010): 307–321.

75. A. J. Carr et al., "Effect of Sodium Bicarbonate On [HCO3-], pH, and Gastrointestinal Symptoms," *International Journal of Sport Nutrition and Exercise Metabolism* 21, no. 3 (2011): 189–194.

76. L. McNaughton et al., "Effects of Chronic Bicarbonate Ingestion on the Performance of High-Intensity Work," *European Journal of Applied Physiology and Occupational Physiology* 80, no. 4 (1999): 333–336.

77. L. McNaughton and D. Thompson, "Acute Versus Chronic Sodium Bicarbonate Ingestion and Anaerobic Work and Power Output," *Journal of Sports Medicine and Physical Fitness* 41, no. 4 (2001): 456–462.

78. A. H. Manninen, "Metabolic Effects of the Very-Low-Carbohydrate Diets: Misunderstood 'Villains' of Human Metabolism," *Journal of the International Society of Sports Nutrition* 1, no. 2 (2004): 7–11, https://doi.org/10.1186/1550-2783-1-2-7.

79. E. Brodwin and M. Robinson, "Scientists Think They've Discovered a Fourth Type of Fuel for Humans—Beyond Carbs, Fat, and Protein," *Business Insider*, November 8, 2017, http://www.businessinsider.com/ketones-fuel-athletic-performance-sports-2017-11.

80. M. Evans, K. E. Cogan, and B. Egan, "Metabolism of Ketone Bodies During Exercise and Training: Physiological Basis for Exogenous Supplementation," *Journal of Physiology* 595, no. 9 (2017): 2857–2871.

81. P. J. Pinckaers et al., "Ketone Bodies and Exercise Performance: The Next Magic Bullet or Merely Hype?" *Sports Medicine* 47, no. 3 (2017): 383–391.

82. T. O'Malley et al., "Nutritional Ketone Salts Increase Fat Oxidation but Impair High-Intensity Exercise Performance in Healthy Adult Males," *Applied Physiology, Nutrition, and Metabolism* 42, no. 10 (2017): 1031–1035.

83. J. J. Leckey et al., "Ketone Diester Ingestion Impairs Time-Trial Performance in Professional Cyclists," *Frontiers in Physiology* 8 (2017): 806, https://doi.org/10.3389/fphys.2017.00806.

84. K. Clarke et al., "Kinetics, Safety and Tolerability of (R)-3-Hydroxybutyl (R)-3-Hydroxybutyrate in Healthy Adult Subjects," *Regulatory Toxicology and Pharmacology* 63, no. 3 (2012): 401–408.

Chapter 11

1. B. Plaschke, "While Playing in the Biggest Game of His Life Eagles Guard Brandon Brooks Will Also Take On His Anxiety Disorder," *Los Angeles Times*, February 2, 2018, http://www.latimes.com/sports/la-sp-super-bowl-anxiety-plaschke-20180202-story.html.

2. "Bill Russell Tosses His Cookies," New England Historical Society, http://www.newenglandhistoricalsociety.com/bill-russell-tosses-cookies/.

3. E. Branch, "In a New Book, Ex-49er Steve Young Details His Battle with Anxiety," *San Francisco Chronicle*, October 28, 2016, https://www.sfchronicle.com/49ers/article/In-new-book-ex-49er-Steve-Young-details-his-10421195.php.

4. G. Fink, "Stress: Concepts, Definition and History," in *Reference Module in Neuroscience and Biobehavioral Psychology*, ed. J. Stein (Amsterdam: Elsevier, 2017).

5. H. Selye, *Stress in Health and Disease* (Oxford: Butterworth-Heinemann, 1976), 15.

6. J. Booth et al., "Evidence of Perceived Psychosocial Stress as a Risk Factor for Stroke in Adults: A Meta-Analysis," *BMC Neurology* 15 (2015): 233, https://doi.org/10.1186/s12883-015-0456-4.

7. S. J. Kelly and M. Ismail, "Stress and Type 2 Diabetes: A Review of How Stress Contributes to the Development of Type 2 Diabetes," *Annual Review of Public Health* 36 (2015): 441–462.

8. N. Bergmann, F. Gyntelberg, and J. Faber, "The Appraisal of Chronic Stress and the Development of the Metabolic Syndrome: A Systematic Review of Prospective Cohort Studies," *Endocrine Connections* 3, no. 2 (2014): R55–R80.

9. A. Junge, "The Influence of Psychological Factors on Sports Injuries. Review of the Literature," *American Journal of Sports Medicine* 28, no. 5 supplement (2000): 10–15.

10. American College of Sports Medicine et al., "Psychological Issues Related to Injury in Athletes and the Team Physician: A Consensus Statement," *Medicine and Science in Sports and Exercise* 38, no. 11 (2006): 2030–2034.

11. C. M. Janelle and B. D. Hatfield, "Visual Attention and Brain Processes That Underlie Expert Performance: Implications for Sport and Military Psychology," *Military Psychology* 20, no. S1 (2008): S39–S69.

12. C. Berglund, "Cortisol: Why the 'Stress Hormone' Is Public Enemy No. 1: 5 Simple Ways to Lower Your Cortisol Levels Without Drugs," *Psychology Today*, January 22, 2013, https://www.psychologytoday.com /us/blog/the-athletes-way/201301/cortisol-why-the-stress-hormone-is-public-enemy-no-1.

13. S. M. Staufenbiel et al., "Hair Cortisol, Stress Exposure, and Mental Health in Humans: A Systematic Review," *Psychoneuroendocrinology* 38, no. 8 (2013): 1220–1235.

14. A. Lehrner, N. Daskalakis, and R. Yehuda, "Cortisol and the Hypothalamic–Pituitary–Adrenal Axis in PTSD," in *Posttraumatic Stress Disorder: From Neurobiology to Treatment*, ed. J. D. Bremner (Hoboken, NJ: John Wiley and Sons, 2016).

15. H. Singh and D. E. Conroy, "Systematic Review of Stress-Related Injury Vulnerability in Athletic and Occupational Contexts," *Psychology of Sport and Exercise* 33 (2017): 37–44.

16. R. H. Rahe, "Life-Change Measurement as a Predictor of Illness," *Proceedings of the Royal Society of Medicine* 61, no. 11 (1968): 1124–1126.

17. R. H. Rahe and R. J. Arthur, "Life-Change Patterns Surrounding Illness Experience," *Journal of Psychosomatic Research* 11, no. 4 (1968): 341–345.

18. S. C. Segerstrom and G. E. Miller, "Psychological Stress and the Human Immune System: A Meta-Analytic Study of 30 Years of Inquiry," *Psychological Bulletin* 130, no. 4 (2004): 601–630.

19. F. S. Dhabhar, "Effects of Stress on Immune Function: The Good, the Bad, and the Beautiful," *Immunologic Research* 58, no. 2–3 (2014): 193–210.

20. P. T. Marucha, J. K. Kiecolt-Glaser, and M. Favagehi, "Mucosal Wound Healing Is Impaired by Examination Stress," *Psychosomatic Medicine* 60, no. 3 (1998): 362–365.

21. J. Walburn et al., "Psychological Stress and Wound Healing in Humans: A Systematic Review and Meta-Analysis," *Journal of Psychosomatic Research* 67, no. 3 (2009): 253–271.

22. B. Linde et al., "Adipose Tissue and Skeletal Muscle Blood Flow During Mental Stress," *American Journal of Physiology* 256, no. 1 Part 1 (1989): E12–E18.

23. C. D. Murray et al., "Effect of Acute Physical and Psychological Stress on Gut Autonomic Innervation in Irritable Bowel Syndrome," *Gastroenterology* 127, no. 6 (2004): 1695–1703.

24. N. Hayashi et al., "Vasoconstriction and Blood Flow Responses in Visceral Arteries to Mental Task in Humans," *Experimental Physiology* 91, no. 1 (2006): 215–220.

25. T. Ghose, "Man with Hole in Stomach Revolutionized Medicine," LiveScience, April 24, 2013, https://www .livescience.com/28996-hole-in-stomach-revealed-digestion.html.

26. W. Beaumont, *Experiments and Observations on the Gastric Juice and the Physiology of Digestion* (Edinburgh: Maclachlan and Stewart, 1838).

27. S. Wolf, "The Psyche and the Stomach: A Historical Vignette," *Gastroenterology* 80, no. 3 (1981): 605–614.

28. Y. Taché et al., "III. Stress-Related Alterations of Gut Motor Function: Role of Brain Corticotropin-Releasing Factor Receptors," *American Journal of Physiology-Gastrointestinal and Liver Physiology* 280, no. 2 (2001): G173–G177.

29. W. B. Cannon, "The Effect of the Emotions on Digestion," in *Bodily Changes in Pain, Hunger, Fear, and Rage: An Account of Recent Researches into the Function of Emotional Excitement* (New York: D. Appleton and Company, 1916).

30. W. B. Cannon and D. de la Paz., "Emotional Stimulation of Adrenal Secretion," *American Journal of Physiology -Legacy Content* 28, no. 1 (1911): 64–70.

31. T. P. Almy et al., "Alterations in Colonic Function in Man Under Stress: III. Experimental Production of Sigmoid Spasm in Patients with Spastic Constipation," *Gastroenterology* 12, no. 3 (1949): 437–449.

32. T. P. Almy, F. Kern, and M. Tulin, "Alterations in Colonic Function in Man Under Stress: II. Experimental Production of Sigmoid Spasm in Healthy Persons," *Gastroenterology* 12, no. 3 (1949): 425–436.

33. M. J. Ford et al., "Psychosensory Modulation of Colonic Sensation in the Human Transverse and Sigmoid Colon," *Gastroenterology* 109, no. 6 (1995): 1772–1780.

34. P. Welgan, H. Meshkinpour, and M. Beeler, "Effect of Anger on Colon Motor and Myoelectric Activity in Irritable Bowel Syndrome," *Gastroenterology* 94, no. 5 (1988): 1150–1156.

35. C. S. Hall, "Emotional Behavior in the Rat. I. Defecation and Urination as Measures of Individual Differences in Emotionality," *Journal of Comparative Psychology* 18, no. 3 (1934): 385–403.

36. Y. Taché and B. Bonaz, "Corticotropin-Releasing Factor Receptors and Stress-Related Alterations of Gut Motor Function," *Journal of Clinical Investigation* 117, no. 1 (2007): 33–40.
37. A.J. Dunn and C. W. Berridge, "Physiological and Behavioral Responses to Corticotropin-Releasing Factor Administration: Is CRF a Mediator of Anxiety or Stress Responses?" *Brain Research Reviews* 15, no. 2 (1990): 71–100.
38. D. Grossman and B. Siddle, "Psychological Effects of Combat," in *Encyclopedia of Violence, Peace, and Conflict*, 2nd ed., ed. L. Kurtz (San Diego, CA: Academic Press, 2008).
39. N. Rohleder et al., "Psychosocial Stress-Induced Activation of Salivary Alpha-Amylase: An Indicator of Sympathetic Activity?" *Annals of the New York Academy of Sciences* 1032, no. 1 (2004): 258–263.
40. A. Ferrauti et al., "Urine Catecholamine Concentrations and Psychophysical Stress in Elite Tennis Under Practice and Tournament Conditions," *Journal of Sports Medicine and Physical Fitness* 41, no. 2 (2001): 269–274.
41. G. P. Lambert, "Stress-Induced Gastrointestinal Barrier Dysfunction and Its Inflammatory Effects," *Journal of Animal Science* 87, no. supplement 14 (2009): E101–E108.
42. A. A. Siddiqui and P. B. Miner, "The Role of Mast Cells in Common Gastrointestinal Diseases," *Current Allergy and Asthma Reports* 4, no. 1 (2004): 47–54.
43. T. Vanuytsel et al., "Psychological Stress and Corticotropin-Releasing Hormone Increase Intestinal Permeability in Humans by a Mast Cell-Dependent Mechanism," *Gut* 63, no. 8 (2014): 1293–1299.
44. American Psychiatric Association, *Diagnostic and Statistical Manual of Mental Disorders*, 5th ed. (Washington, DC: American Psychiatric Association, 2013), 829, 818.
45. D. F. Grös et al., "Psychometric Properties of the State-Trait Inventory for Cognitive and Somatic Anxiety (STICSA): Comparison to the State-Trait Anxiety Inventory (STAI)," *Psychological Assessment* 19, no. 4 (2007): 369–381.
46. B. Geeraerts et al., "Influence of Experimentally Induced Anxiety on Gastric Sensorimotor Function in Humans," *Gastroenterology* 129, no. 5 (2005): 1437–1444.
47. B. Geeraerts et al., "Influence of Experimentally Induced Anxiety on Rectal Sensorimotor Function in Healthy Humans," *Neurogastroenterology and Motility* 20, no. 11 (2008): 1227–1233.

Chapter 12

1. E. R. Muth, "Motion and Space Sickness: Intestinal and Autonomic Correlates," *Autonomic Neuroscience* 129, no. 1–2 (2006): 58–66.
2. P. J. Gianaros et al., "Relationship Between Temporal Changes in Cardiac Parasympathetic Activity and Motion Sickness Severity," *Psychophysiology* 40, no. 1 (2003): 39–44.
3. R. Jerath et al., "Physiology of Long Pranayamic Breathing: Neural Respiratory Elements May Provide a Mechanism That Explains How Slow Deep Breathing Shifts the Autonomic Nervous System," *Medical Hypotheses* 67, no. 3 (2006): 566–571.
4. M. D. Jokerst et al., "Slow Deep Breathing Prevents the Development of Tachygastria and Symptoms of Motion Sickness," *Aviation, Space, and Environmental Medicine* 70, no. 12 (1999): 1189–1192.
5. M. E. Russell et al., "Use of Controlled Diaphragmatic Breathing for the Management of Motion Sickness in a Virtual Reality Environment," *Applied Psychophysiology and Biofeedback* 39, no. 3–4 (2014): 269–277.
6. S. E. Stromberg, M. E. Russell, and C. R. Carlson, "Diaphragmatic Breathing and Its Effectiveness for the Management of Motion Sickness," *Aerospace Medicine and Human Performance* 86, no. 5 (2015): 452–457.
7. B. Plaschke, "While Playing in the Biggest Game of His Life Eagles Guard Brandon Brooks Will Also Take On His Anxiety Disorder," February 2, 2018, http://www.latimes.com/sports/la-sp-super-bowl-anxiety -plaschke-20180202-story.html.
8. V. Stanghellini et al., "Gastroduodenal Disorders," *Gastroenterology* 150, no. 6 (2016): 1380–1392.
9. S. Mahadeva and K. Goh, "Epidemiology of Functional Dyspepsia: A Global Perspective," *World Journal of Gastroenterology* 12, no. 17 (2006): 2661–2666.
10. J. Tack, R. Bisschops, and G. Sarnelli, "Pathophysiology and Treatment of Functional Dyspepsia," *Gastroenterology* 127, no. 4 (2004): 1239–1255.
11. I. E. Hjelland et al., "Breathing Exercises with Vagal Biofeedback May Benefit Patients with Functional Dyspepsia," *Scandinavian Journal of Gastroenterology* 42, no. 9 (2007): 1054–1062.
12. L. A. Martínez-Martínez et al., "Sympathetic Nervous System Dysfunction in Fibromyalgia, Chronic Fatigue Syndrome, Irritable Bowel Syndrome, and Interstitial Cystitis: A Review of Case-Control Studies," *Journal of Clinical Rheumatology* 20, no. 3 (2014): 146–150.

13. S. G. Hofmann et al., "The Effect of Mindfulness-Based Therapy on Anxiety and Depression: A Meta-Analytic Review," *Journal of Consulting and Clinical Psychology* 78, no. 2 (2010): 169-183.
14. S. K. Singh and K. M. Gorey, "Relative Effectiveness of Mindfulness and Cognitive Behavioral Interventions for Anxiety Disorders: Meta-Analytic Review," *Social Work in Mental Health* 16, no. 2 (2018): 238-251.
15. J. Gu et al., "How Do Mindfulness-Based Cognitive Therapy and Mindfulness-Based Stress Reduction Improve Mental Health and Wellbeing? A Systematic Review and Meta-Analysis of Mediation Studies," *Clinical Psychology Review* 37 (2015): 1-12.
16. B. Ditto, M. Eclache, and N. Goldman, "Short-Term Autonomic and Cardiovascular Effects of Mindfulness Body Scan Meditation," *Annals of Behavioral Medicine* 32, no. 3 (2006): 227-234.
17. M. A. Braeken et al., "Potential Benefits of Mindfulness During Pregnancy on Maternal Autonomic Nervous System Function and Infant Development," *Psychophysiology* 54, no. 2 (2017): 279-288.
18. M. Aucoin, M. J. Lalonde-Parsi, and K. Cooley, "Mindfulness-Based Therapies in the Treatment of Functional Gastrointestinal Disorders: A Meta-Analysis," *Evidence-Based Complementary and Alternative Medicine* 2014 (2014): 140724, https://doi.org/10.1155/2014/140724.
19. F. Asare, S. Störsrud, and M. Simrén, "Meditation over Medication for Irritable Bowel Syndrome? On Exercise and Alternative Treatments for Irritable Bowel Syndrome," *Current Gastroenterology Reports* 14, no. 4 (2012): 283-289.
20. R. M. McAllister, "Adaptations in Control of Blood Flow with Training: Splanchnic and Renal Blood Flows," *Medicine and Science in Sports and Exercise* 30, no. 3 (1998): 375-381.
21. D. S. ten Haaf et al., "Nutritional Indicators for Gastrointestinal Symptoms in Female Runners: The 'Marikenloop Study,'" *BMJ Open* 4, no. 8 (2014): e005780, https://doi.org/10.1136/bmjopen-2014-005780.
22. R. W. ter Steege, J. Van Der Palen, and J. J. Kolkman, "Prevalence of Gastrointestinal Complaints in Runners Competing in a Long-Distance Run: An Internet-Based Observational Study in 1281 Subjects," *Scandinavian Journal of Gastroenterology* 43, no. 12 (2008): 1477-1482.
23. P. B. Wilson, "Perceived Life Stress and Anxiety Correlate with Chronic Gastrointestinal Symptoms in Runners," *Journal of Sports Sciences* 36, no. 15 (2018): 1713-1719.
24. A. L. Rebar et al., "A Meta-Meta-Analysis of the Effect of Physical Activity on Depression and Anxiety in Non-clinical Adult Populations," *Health Psychology Review* 9, no. 3 (2015): 366-378.
25. B. Stubbs et al., "An Examination of the Anxiolytic Effects of Exercise for People with Anxiety and Stress-Related Disorders: A Meta-Analysis," *Psychiatry Research* 249 (2017): 102-108.
26. B. R. Gordon et al., "The Effects of Resistance Exercise Training on Anxiety: A Meta-Analysis and Meta-Regression Analysis of Randomized Controlled Trials," *Sports Medicine* 47, no. 12 (2017): 2521-2532.
27. H. Cramer et al., "Yoga for Anxiety: A Systematic Review and Meta-Analysis of Randomized Controlled Trials," *Depression and Anxiety* 35, no. 9 (2018): 830-843.
28. J. Yin and R. K. Dishman, "The Effect of Tai Chi and Qigong Practice on Depression and Anxiety Symptoms: A Systematic Review and Meta-Regression Analysis of Randomized Controlled Trials," *Mental Health and Physical Activity* 7, no. 3 (2014): 135-146.
29. A. J. Daley et al., "The Effects of Exercise Upon Symptoms and Quality of Life in Patients Diagnosed with Irritable Bowel Syndrome: A Randomised Controlled Trial," *International Journal of Sports Medicine* 29, no. 9 (2008): 778-782.
30. E. Johannesson et al., "Physical Activity Improves Symptoms in Irritable Bowel Syndrome: A Randomized Controlled Trial," *American Journal of Gastroenterology* 106, no. 5 (2011): 915-922.
31. D. Schumann et al., "Effect of Yoga in the Therapy of Irritable Bowel Syndrome: A Systematic Review," *Clinical Gastroenterology and Hepatology* 14, no. 12 (2016): 1720-1731.
32. D. C. Hammond, "A Review of the History of Hypnosis Through the Late 19th Century," *American Journal of Clinical Hypnosis* 56, no. 2 (2013): 174-191.
33. D. M. Eisenberg et al., "Trends in Alternative Medicine Use in the United States, 1990-1997: Results of a Follow-Up National Survey," *JAMA* 280, no. 18 (1998): 1569-1575.
34. T. C. Clarke et al., "Trends in the Use of Complementary Health Approaches Among Adults: United States, 2002-2012," *National Health Statistics Reports* no. 79 (2015): 1-16.
35. H. F. Coelho, P. H. Canter, and E. Ernst, "The Effectiveness of Hypnosis for the Treatment of Anxiety: A Systematic Review," *Primary Care and Community Psychiatry* 12, no. 2 (2008): 49-63.
36. R. Schaefert, et al., "Efficacy, Tolerability, and Safety of Hypnosis in Adult Irritable Bowel Syndrome: Systematic Review and Meta-Analysis," *Psychosomatic Medicine* 76, no. 5 (2014): 389-398.

37. A. C. Ford et al., "Effect of Antidepressants and Psychological Therapies, Including Hypnotherapy, in Irritable Bowel Syndrome: Systematic Review and Meta-Analysis," *American Journal of Gastroenterology* 109, no. 9 (2014): 1350–1365.

38. M. Landry, M. Lifshitz, and A. Raz, "Brain Correlates of Hypnosis: A Systematic Review and Meta-Analytic Exploration," *Neuroscience and Biobehavioral Reviews* 81, Part A (2017): 75–98.

39. M. J. Peebles, "Harm in Hypnosis: Three Understandings from Psychoanalysis That Can Help," *American Journal of Clinical Hypnosis* 60, no. 3 (2018): 239–261.

40. T. Parker-Pope, "For Snowboarders, the Music Matters as Much as the Gear," *New York Times*, February 20, 2018, https://www.nytimes.com/2018/02/20/sports/olympics/snowboarding-music.html.

41. P. C. Terry et al., "Use and Perceived Effectiveness of Pre-competition Mood Regulation Strategies Among Athletes," in *Psychology Bridging the Tasman: Science, Culture and Practice—Proceedings of the Joint Conference of the Australian Psychological Society and the New Zealand Psychological Society*, ed. M. Katsikitis (Melbourne: Australian Psychological Society, 2006).

42. P. Laukka and L. Quick, "Emotional and Motivational Uses of Music in Sports and Exercise: A Questionnaire Study Among Athletes," *Psychology of Music* 41, no. 2 (2013): 198–215.

43. J. Lanzillo, "The Effects of Music on the Intensity and Direction of Pre-competitive Cognitive and Somatic State Anxiety and State Self-Confidence in Collegiate Athletes," *Legacy ETDs* (2000), https://digitalcommons.georgiasouthern.edu/etd_legacy/318.

44. D. Elliott, R. Polman, and J. Taylor, "The Effects of Relaxing Music for Anxiety Control on Competitive Sport Anxiety," *European Journal of Sport Science* 14, no. S1 (2014): S296–S301.

45. Y. Panteleeva et al., "Music for Anxiety? Meta-Analysis of Anxiety Reduction in Non-clinical Samples," *Psychology of Music* 46, no. 4 (2018): 473–487.

46. E. Daniel, "Music Used as Anti-anxiety Intervention for Patients During Outpatient Procedures: A Review of the Literature," *Complementary Therapies in Clinical Practice* 22 (2016): 21–23.

47. J. P. Jayakar and D. A. Alter, "Music for Anxiety Reduction in Patients Undergoing Cardiac Catheterization: A Systematic Review and Meta-Analysis of Randomized Controlled Trials," *Complementary Therapies in Clinical Practice* 28 (2017): 122–130.

48. O. S. Palsson and W. E. Whitehead, "Psychological Treatments in Functional Gastrointestinal Disorders: A Primer for the Gastroenterologist," *Clinical Gastroenterology and Hepatology* 11, no. 3 (2013): 208–216.

49. S. G. Hofmann et al., "The Efficacy of Cognitive Behavioral Therapy: A Review of Meta-Analyses," *Cognitive Therapy and Research* 36, no. 5 (2012): 427–440.

50. S. G. Hofmann et al., "The Effect of Mindfulness-Based Therapy on Anxiety and Depression: A Meta-Analytic Review," *Journal of Consulting and Clinical Psychology* 78, no. 2 (2010): 169–183.

51. M. J. Turner, "Rational Emotive Behavior Therapy (REBT), Irrational and Rational Beliefs, and the Mental Health of Athletes," *Frontiers in Psychology* 7 (2016): 1423, https://doi.org/10.3389/fpsyg.2016.01423.

52. C. Cullen, "Acceptance and Commitment Therapy (ACT): A Third Wave Behaviour Therapy," *Behavioural and Cognitive Psychotherapy* 36, no. 6 (2008): 667–673.

53. P. Bach and S. C. Hayes, "The Use of Acceptance and Commitment Therapy to Prevent the Rehospitalization of Psychotic Patients: A Randomized Controlled Trial," *Journal of Consulting and Clinical Psychology* 70, no. 5 (2002): 1129–1139.

54. J. G. L. A-Tjak et al., "A Meta-Analysis of the Efficacy of Acceptance and Commitment Therapy for Clinically Relevant Mental and Physical Health Problems," *Psychotherapy and Psychosomatics* 84 (2015): 30–36.

55. B. Sebastián Sánchez et al., "New Psychological Therapies for Irritable Bowel Syndrome: Mindfulness, Acceptance and Commitment Therapy (ACT)," *Revista Española de Enfermedades Digestivas* 109, no. 9 (2017): 648–657.

56. M. Oaklander, "New Hope for Depression," *Time*, July 27, 2017, http://time.com/magazine/us/4876068/august-7th-2017-vol-190-no-6-u-s/.

57. H. P. Loomer, J. C. Saunders, and N. S. Kline, "A Clinical and Pharmacodynamic Evaluation of Iproniazid as a Psychic Energizer," *Psychiatric Research Reports* 8 (1957): 129–141.

58. T. A. Ban, "Fifty Years Chlorpromazine: A Historical Perspective," *Neuropsychiatric Disease and Treatment* 3, no. 4 (2007): 495–500.

59. W. A. Brown and M. Rosdolsky, "The Clinical Discovery of Imipramine," *American Journal of Psychiatry* 172, no. 5 (2015): 426–429.

60. D. S. Baldwin et al., "Evidence-Based Pharmacological Treatment of Anxiety Disorders, Post-Traumatic Stress Disorder and Obsessive-Compulsive Disorder: A Revision of the 2005 Guidelines from the British Association for Psychopharmacology," *Journal of Psychopharmacology* 28, no. 5 (2014): 403–439.

61. M. B. Stein and M. G. Craske, "Treating Anxiety in 2017: Optimizing Care to Improve Outcomes," *JAMA* 318, no. 3 (2017): 235–236.

62. A. C. Ford et al., "Efficacy of Psychotropic Drugs in Functional Dyspepsia: Systematic Review and Meta-Analysis," *Gut* 66, no. 3 (2017): 411–420.

63. A. White and E. Ernst, "A Brief History of Acupuncture," *Rheumatology* 43, no. 5 (2004): 662–663.

64. G. Chao and S. Zhang, "Effectiveness of Acupuncture to Treat Irritable Bowel Syndrome: A Meta-Analysis," *World Journal of Gastroenterology* 20, no. 7 (2014): 1871–1877.

65. L. Lan et al., "Acupuncture for Functional Dyspepsia," *Cochrane Database of Systematic Reviews*, no. 10 (2014): CD008487, https://doi.org/10.1002/14651858.CD008487.pub2.

66. J. A. Chalmers et al., "Anxiety Disorders Are Associated with Reduced Heart Rate Variability: A Meta-Analysis," *Frontiers in Psychiatry* 5 (2014): 80, https://doi.org/10.3389/fpsyt.2014.00080.

67. P. L. Schoenberg and A. S. David, "Biofeedback for Psychiatric Disorders: A Systematic Review," *Applied Psychophysiology and Biofeedback* 39, no. 2 (2014): 109–135.

68. V. C. Goessl, J. E. Curtiss, and S. G. Hofmann, "The Effect of Heart Rate Variability Biofeedback Training on Stress and Anxiety: A Meta-Analysis," *Psychological Medicine* 47, no. 15 (2017): 2578–2586.

69. J. V. Schurman et al., "A Pilot Study to Assess the Efficacy of Biofeedback-Assisted Relaxation Training as an Adjunct Treatment for Pediatric Functional Dyspepsia Associated with Duodenal Eosinophilia," *Journal of Pediatric Psychology* 35, no. 8 (2010): 837–847.

70. A. Dobbin et al., "Randomised Controlled Trial of Brief Intervention with Biofeedback and Hypnotherapy in Patients with Refractory Irritable Bowel Syndrome," *Journal of the Royal College of Physicians of Edinburgh* 43, no. 1 (2013): 15–23.

71. J. A. Foster and K. A. McVey Neufeld, "Gut–Brain Axis: How the Microbiome Influences Anxiety and Depression," *Trends in Neurosciences* 36, no. 5 (2013): 305–312.

72. B. Liu et al., "Efficacy of Probiotics on Anxiety—A Meta-Analysis of Randomized Controlled Trials," *Depression and Anxiety* 35, no. 10 (2018): 935–945.

73. A. C. Ford et al., "Efficacy of Prebiotics, Probiotics, and Synbiotics in Irritable Bowel Syndrome and Chronic Idiopathic Constipation: Systematic Review and Meta-Analysis," *American Journal of Gastroenterology* 109, no. 10 (2014): 1547–1561.

Appendix A

1. C. Catassi, S. Gatti, and E. Lionetti, "World Perspective and Celiac Disease Epidemiology," *Digestive Diseases* 33, no. 2 (2015): 141–146.

2. B. Lebwohl, J. F. Ludvigsson, and P. H. R. Green, "Celiac Disease and Non-celiac Gluten Sensitivity," *BMJ* 351 (2015): h4347, https://doi.org/10.1136/bmj.h4347.

3. A. Fasano, "Celiac Disease: How to Handle a Clinical Chameleon," *New England Journal of Medicine* 348, no. 25 (2003): 2568–2570.

4. S. Perry, "Gluten-Free-Diet Fad Poses Risks, Particularly for Children, Expert Says," *MinnPost*, May 20, 2016, https://www.minnpost.com/second-opinion/2016/05/gluten-free-diet-fad-poses-risks-particularly-children-expert-says.

5. D. M. Lis et al., "Exploring the Popularity, Experiences, and Beliefs Surrounding Gluten-Free Diets in Nonceliac Athletes," *International Journal of Sport Nutrition and Exercise Metabolism* 25, no. 1 (2015): 37–45.

6. P. B. Wilson, "Nutrition Behaviors, Perceptions, and Beliefs of Recent Marathon Finishers," *The Physician and Sportsmedicine* 44, no. 3 (2016): 242–251.

7. D. Epstein, "Running Away from Gluten," *Sports Illustrated*, November 7, 2011, https://www.si.com/vault/2011/11/07/106127599/running-away-from-gluten.

8. C. Catassi et al., "Non-celiac Gluten Sensitivity: The New Frontier of Gluten Related Disorders," *Nutrients* 5, no. 10 (2013): 3839–3853.

9. M. M. Leonard et al., "Celiac Disease and Nonceliac Gluten Sensitivity: A Review," *JAMA* 318, no. 7 (2017): 647–656.

10. J. Molina-Infante and A. Carroccio, "Suspected Nonceliac Gluten Sensitivity Confirmed in Few Patients After Gluten Challenge in Double-Blind, Placebo-Controlled Trials," *Clinical Gastroenterology and Hepatology* 15, no. 3 (2017): 339–348.

11. G. I. Skodje et al., "Fructan, Rather Than Gluten, Induces Symptoms in Patients with Self-Reported Non-celiac Gluten Sensitivity," *Gastroenterology* 154, no. 3 (2018): 529–539.e2.

12. R. Caprilli, "Why Does Crohn's Disease Usually Occur in Terminal Ileum?" *Journal of Crohn's and Colitis* 2, no. 4 (2008): 352–356.

13. F. Gomollón et al., "3rd European Evidence-Based Consensus on the Diagnosis and Management of Crohn's Disease 2016: Part 1: Diagnosis and Medical Management," *Journal of Crohn's and Colitis* 11, no. 1 (2016): 3–25.

14. S. C. Ng et al., "Worldwide Incidence and Prevalence of Inflammatory Bowel Disease in the 21st Century: A Systematic Review of Population-Based Studies," *The Lancet* 390, no. 10114 (2017): 2769–2778.

15. D. N. Floyd et al., "The Economic and Quality-of-Life Burden of Crohn's Disease in Europe and the United States, 2000 to 2013: A Systematic Review," *Digestive Diseases and Sciences* 60, no. 2 (2015): 299–312.

16. T. M. Connelly and E. Messaris, "Predictors of Recurrence of Crohn's Disease After Ileocolectomy: A Review," *World Journal of Gastroenterology* 20, no. 39 (2014): 14393–14406.

17. L. Nance Jr., "Trust Me, Being an NBA Legacy Son Is a Lot Harder Than It Looks," *The Cauldron*, December 29, 2015, https://the-cauldron.com/trust-me-being-an-nba-legacy-son-is-a-lot-harder-than-it-looks-544b78e2d674.

18. M. Reiss, "Matt Light Reveals Battle with Crohn's," *ESPN*, May 14, 2012, http://www.espn.com/boston/nfl/story/_/id/7903017/matt-light-reveals-decade-long-battle-crohns.

19. C. Hwang, V. Ross, and U. Mahadevan, "Micronutrient Deficiencies in Inflammatory Bowel Disease: From A to Zinc," *Inflammatory Bowel Diseases* 18, no. 10 (2012): 1961–1981.

20. S. V. Rana and A. Malik, "Hydrogen Breath Tests in Gastrointestinal Diseases," *Indian Journal of Clinical Biochemistry* 29, no. 4 (2014): 398–405.

21. H. F. Jones, R. N. Butler, and D. A. Brooks, "Intestinal Fructose Transport and Malabsorption in Humans," *American Journal of Physiology-Gastrointestinal and Liver Physiology* 300, no. 2 (2010): G202–G206.

22. P. R. Gibson et al., "Fructose Malabsorption and the Bigger Picture," *Alimentary Pharmacology and Therapeutics* 25, no. 4 (2007): 349–363.

23. V. Stanghellini et al., "Gastroduodenal Disorders," *Gastroenterology* 150, no. 6 (2016): 1380–1392.

24. N. J. Talley and A. C. Ford, "Functional Dyspepsia," *New England Journal of Medicine* 373, no. 19 (2015): 1853–1863.

25. S. Mahadeva and K. L. Goh, "Epidemiology of Functional Dyspepsia: A Global Perspective," *World Journal of Gastroenterology* 12, no. 17 (2006): 2661–2666.

26. R. A. Brook et al., "Functional Dyspepsia Impacts Absenteeism and Direct and Indirect Costs," *Clinical Gastroenterology and Hepatology* 8, no. 6 (2010): 498–503.

27. P. Aro et al., "Functional Dyspepsia Impairs Quality of Life in the Adult Population," *Alimentary Pharmacology and Therapeutics* 33, no. 11 (2011): 1215–1224.

28. R. M. Donaldson, "Dyspepsia: The Broad Etiologic Spectrum," *Hospital Practice* 22, no. 9A (1987): 41–9, 53.

29. N. J. Talley, M. M. Walker, and G. Holtmann, "Functional Dyspepsia," *Current Opinion in Gastroenterology* 32, no. 6 (2016): 467–473.

30. A. C. Ford et al., "Efficacy of Psychotropic Drugs in Functional Dyspepsia: Systematic Review and Meta-Analysis," *Gut* 66, no. 3 (2017): 411–420.

31. A. Tursi, A. Papa, and S. Danese, "Review Article: The Pathophysiology and Medical Management of Diverticulosis and Diverticular Disease of the Colon," *Alimentary Pharmacology and Therapeutics* 42, no. 6 (2015): 664–684.

32. L. Lamanna and P. E. Moran, "Diverticular Disease," *Gastroenterology Nursing* 41, no. 2 (2018): 111–119.

33. M. Delvaux, "Diverticular Disease of the Colon in Europe: Epidemiology, Impact on Citizen Health and Prevention," *Alimentary Pharmacology and Therapeutics* 18 (2003): 71–74.

34. J. Granlund et al., "The Genetic Influence on Diverticular Disease: A Twin Study," *Alimentary Pharmacology and Therapeutics* 35, no. 9 (2012): 1103–1107.

35. J. H. Cummings and A. Engineer, "Denis Burkitt and the Origins of the Dietary Fibre Hypothesis," *Nutrition Research Reviews* 31, no. 1 (2018): 1–15.

36. N. S. Painter, "Diverticulosis of the Colon," (Master of Surgery thesis, University of London, 1962).

37. N. S. Painter, A. Z. Almeida, and K. W. Colebourne, "Unprocessed Bran in Treatment of Diverticular Disease of the Colon," *British Medical Journal* 2, no. 5806 (1972): 137–140.

38. N. S. Painter and D. P. Burkitt, "Diverticular Disease of the Colon: A Deficiency Disease of Western Civilization," *British Medical Journal* 2, no. 5759 (1971): 450–454.

39. L. L. Strate, "Diverticulosis and Dietary Fiber: Rethinking the Relationship," *Gastroenterology* 142, no. 2 (2012): 205–207.

40. A. Tursi, "Dietary Pattern and Colonic Diverticulosis," *Current Opinion in Clinical Nutrition and Metabolic Care* 20, no. 5 (2017): 409–413.

41. J. D. Feuerstein and K. R. Falchuk, "Diverticulosis and Diverticulitis," *Mayo Clinic Proceedings*, 91, no. 8 (2016): 1094–1104.

42. D. Aune et al., "Tobacco Smoking and the Risk of Diverticular Disease—a Systematic Review and Meta-Analysis of Prospective Studies," *Colorectal Disease* 19, no. 7 (2017): 621–633.

43. D. Aune et al., "Body Mass Index and Physical Activity and the Risk of Diverticular Disease: A Systematic Review and Meta-Analysis of Prospective Studies," *European Journal of Nutrition* 56, no. 8 (2017): 2423–2438.

44. N. Stollman et al., "American Gastroenterological Association Institute Guideline on the Management of Acute Diverticulitis," *Gastroenterology* 149, no. 7 (2015): 1944–1949.

45. S. Sethi and J. E. Richter, "Diet and Gastroesophageal Reflux Disease: Role in Pathogenesis and Management," *Current Opinion in Gastroenterology* 33, no. 2 (2017): 107–111.

46. P. O. Katz, L. B. Gerson, and M. F. Vela, "Guidelines for the Diagnosis and Management of Gastroesophageal Reflux Disease," *American Journal of Gastroenterology* 108, no. 3 (2013): 308–328.

47. H. B. El-Serag et al., "Update on the Epidemiology of Gastro-Oesophageal Reflux Disease: A Systematic Review," *Gut* 63, no. 6 (2014): 871–880.

48. P. W. Brown, "The Irritable Bowel Syndrome," *Rocky Mountain Medical Journal* 47, no. 5 (1950): 343–346.

49. S. Stossel, *My Age of Anxiety: Fear, Hope, Dread, and the Search for Peace of Mind* (New York: Alfred A. Knopf, 2014).

50. A. D. Sperber et al., "The Global Prevalence of IBS in Adults Remains Elusive Due to the Heterogeneity of Studies: A Rome Foundation Working Team Literature Review," *Gut* 66, no. 6 (2017): 1075–1082.

51. S. Fukudo et al., "Evidence-Based Clinical Practice Guidelines for Irritable Bowel Syndrome," *Journal of Gastroenterology* 50, no. 1 (2015): 11–30.

52. L. A. Killian and S. Y. Lee, "Irritable Bowel Syndrome Is Underdiagnosed and Ineffectively Managed Among Endurance Athletes," *Applied Physiology, Nutrition, and Metabolism* 44, no. 12 (2019): 1329–1338, https://doi.org/10.1139/apnm-2019-0261.

53. G. Fond et al., "Anxiety and Depression Comorbidities in Irritable Bowel Syndrome (IBS): A Systematic Review and Meta-Analysis," *European Archives of Psychiatry and Clinical Neuroscience* 264, no. 8 (2014): 651–660.

54. F. H. Kruse, "Functional Disorders of the Colon: The Spastic Colon, the Irritable Colon, and Mucous Colitis," *California and Western Medicine* 39, no. 2 (1933): 97–103.

55. M. C. F. Passos et al., "Adequate Relief in a Treatment Trial with IBS Patients: A Prospective Assessment," *American Journal of Gastroenterology* 104, no. 4 (2009): 912–919.

56. A. J. Lembo et al., "Eluxadoline for Irritable Bowel Syndrome with Diarrhea," *New England Journal of Medicine* 374, no. 3 (2016): 242–253.

57. Y. Deng et al., "Lactose Intolerance in Adults: Biological Mechanism and Dietary Management," *Nutrients* 7, no. 9 (2015): 8020–8035.

58. S. R. Hertzler and D. A. Savaiano, "Colonic Adaptation to Daily Lactose Feeding in Lactose Maldigesters Reduces Lactose Intolerance," *American Journal of Clinical Nutrition* 64, no. 2 (1996): 232–236.

59. L. S. Stephenson and M. C. Latham, "Lactose Intolerance and Milk Consumption: The Relation of Tolerance to Symptoms," *American Journal of Clinical Nutrition* 27, no. 3 (1974): 296–303.

60. M. C. E. Lomer, G. C. Parkes, and J. D. Sanderson, "Review Article: Lactose Intolerance in Clinical Practice—Myths and Realities," *Alimentary Pharmacology and Therapeutics* 27, no. 2 (2008): 93–103.

61. R. P. Heaney, "Dairy Intake, Dietary Adequacy, and Lactose Intolerance," *Advances in Nutrition* 4, no. 2 (2013): 151–156.

62. K. Schwarz, "Ueber penetrierende Magen-und Jejunalgeschwüre" [About penetrating gastric and jejunal ulcers], *Beitrage zur Klinischen Chirurgie* 67 (1910): 96–128.

63. J. Gustafson and D. Welling, "'No Acid, No Ulcer'—100 Years Later: A Review of the History of Peptic Ulcer Disease," *Journal of the American College of Surgeons* 210, no. 1 (2010): 110–116.

64. B. W. Sippy, "Gastric and Duodenal Ulcer," *Transactions of the Association of American Physicians* 30 (1915): 129–148.

65. A. Lanas and F. K. L. Chan, "Peptic Ulcer Disease," *The Lancet* 390, no. 10094 (2017): 613–624.

66. J. R. Warren. "*Helicobacter*: The Ease and Difficulty of a New Discovery (Nobel Lecture)," *ChemMedChem: Chemistry Enabling Drug Discovery* 1, no. 7 (2006): 672–685.

67. B. Marshall and J. R. Warren, "Unidentified Curved Bacilli in the Stomach of Patients with Gastritis and Peptic Ulceration," *The Lancet* 323, no. 8390 (1984): 1311–1315.
68. B. Marshall and P. C. Adams, "*Helicobacter pylori*: A Nobel Pursuit?" *Canadian Journal of Gastroenterology and Hepatology* 22, no. 11 (2008): 895–896.
69. B. J. Marshall et al., "Attempt to Fulfil Koch's Postulates for Pyloric Campylobacter," *Medical Journal of Australia* 142, no. 8 (1985): 436–439.
70. B. Marshall et al., "Prospective Double-Blind Trial of Duodenal Ulcer Relapse After Eradication of *Campylobacter pylori*," *The Lancet* 332, no. 8626–8627 (1988): 1437–1442.
71. R. M. Zagari et al., "Treatment of *Helicobacter pylori* Infection: A Clinical Practice Update," *European Journal of Clinical Investigation* 48, no. 1 (2018): e12857, https://doi.org/10.1111/eci.12857.
72. J. Q. Yuan et al., "Systematic Review with Network Meta-Analysis: Comparative Effectiveness and Safety of Strategies for Preventing NSAID-Associated Gastrointestinal Toxicity," *Alimentary Pharmacology and Therapeutics* 43, no. 12 (2016): 1262–1275.
73. Y. Yuan, I. T. Padol, and R. H. Hunt, "Peptic Ulcer Disease Today," *Nature Reviews Gastroenterology and Hepatology* 3, no. 2 (2006): 80–89.
74. G. B. Eusterman, "Surgical and Nonsurgical Aspects of Chronic Gastric Duodenal Ulcers," *Collected Papers by the Staff of Saint Mary's Hospital, Mayo Clinic* 12 (1921): 54–59.
75. S. Levenstein et al., "Psychological Stress Increases Risk for Peptic Ulcer, Regardless of *Helicobacter pylori* Infection or Use of Nonsteroidal Anti-inflammatory Drugs," *Clinical Gastroenterology and Hepatology* 13, no. 3 (2015): 498–506.
76. A. Rezaie, M. Pimentel, and S. S. Rao, "How to Test and Treat Small Intestinal Bacterial Overgrowth: An Evidence-Based Approach," *Current Gastroenterology Reports* 18, no. 2 (2016): 8, https://doi.org/10.1007/s11894-015-0482-9.
77. R. Sender, S. Fuchs, and R. Milo, "Revised Estimates for the Number of Human and Bacteria Cells in the Body," *PLoS Biology* 14, no. 8 (2016): e1002533, https://doi.org/10.1371/journal.pbio.1002533.
78. J. Bures et al., "Small Intestinal Bacterial Overgrowth Syndrome," *World Journal of Gastroenterology* 16, no. 24 (2010): 2978–2990.
79. E. Grace et al., "Review Article: Small Intestinal Bacterial Overgrowth–Prevalence, Clinical Features, Current and Developing Diagnostic Tests, and Treatment," *Alimentary Pharmacology and Therapeutics* 38, no. 7 (2013): 674–688.
80. T. E. Lawrence, *Seven Pillars of Wisdom* (London: Black House Publishing, 2013), 193.
81. C. Troeger et al., "Estimates of Global, Regional, and National Morbidity, Mortality, and Aetiologies of Diarrhoeal Diseases: A Systematic Analysis for the Global Burden of Disease Study 2015," *The Lancet Infectious Diseases* 17, no. 9 (2017): 909–948.
82. D. R. Hill and N. J. Beeching, "Travelers' Diarrhea," *Current Opinion in Infectious Diseases* 23, no. 5 (2010): 481–487.
83. R. Steffen, D. R. Hill, and H. L. DuPont, "Traveler's Diarrhea: A Clinical Review," *JAMA* 313, no. 1 (2015): 71–80.
84. B. H. Kean and S. Waters, "The Diarrhea of Travelers: I. Incidence in Travelers Returning to the United States from Mexico," *Archives of Industrial Health* 18, no. 2 (1958): 148–150.
85. "Traveler's Diarrhea," Centers for Disease Control and Prevention, https://wwwnc.cdc.gov/travel/page/travelers-diarrhea.
86. M. S. Riddle et al., "Guidelines for the Prevention and Treatment of Travelers' Diarrhea: A Graded Expert Panel Report," *Journal of Travel Medicine* 24, no. S1 (2017): S63–S80.
87. X. Qin, "Why Is Damage Limited to the Mucosa in Ulcerative Colitis but Transmural in Crohn's Disease?" *World Journal of Gastrointestinal Pathophysiology* 4, no. 3 (2013): 63–64.
88. A. Dignass et al., "Second European Evidence-Based Consensus on the Diagnosis and Management of Ulcerative Colitis Part 1: Definitions and Diagnosis," *Journal of Crohn's and Colitis* 6, no. 10 (2012): 965–990.
89. R. Shivashankar et al., "Incidence and Prevalence of Crohn's Disease and Ulcerative Colitis in Olmsted County, Minnesota from 1970 Through 2010," *Clinical Gastroenterology and Hepatology* 15, no. 6 (2017): 857–863.
90. A. N. Ananthakrishnan, "Epidemiology and Risk Factors for IBD," *Nature Reviews Gastroenterology and Hepatology* 12, no. 4 (2015): 205–217.
91. F. Pisani, "Fernando Pisani: Battling Back from Ulcerative Colitis," *The Hockey News*, May 6, 2008, https://thehockeynews.com/news/article/fernando-pisani-battling-back-from-ulcerative-colitis.

92. D. Chan et al., "Inflammatory Bowel Disease and Exercise: Results of a Crohn's and Colitis UK Survey," *Frontline Gastroenterology* 5, no. 1 (2014): 44–48.
93. A. Dignass et al., "Second European Evidence-Based Consensus on the Diagnosis and Management of Ulcerative Colitis Part 2: Current Management," *Journal of Crohn's and Colitis* 6, no. 10 (2012): 991–1030.
94. C. Rungoe et al., "Changes in Medical Treatment and Surgery Rates in Inflammatory Bowel Disease: A Nationwide Cohort Study 1979–2011," *Gut* 63, no. 10 (2014): 1607–1616.
95. H. Ross et al., "Practice Parameters for the Surgical Treatment of Ulcerative Colitis," *Diseases of the Colon and Rectum* 57, no. 1 (2014): 5–22.
96. H. E. Mardini and A. Y. Grigorian, "Probiotic Mix VSL#3 Is Effective Adjunctive Therapy for Mild to Moderately Active Ulcerative Colitis: A Meta-Analysis," *Inflammatory Bowel Diseases* 20, no. 9 (2014): 1562–1567.

Appendix B

1. T. K. Machu, "Therapeutics of 5-HT3 Receptor Antagonists: Current Uses and Future Directions," *Pharmacology and Therapeutics* 130, no. 3 (2011): 338–347.
2. H. S. Smith, L. R. Cox, and E. J. Smith, "5-HT3 Receptor Antagonists for the Treatment of Nausea/Vomiting," *Annals of Palliative Medicine* 1, no. 2 (2012): 115–120.
3. A. Pasternak, D. Fiore, and A. Islas, "Use of Ondansetron for Nausea and Vomiting During an Ultra-Endurance Run," *International Journal of Sports Physiology and Performance* 13, no. S1 (2018): S1-1–S1-9.
4. M. D. Hoffman et al., "Medical Services at Ultra-Endurance Foot Races in Remote Environments: Medical Issues and Consensus Guidelines," *Sports Medicine* 44, no. 8 (2014): 1055–1069.
5. M. A. Kwiatek et al., "An Alginate-Antacid Formulation (Gaviscon Double Action Liquid) Can Eliminate or Displace the Postprandial 'Acid Pocket' in Symptomatic GERD Patients," *Alimentary Pharmacology and Therapeutics* 34, no. 1 (2011): 59–66.
6. P. M. Christensen et al., "Caffeine and Bicarbonate for Speed. A Meta-Analysis of Legal Supplements Potential for Improving Intense Endurance Exercise Performance," *Frontiers in Physiology* 8 (2017): 240, https://doi.org/10.3389/fphys.2017.00240.
7. K. E. Fleming-Dutra et al., "Prevalence of Inappropriate Antibiotic Prescriptions Among US Ambulatory Care Visits, 2010–2011," *JAMA* 315, no. 17 (2016): 1864–1873.
8. J. G. Bartlett, "Antibiotic-Associated Diarrhea," *New England Journal of Medicine* 346, no. 5 (2002): 334–339.
9. S. Hempel et al., "Probiotics for the Prevention and Treatment of Antibiotic-Associated Diarrhea: A Systematic Review and Meta-Analysis," *JAMA* 307, no. 18 (2012): 1959–1969.
10. L. V. McFarland, C. T. Evans, and E. J. C. Goldstein, "Strain-Specificity and Disease-Specificity of Probiotic Efficacy: A Systematic Review and Meta-Analysis," *Frontiers in Medicine* 5 (2018): 124, https://doi.org/10.3389/fmed.2018.00124.
11. M. S. Riddle et al., "Guidelines for the Prevention and Treatment of Travelers' Diarrhea: A Graded Expert Panel Report," *Journal of Travel Medicine* 24, no. S1 (2017): S63–S80.
12. D. E. Baker, "Loperamide: A Pharmacological Review," *Reviews in Gastroenterological Disorders* 7, no. S3 (2007): S11–18.
13. M. L. Bechtold et al., "The Pharmacologic Treatment of Short Bowel Syndrome: New Tricks and Novel Agents," *Current Gastroenterology Reports* 16, no. 7 (2014): 392, https://doi.org/10.1007/s11894-014-0392-2.
14. S. L. Gorbach, "Bismuth Therapy in Gastrointestinal Diseases," *Gastroenterology* 99, no. 3 (1990): 863–875.
15. C. Regnard et al., "Loperamide," *Journal of Pain and Symptom Management* 42, no. 2 (2011): 319–323.
16. R. Steffen et al., "Prevention of Traveler's Diarrhea by the Tablet Form of Bismuth Subsalicylate," *Antimicrobial Agents and Chemotherapy* 29, no. 4 (1986): 625–627.
17. S. L. Giddings, A. M. Stevens, and D. T. Leung, "Traveler's Diarrhea," *Medical Clinics* 100, no. 2 (2016): 317–330.
18. H. S. Smith, L. R. Cox, and B. R. Smith, "Dopamine Receptor Antagonists," *Annals of Palliative Medicine* 1, no. 2 (2012): 137–142.
19. B. J. Pleuvry, "Physiology and Pharmacology of Nausea and Vomiting," *Anaesthesia and Intensive Care Medicine* 13, no. 12 (2012): 598–602.
20. F. E. R. Simons and K. J. Simons, "Histamine and H1-Antihistamines: Celebrating a Century of Progress," *Journal of Allergy and Clinical Immunology* 128, no. 6 (2011): 1139–1150.
21. "H2 Blockers," MedlinePlus, last reviewed April 24, 2017, https://medlineplus.gov/ency/patientinstructions/000382.htm.

22. B. B. Kraus, J. W. Sinclair, and D. O. Castell, "Gastroesophageal Reflux in Runners: Characteristics and Treatment," *Annals of Internal Medicine* 112, no. 6 (1990): 429–433.

23. R. S. Baska, F. M. Moses, and P. A. Deuster, "Cimetidine Reduces Running-Associated Gastrointestinal Bleeding," *Digestive Diseases and Sciences* 35, no. 8 (1990): 956–960.

24. F. M. Moses et al., "Effect of Cimetidine on Marathon-Associated Gastrointestinal Symptoms and Bleeding," *Digestive Diseases and Sciences* 36, no. 10 (1991): 1390–1394.

25. K. Krogh, G. Chiarioni, and W. Whitehead, "Management of Chronic Constipation in Adults," *United European Gastroenterology Journal* 5, no. 4 (2017): 465–472.

26. E. H. Baker and G. I. Sandle, "Complications of Laxative Abuse," *Annual Review of Medicine* 47, no. 1 (1996): 127–134.

27. C. Greenleaf et al., "Female Collegiate Athletes: Prevalence of Eating Disorders and Disordered Eating Behaviors," *Journal of American College Health* 57, no. 5 (2009): 489–496.

28. M. Nagari, "Diagnosis and Management of Irritable Bowel Syndrome," *Prescriber* 25, no. 6 (2014): 17–23.

29. A. Spinks and J. Wasiak, "Scopolamine (Hyoscine) for Preventing and Treating Motion Sickness," *Cochrane Database of Systematic Reviews* no. 6 (2011): CD002851, https://doi.org/10.1002/14651858.CD002851.pub4.

30. G. W. Ho, "Lower Gastrointestinal Distress in Endurance Athletes," *Current Sports Medicine Reports* 8, no. 2 (2009): 85–91.

31. J. Jin, "Nonsteroidal Anti-inflammatory Drugs," *JAMA* 314, no. 10 (2015): 1084–1084.

32. K. Van Wijck et al., "Aggravation of Exercise-Induced Intestinal Injury by Ibuprofen in Athletes," *Medicine and Science in Sports and Exercise* 44, no. 12 (2012): 2257–2262.

33. M. Küster et al., "Consumption of Analgesics Before a Marathon and the Incidence of Cardiovascular, Gastrointestinal and Renal Problems: A Cohort Study," *BMJ Open* 3, no. 4 (2013): e002090, https://doi.org/10.1136/bmjopen-2012-002090.

34. P. C. Wharam et al., "NSAID Use Increases the Risk of Developing Hyponatremia During an Ironman Triathlon," *Medicine and Science in Sports and Exercise* 38, no. 4 (2006): 618–622.

35. M. Lilja et al., "High Doses of Anti-inflammatory Drugs Compromise Muscle Strength and Hypertrophic Adaptations to Resistance Training in Young Adults," *Acta Physiologica* 222, no. 2 (2018): e12948, https://doi.org/10.1111/apha.12948.

36. B. J. Schoenfeld, "The Use of Nonsteroidal Anti-inflammatory Drugs for Exercise-Induced Muscle Damage," *Sports Medicine* 42, no. 12 (2012): 1017–1028.

37. D. R. Morales et al., "NSAID-Exacerbated Respiratory Disease: A Meta-Analysis Evaluating Prevalence, Mean Provocative Dose of Aspirin and Increased Asthma Morbidity," *Allergy* 70, no. 7 (2015): 828–835.

38. G. Sigthorsson et al., "COX-2 Inhibition with Rofecoxib Does Not Increase Intestinal Permeability in Healthy Subjects: A Double Blind Crossover Study Comparing Rofecoxib with Placebo and Indomethacin," *Gut* 47, no. 4 (2000): 527–532.

39. J. Baker et al., "Effects of Indomethacin and Celecoxib on Renal Function in Athletes," *Medicine and Science in Sports and Exercise* 37, no. 5 (2005): 712–717.

40. B. J. Schoenfeld, "Non-steroidal Anti-inflammatory Drugs May Blunt More Than Pain," *Acta Physiologica* 222, no. 2 (2018): e12990. https://doi.org/10.1111/apha.12990.

41. G. W. Pasternak, "Pharmacological Mechanisms of Opioid Analgesics," *Clinical Neuropharmacology* 16, no. 1 (1993): 1–18.

42. R. Benyamin et al., "Opioid Complications and Side Effects," *Pain Physician* 11, no. S2 (2008): S105–S120.

43. S. F. Cook et al., "Gastrointestinal Side Effects in Chronic Opioid Users: Results From a Population-Based Survey," *Alimentary Pharmacology and Therapeutics* 27, no. 12 (2008): 1224–1232.

44. T. J. Bell et al., "The Prevalence, Severity, and Impact of Opioid-Induced Bowel Dysfunction: Results of a US and European Patient Survey (PROBE 1)," *Pain Medicine* 10, no. 1 (2009): 35–42.

45. L. B. Cottler et al., "Injury, Pain, and Prescription Opioid Use Among Former National Football League (NFL) Players," *Drug and Alcohol Dependence* 116, no. 1–3 (2011): 188–194.

46. P. Veliz et al., "Opioid Use Among Interscholastic Sports Participants: An Exploratory Study From a Sample of College Students," *Research Quarterly for Exercise and Sport* 86, no. 2 (2015): 205–211.

47. B. Hainline et al., "International Olympic Committee Consensus Statement on Pain Management in Elite Athletes," *British Journal of Sports Medicine* 51, no. 17 (2017): 1245–1258.

48. R. Schey and S. S. Rao, "Lubiprostone for the Treatment of Adults with Constipation and Irritable Bowel Syndrome," *Digestive Diseases and Sciences* 56, no. 6 (2011): 1619–1625.

49. P. Layer and V. Stanghellini, "Linaclotide for the Management of Irritable Bowel Syndrome with Constipation," *Alimentary Pharmacology and Therapeutics* 39, no. 4 (2014): 371–384.
50. K. M. Fock et al., "Proton Pump Inhibitors," *Clinical Pharmacokinetics* 47, no. 1 (2008): 1–6.
51. P. W. Ament, D. B. Dicola, and M. E. James, "Reducing Adverse Effects of Proton Pump Inhibitors," *American Family Physician* 86, no. 1 (2012): 66–70.
52. M. Thalmann et al., "Proton Pump Inhibition Prevents Gastrointestinal Bleeding in Ultramarathon Runners: A Randomised, Double Blinded, Placebo Controlled Study," *British Journal of Sports Medicine* 40, no. 4 (2006): 359–362.
53. H. P. Peters et al., "The Effect of Omeprazole on Gastro-Oesophageal Reflux and Symptoms During Strenuous Exercise," *Alimentary Pharmacology and Therapeutics* 13, no. 8 (1999): 1015–1022.
54. C. M. Dording et al., "The Pharmacologic Management of SSRI-Induced Side Effects: A Survey of Psychiatrists," *Annals of Clinical Psychiatry* 14, no. 3 (2002): 143–147.
55. E. Cascade, A. H. Kalali, and S. H. Kennedy, "Real-World Data on SSRI Antidepressant Side Effects," *Psychiatry (Edgmont)* 6, no. 2 (2009): 16–18.
56. S. M. Wang et al., "Addressing the Side Effects of Contemporary Antidepressant Drugs: A Comprehensive Review," *Chonnam Medical Journal* 54, no. 2 (2018): 101–112.
57. A. C. Ford et al., "American College of Gastroenterology Monograph on Management of Irritable Bowel Syndrome," *American Journal of Gastroenterology* 113, no. S2 (2018): 1–18.
58. C. L. Reardon and R. M. Factor, "Sport Psychiatry: A Systematic Review of Diagnosis and Medical Treatment of Mental Illness in Athletes," *Sports Medicine* 40, no. 11 (2010): 961–980.
59. C. L. Reardon, "The Sports Psychiatrist and Psychiatric Medication," *International Review of Psychiatry* 28, no. 6 (2016): 606–613.
60. A. Plattner and B. Dantz, "Tricyclic Antidepressants: An Underutilized Treatment? Part II," *Psychopharm Review* 46, no. 3 (2011): 17–23.
61. "Comparing Selective Serotonin Reuptake Inhibitors (SSRIs) to Tricyclic Antidepressants (TCAs)," eMed Expert, May 7, 2007, last modified December 22, 2018, https://www.emedexpert.com/compare/ssris-vs-tca.shtml#3.
62. D. Taylor, "Antidepressant Drugs and Cardiovascular Pathology: A Clinical Overview of Effectiveness and Safety," *Acta Psychiatrica Scandinavica* 118, no. 6 (2008): 434–442.

INDEX

abdominal cavity, 13, 31, 53
absorption, 3, 62; carbohydrate, 17, 22
acceptance and commitment therapy (ACT), 221, 225
acetyl-CoA, 186
acids, 10; neutralizing, 185; secretion of, 203; small intestine and, 14; stomach, 14. *See also* amino acids; fatty acids; gastric acid; hydrochloric acid
Acosta, José de, 34, 35
ACT. *See* acceptance and commitment therapy
acupuncture, 223, 225
adaptation process, 68, 155, 164
adenosine triphosphate (ATP), 77, 78, 89, 90, 91, 110, 132, 134, 155
adrenaline, 33, 205
aerobics, 37, 52, 217
aerophagia, 57
Afremow, Jim, 209
alimentary canal, x, xiii, 3, 6, 9, 15, 28
Almy, Thomas, 201–202
altitude sickness, 37, 38
American College of Sports Medicine, 94, 98, 101, 107, 125, 136, 137, 163, 195
amino acids, 11, 22, 123, 125, 178, 179; branched-chain, 17, 131, 132; essential/nonessential, 17
amygdala, 47
amylase, 5, 10, 14, 96
anabolic steroids, 172
anemia, 64, 66
ankyrins, 152, 153, 154, 165
anorexia nervosa, 82, 83, 160
antacids, 63, 254 (table)
antibiotics, 59, 60, 255 (table)
antidepressants, 222–223, 225
antidiarrheals, 256 (table)
anti-inflammatories, 259 (table), 260 (table)
antipsychotics, 222
anus, 24–25, 28
anxiety, 60, 84, 196, 203, 206–209, 214, 215, 216, 224; ACT and, 221; cardiovascular/respiratory manifestations of, 192; colonic function and, 210; colorectal function and, 210; competition-related, 191, 193, 194; gut function and, 208, 209–210, 221; hypnosis and, 218; managing, 208, 225; music and, 219; performance and, 194, 208; pharmaceutical drugs and, 222–223; psychological, 216; reducing, 217, 225; state, 207, 208; stress and, 49, 61, 194, 206, 211, 213; trait, 207, 208; treatments for, 224; vomiting and, 193, 194
aorta, 10

apical membrane, 96
arginine vasopressin (AVP), 41, 131, 132; dehydration and, 39; surges in, 38
asthma, 173, 214
Athlete Biological Passport, 143
ATP. *See* adenosine triphosphate
atropine, 38
Aucouturier, Hippolyte, 49
Auerbach, Red, 194
Australian Institute of Sport, 158, 159
AVP. *See* arginine vasopressin

bacteria, 39, 48, 56, 97, 172, 175; butyrate-producing, 24; colonic, 23, 24; gut function and, 173; health and, 23, 173; intestinal, 55; metabolization by, 24
barrier integrity, 179
basal metabolic rate, 79
basolateral membrane, 96
Bayliss, William M., 26
Bearden, Shawn, 29
Beaumont, William, 199–200
Bechler, Steve, 171
beverages: hypertonic/hypotonic, 20, 54, 99; pre-exercise, 143; sodium-rich, 144, 146, 148, 150. *See also* carbohydrate beverages
Bifidobacterium, 117, 174, 175
bile, 14, 23
biofeedback, 64, 224
Bitter, Zach, 116
bleeding, 66; disorders, 183
bloating, 82, 84, 97, 109, 117, 131, 132, 144, 174, 201; avoiding, 130; fullness and, 46–49; prevalence/ development of, 71 (table); severity of, 209; stress and, 49; blood, 134; components, 64–65; delivery, 133; occult, 64, 65; oxygen and, 191
blood ammonia, 181
blood-brain barrier, 31
blood flow, 26, 102, 134, 135, 165, 191; absolute amount of, 157; changes in, 48, 73, 199; exercise and, 68; fluid and, 139; fluid loss and, 136; gut, 67, 157, 199, 200, 201, 217; redistribution of, 156
blood loss, 65, 66
blood pressure, 84, 108, 133, 170; sodium and, 147
blood volume, 103, 138, 148–149, 150, 165; increasing, 133, 155; loss of, 134, 142
body mass, 138, 146, 165; loss of, 135, 139
body weight, 8, 92, 141, 150
Bogues, Muggsy, 5, 6, 7
Bolt, Usain, 34

bolus, 6, 7, 25, 26, 28
bomb calorimeter, 78
bovine colostrum, 175-178, 181, 188
bowel issues, 54, 59, 104
bowel movements, 56, 69, 62, 108, 202
bowels, 18, 23, 48; angry, 58; controlling, 25; emotional responses and, 203; in-race disaster with, 58
brain, xi, 25, 26, 134; activity, 47, 218, 224; blood delivery to, 133; blood glucose and, 41; exercise and, 155; gut and, xi; second, 28, 191; training and, 155
brain scans, xii, 27
breathing: shortness of, 34, 66; slow deep, 54, 206, 213-214, 215, 216, 224, 225
Brooks, Brandon, 193, 194, 205, 215
bulimia, 8, 9, 10
Burke, Louise, 116
Bush, George W., 31
butyrate production, 129, 132

caffeine, 188, 211; colon and, 184; consuming, 42, 120, 185; gut problems and, 185; limiting, 206, 208; muscular contraction and, 185; nausea and, 42; performance and, 62, 184; sodium bicarbonate and, 62
Caine, Sir Michael, 5, 14, 16
calcium, 63, 169
cancer, 29, 45, 108; colon, 64, 109; colorectal, 24, 108, 129
Cannon, Walter Bradford, 201
carbohydrate beverages, 48, 81, 89, 94, 99, 103, 120, 127, 160, 163, 181; drinking, 138-139; glucose-fructose, 50; gut symptoms and, 100; hydrogel-based, 101; hypertonic, 36; performance and, 139
carbohydrate loading, 142
carbohydrates, 16, 20, 28, 40, 45, 48, 78, 92, 106, 113, 126, 163, 165, 187, 206; absorbing, 17, 22, 51, 158; accumulation of, 96-97; burning, xi, 90, 93, 116, 121, 159, 160; concentration of, 22, 51, 99; consuming, 50, 56, 93, 94, 95, 89, 99, 102, 104, 110, 127, 129, 132, 158, 208; daily need of, 92 (table); digesting, 10, 14, 17, 18, 24, 96; emptying, 12, 160; encapsulated, 100; exercise and, 89, 90, 93-95, 98, 101, 102 (table), 110, 156, 160, 180-181; fat and, 186; fermentable, 129; fiber and, 105; gastrointestinal integrity and, 102-104; gel, 100; ingesting, 89, 93-94, 101, 103, 114, 120, 132, 157-160, 159 (fig.), 160, 162, 180-181; liquid, 100; long-chain, 95, 99; malabsorption of, 97 (fig.), 120; performance and, 110, 114, 120, 132, 159, 161; recommendations for, 93-95; restriction on, 186, 187; short-chain, 55; solids, 100; storing, 90, 91
carbon dioxide, 24, 55, 57, 77, 106, 117
cardiac output, 133, 134, 157
cardiovascular disease, 108, 143, 170
carnitine, 91
Carrell, Steve, 36
catecholamines, 33, 34, 42, 68, 204, 211; hypersection of, 35; release of, 206; stress and, 205
CBT. See cognitive behavioral therapy
cecum, 66, 162
celiac disease, 24, 59; described, 227-228

cells: animal, 23; bacterial, 23; epithelial, 16, 123, 179; gastrointestinal, 179; gut, 102; immune, 179, 180; intestinal, 17, 24, 39, 96, 102; parietal, 10; white blood, 176
cerebral edema, 34
chemoreceptor triggers, 31, 32
Chestnut, Joey, 9, 155, 156
chloride, 147
chlorpromazine, 222
cholecystokinin, 14, 36, 113, 123
cholesterol, 17, 108, 170
Christensen, Peter, 185
chylomicrons, 17, 114, 118
chyme, 12, 14, 23, 25, 28
chymotrypsin, 14, 124
chymotrypsinogen, 14
cimetidine, 66
Clayton, Derek, 64
cognitive behavioral therapy (CBT), 220-221, 223, 225
colon, 22, 23, 28, 61, 66; activity, 184, 185; anxiety and, 210; caffeine and, 184; digestive material and, 63; spasm of, 201-202
colostrum, 176
competition, 95, 107, 117, 144, 193, 223; bowel movements and, 59; carbohydrates and, 160; energy needs and, 81; music for, 219; nausea and, 205; stressful, 46, 205, 210; ultraendurance, 121, 165
constipation, 55, 69, 84, 108, 130, 202; disordered eating and, 83; fluid intake and, 63; prevalence/development of, 72, 72 (table)
ConsumerLab.com, 169, 172
corticotropin-releasing factor (CRF), 203, 203-204, 206, 211
cortisol, 196, 197
Cox, Madisyn, 168-169
cramps, 48, 54, 60, 61, 165, 202; abdominal, 12, 50, 52, 73, 97, 105, 119, 121, 153, 158, 191; electrolyte imbalances and, 151; exercise-associated, 150; intestinal, 49-52, 71 (table); NSAIDs and, 51; pickle juice and, 151; prevalence/development of, 71 (table); preventing, 148, 152; sodium and, 150-152; stomach, 49, 50, 51
CRF. See corticotropin-releasing factor
Crohn's disease, 59, 230-232
curcumin, 181, 244
cystic fibrosis, 62

dairy, 60; diarrhea and, 62; protein from, 129
defecation, 109; diarrhea and, 58-62; prevalence/development of, 72 (table)
dehydration, 38, 41, 51, 83, 133, 134-135, 137, 138, 144, 148, 150, 211; avoiding, 206, 208; AVP and, 39; blood flow and, 48; gut and, 135 (fig.); minimizing, 139; moderate-to-severe, 135, 136; nausea and, 37; performance and, 140; sweating and, 140
depression, 84, 170, 197, 214, 216, 222, 225
DHA, 170
Dhabhar, Firdaus, 198
diabetes, 59, 64, 143, 195

Diagnostic and Statistical Manual of Mental Disorders (DSM-5), 206, 207
diarrhea, x, 12, 49, 73, 97, 119, 121, 132, 158, 178; black, 64; chronic, 59; dairy foods and, 62; defecation and, 58–62; explosive, 62, 185; prevalence/development of, 72 (table); short-lived, 59; as side effect, 131; traveler's, 60, 246–249
diet: energy-restricted, 128, 129; fat-rich, 161, 165; fiber-free, 55; high-carbohydrate, 156, 158, 159, 160, 161, 165; high-fat, 90, 111, 112, 115–116, 116–117, 121, 161, 162; high-protein, 128, 128–130, 129, 130, 132, 162, 163; low-carbohydrate, 116, 117, 129, 130, 132, 186; low-fat, 130; low-fiber, 130; low-FODMAP, 117; moderate-carbohydrate, 158, 159; protein-rich, 162–163; weight-loss, 80
Dietary Supplement and Health Education Act (DSHEA) (1994), 167
digestion, 6, 19, 93; chemical, 5; fiber and, 106; growth factors and, 178; location for, 15; mechanical, 10; problems with, 82, 217; protein, 12; side effects on, 131
digestive process, 3, 5, 10, 14, 23, 64, 83
digestive symptoms, 70, 157, 160
digestive tract, ix, 14, 31, 33, 84, 199; exercise and, 68; overview of, 3
dissaccharides, 17, 95
diverticulosis, described, 235–237
dopamine-receptor antagonists, 257 (table)
doping, 143, 168, 178, 188
drinking: exercise and, 142, 144; frequency of, 145; stomach emptying and, 163; sweat rates and, 137; thirst and, 146; training and, 164; volume of, 145
DSHEA. *See* Dietary Supplement and Health Education Act
DSM-5. *See Diagnostic and Statistical Manual of Mental Disorders*
Dumoulin, Tom, 59, 106
Dunne, Harry, 58
duodenum, 13–14, 14, 28
dyspepsia, functional, 215, 220, 221, 223, 224, 225, 233–235

E. coli, 60
eating disorders, 9, 83, 84, 86
eczema, 173
electrolytes, 20, 22, 23, 28, 142, 147, 148, 149, 150; cramps and, 151; supplementing with, 153
emulsifiers, 14–15, 17, 112
endotoxins, 39, 41, 103, 174
endurance events, 30, 94; bowel disasters and, 58; ketones and, 187; nausea and, 31; stress and, 203
energy, x, 47, 127, 133; balance, 79–80; boosting, 172, 188; dietary, 81, 83, 108, 162; fat and, 118; food and, 118, 161; overconsuming, 77, 78; physical work and, 77; production of, 22, 90, 157, 163, 187; restricting, 87, 187; underconsuming, 82–84, 87
energy density: dietary, 82 (table); spectrum, 80
energy expenditure, 79, 84; daily, 80, 86; overestimating, 85
energy intake, 47, 81, 160; low, 84; regulating, 79

energy needs, 77, 79–80, 81, 82; daily, 81 (fig.), 86 (table); determining, 84–85; total, 87
enzymes, 5, 10, 28, 42, 51, 91, 124, 147, 155; pancreatic, 17, 123; protein-digesting, 11
EPA, 170
ephedrine, 42
epiglottis, 6
epinephrine, 33, 35, 41
esophagus, 8, 28; function of, 6–7, 43–44; gastric secretions in, 42; pH changes in, 46
ETAP. *See* exercise-related transient abdominal pain
exercise, 50, 69, 111, 135, 179, 198, 217, 220; acute, 68; aerobic, 146, 155, 157; blood flow and, 48, 68; brain and, 155; carbohydrates and, 89, 90, 93–95, 98, 101, 102 (fig.), 156, 180–181; digestion during, 68, 104; drinking during, 142, 144; fat consumption and, 36–37, 45, 113, 115 (fig.); fiber and, 107–108; fluids and, 54, 136–142; fuels for, 89–93, 91 (fig.); gut function and, xi, 1, 109, 181; gut problems and, 67, 125, 138; heart rate and, 133; high-fat diets and, 115; hydration and, 136, 137; intense, ix, 12, 33, 41, 44, 67–68, 90, 91, 93, 134, 141, 157–158, 199, 204; leaky gut and, 103; moderate-to-intense, 91–92, 101, 105; nausea and, 30, 31, 33, 35, 41, 42, 125, 215; peptic problems and, 67; prolonged, 137, 157–158, 174, 199; protein and, 45, 125, 127–128, 132; sodium and, 165; ultraendurance, 67, 215
exercise duration, 65, 67–68, 93, 94, 126, 137; increase in, 37
exercise-related transient abdominal pain (ETAP), 52, 53–54
Experiments and Observations on the Gastric Juice and the Physiology of Digestion (St. Martin and Beaumont), 200

Farah, Mo, 34
fat, x, 15, 48, 62, 78, 83, 89, 147, 163, 187; absorption of, 17; burning, 90, 91, 119, 121; carbohydrates and, 186; defining, 112–113; dietary, 47, 77, 111, 112, 152, 161; digestion of, 5, 6, 10, 14; energy and, 113, 116, 118, 162; exercise and, 115 (fig.); gut symptoms and, 13; limiting, 126; long-chain, 22; mass worth of, 15; moderate, 114; oxidation of, 161; performance and, 161; quantities of, 90; removing, 112; stomach emptying and, 161, 162; traces of, 127; unsaturated, 130
fat consumption, 103, 113–115, 127, 129, 165; adaptation to, 160–162; exercise and, 36–37, 45, 113, 115 (fig.)
fatigue, 34, 39, 66, 84, 134; delaying, 93, 102, 163; regulation of, 94; sodium and, 148
fatty acids, 17, 36, 91, 157, 186; long-chain, 117, 118, 119 (fig.); medium-chain, 117, 118, 119 (fig.); omega-3, 170; organelles and, 91; short-chain, 24, 117
fermentable oligosaccharides, disaccharides, monosaccharides, and polyols (FODMAPs), 104, 105 (table), 106, 117; research on, 105; restricting, 110
fermentation, 56, 57; fiber, 117, 129
ferritin, 66, 228
fiber, 22, 48, 55, 79, 106–109, 130; avoidance of, 116; carbohydrates and, 105; doses of, 110; exercise

and, 107–108; fermentation of, 117, 129; flatulence and, 55; gut problems and, 108; limiting, 109, 126; supplementing with, 64

fiber ingestion, 10–17, 113

fish oil, 169, 170

5-HT3 receptor antagonists, 254 (table)

flatulence, x, 12, 24, 60, 61, 82, 97, 109, 117, 130, 132, 158, 174, 178, 185; described, 54–57; inducing, 106; prevalence/development of, 72 (table)

fluid: absorption of, 22; blood flow and, 139; consuming, 144, 145, 148, 208; emptying, 12; exercise and, 136–142; hydration and, 146; loading, 142–144; overconsuming/underconsuming of, 140; temperature, 144–145

fluid intake, 103, 136, 139, 141, 149, 155; adaptation to, 163–164; constipation and, 63; optimal, 140 (fig.)

fluoroscopy, 9

FODMAPs. See fermentable oligosaccharides, disaccharides, monosaccharides, and polyols

food, 7, 8, 24, 48, 144, 153; calorically dense, 112; carbohydrate-rich, 94, 95, 160, 186; energy and, 78, 118, 161; energy-dense, 80, 81, 82; fat-rich, 113, 158, 161; gas-forming, 55; high-protein, 130; intake, 136, 155; low-fiber, 110; probiotic-containing, 175; residue, 22; sodium-rich, 150; solid, 95

Food and Drug Administration (FDA), 167, 175; supplements and, 171–172, 188

Franklin, Benjamin, 54

Freud, Sigmund, 220

Froome, Chris, 92–93

fructose, 17, 51, 55, 96, 97; glucose and, 56, 95, 98, 99, 101, 110, 158, 161, 165; lactose and, 59, 106, 110; malabsorption of, 232–233; maltodextrin and, 99

fuel: delivery of, 22; exercise and, 89–93; sources, 104, 157

fullness, 50, 60, 73, 82, 83, 113, 126, 132, 144, 201; bloating and, 46–49; excessive, 114, 138; premature, 84; prevalence/development of, 71 (table); severity of, 209

functional magnetic resonance imaging (functional MRI), 47

galactose, 17, 96

gallbladder, 14, 28

gas, 24, 55, 73, 131; avoiding, 130; dietary source of, 48; fermentation, 57; performance and, 54; production of, 49, 56, 97

gastric acid, 23, 183; reducers, 258 (table), 261 (table)

gastric emptying, 48, 107, 114, 127, 135, 145; regulation of, 13 (fig.); undereating and, 83

gastroesophageal reflux disease (GERD), 8, 42, 46, 70, 238

gastrointestinal discomfort, 29, 69, 102, 136, 145

gastrointestinal disorders, 213; described, 227–251

gastrointestinal integrity, carbohydrates and, 102–104

gastrointestinal issues, 99, 105, 107, 135, 184

gastrointestinal system, ix, 70, 227

Gatorade, 20, 38, 94

Geller, Andrew, 171

gender, gut symptoms and, 69, 73

GERD. See gastroesophageal reflux disease

ghrelin, 123

ginger, 181–184, 188

glucagon, 40, 41

glucose, 12, 17, 51, 97, 107, 114; absorption of, 20, 98, 158; acid-base balance and, 179; brain function and, 41; fructose and, 56, 95, 98, 99, 101, 110, 158, 160, 165; long-chain forms of, 96, 99; nausea and, 40

GLUT5, 17, 96, 98, 158

glutamine, 178–181, 188; gut barrier function and, 180

gluten sensitivity, described, 228–230

glycerol, 117, 143, 144

glycogen, 94; stores of, 91, 93, 187

Goulet, Eric, 137, 138, 143

Grimston, Edward, 34

growth factors, 176, 177, 178

gut: adaptation by, 156–157, 164 (table); anatomy of, 4 (fig.), 28; blood in, 64; carbohydrate ingestion and, 159–160, 159 (fig.); dehydration and, 135 (fig.); exercise and, xi, 1; function of, 3, 77; high-fat diets and, 116–117; nervous system and, 12; physiology of, 27, 93; second brain and, 28, 191; training, 156–157, 159, 160, 165

gut barrier, 177

gut-brain-mood connections, 27, 192

gut distress, 46, 77, 139, 145, 178, 186; competition and, x; documenting, 153; exercise and, 138; experiencing, 87; NSAIDs and, 51–52; prevalence of, ix–x; risks of, 137

gut function, xi, xii–xiii, 117, 136, 161, 172, 213, 220; anxiety and, 209–210; bacteria and, 173; changes in, 211; exercise and, 109, 181; performance and, 112, 162; protein and, 131, 162; sleep and, 70; stress and, 199–206

gut intolerance, 136, 139, 153

gut leakiness, 174, 180, 206, 211; preventing, 103, 181

gut permeability, 174, 180, 181, 206

gut problems, 66, 70, 84, 106, 110, 129, 213, 214; anxiety and, 208; caffeine and, 185; exercise and, 125; fiber and, 108; functional, 221, 225; management strategies for, 73; performance and, 73; preventing, 126; severity of, 67; supplements and, 184–187; volume and, 82

gut symptoms, 29, 49, 52, 83, 114, 115, 125, 126, 145, 146, 153, 180, 181, 183, 188, 211, 227; aging and, 68; anxiety and, 221; carbohydrate beverages and, 100; causes of, 70, 73, 106; debilitating, 217; development of, 71–72 (table); exercise and, 67; experiencing, 173; fat and, 113; frequency of, 64, 69; gender and, 69, 73; managing, 221; nausea and, 215; occurrence/severity of, 67–68; prevalence of, 71–72 (table); protein and, 130; sodium and, 148; stress-induced, 211; worsening, 174

H1 antihistamines, 257 (table)

H2 antagonists, 258 (table)

Haga, Chad, 95

Hayes, Steven, 221

health, xii, 6, 79, 128, 143, 198, 224; bacteria and, 173; fat and, 111; gut, 24; performance and, 108, 136; psychological, 220; stress and, 195

heart, x, 10, 134
heart attacks, 169, 170
heart disease, 111, 169, 214
heart palpitations, 84, 171
heart rate, 34, 84, 133, 171, 224; elevation of, 134, 195
heartburn, 42–46, 69, 70, 183; nausea and, 43; prevalence/development of, 71 (table)
heat: exposure, 137, 175; illnesses, 103, 174; regulation, 136; stress, 41
hemoglobin, 66
hemorrhoids, 64
herbals, 168, 169, 188
Herophilos of Chalcedon, 14
hippocampus, 47
Hippocrates, 54, 227
Hirano, Ayumu, 218
hormones, 14, 31, 33, 47, 118, 204, 205; fluctuations in, 196; glucose-raising, 41; nausea and, 35; sex, 69; stress, 68, 206
Hunt, John N., 152
Hussein, Ibrahim, 50
Hutchinson, Alex, 62
hydration, 20; aggressive, 138; exercise and, 136, 137; fluid and, 146; guidelines for, 136, 137, 140; maintaining, 165; proper, 66, 120; structured, 146
hydrochloric acid, 10–11, 12, 28, 124
hydrogels, 100–101
hydrogen, 24, 55, 57, 106, 117, 185
hydrogen sulfide, 57
hypertonic, 12, 20
hypnosis, 217–218, 225
hypoglycemia, 40, 41, 211; avoiding, 206, 208; nausea and, 40
hyponatremia, 39, 40, 143, 144, 148, 156, 164
hypothalamic-pituitary-adrenal axis, 224
hypothalamus, 47, 197, 204
hypotonic, 12

IBS. See irritable bowel syndrome
ileum, 13, 18, 28
Imahara, Grant, 182
imipramine, 222
immune system, 98, 173, 176, 180, 198, 211; endotoxins and, 103; suppression of, 199; indigestion, 182, 188, 192, 238
infections, 39, 178; gastrointestinal, 173, 175; respiratory, 84, 173, 176
inflammatory bowel disease, 173
Informed-Choice, 172, 178
insomnia, 84
Institute of Medicine, 108, 128
insulin, 41, 107, 114
International Marathon Medical Directors Association, 137
interventions, 223–224; breathing, 214; mindfulness, 216; multicomponent, 215; relaxation, 46, 220
intestine, 14, 19, 20, 51, 96, 179; fluid movement in, 21 (fig.). See also large intestine; small intestine
iproniazid, 222

iron deficiency, 64, 66
irritable bowel syndrome (IBS), 56, 59, 70, 104, 173, 215, 216, 220, 221, 223; described, 239–240; gut symptoms in, 217; living with, 224
ischemia, gut, 66
Ivy, John, 119

James, LeBron, 9
Janus, Tim, 9
jejunum, 13, 18, 28
Jeukendrup, Asker, 118, 158
Journal of the American Medical Association, 44, 130

Kastor, Deena, 53
Kempainen, Bob, 29–30
ketones, 186, 187, 188
kidneys, 133, 134, 143, 171
kilocalories, 78, 79, 84
Kipchoge, Eliud, 99, 100
Kobayashi, Takeru, 156
Kuhn, Roland, 222

l-citrulline, 181
lactase, 51
lactate, 185
Lactobacillus, 174, 175
Lactobacillus acidophilus, 174
Lactobacillus casei, 174
Lactobacillus fermentum, 174
Lactobacillus rhamnosus GG, 173, 174
lactose, 17, 55, 95, 131, 176; fructose and, 59, 106, 110
lactose intolerance, 51, 130, 131, 240–241
lactulose, 61
Lambert, G. Patrick, 163
large intestine, 25, 61, 162; chyme and, 23; function of, 22–24; microorganisms in, 28; water and, 23, 28
laxatives, 59, 61, 64, 258 (table)
Le Clos, Chad, 218
leaky gut, 103, 103 (fig.)
Ledecky, Katie, 34
Liebig, Justus von, 127, 128
Linden, Des, 53
Lindgren, Gerry, 205
lipase, 5, 10, 15
Little, Tom, 200, 201
liver, 22, 28, 41, 134, 157; blood delivery to, 133; damage, 171; disorders, 143; failure, 181; toxicity, 222
lobotomy, 222
lumen, 14, 20, 96–97
lymphocytes, 179

macronutrients, 28, 36, 47, 62, 78, 121, 163
magnesium, 149
maltodextrin, 95, 99
maltose, 95
Marley, Bob, 218
Maurten, 99, 100
MCTs. See triglycerides, medium-chain

medications, 31; acid-suppressing, 45, 66; anticonstipation, 258 (table), 261 (table); anticramping, 259 (table); antihypertensive, 63; antinausea, 183, 254 (table), 257 (table), 259 (table); dyspepsia, 262 (table); irritable bowel syndrome, 225, 262 (table); over-the-counter, 253; pain-relieving, 52; prescription, 253; prosecretory, 64; side effects of, 253
meditation, 206, 216, 220
MedWatch, 171
melena, 64
memory loss, 84
menopause, 69
menstruation, 48, 69, 84
metabolism, 24, 28, 50, 95, 118, 119, 156, 179, 187
metabolites, 23, 132
metformin, 59
methane, 24, 57, 106, 117
methanethiol, 57
microbes, 26, 173, 174
microbiomes, 23, 106, 110, 121
microorganisms, 25, 28, 56, 129, 132, 173, 224; gut, 106; pathogenic, 60; small intestine and, 23
microvilli, 16, 16 (fig.), 17
Mifflin-St. Jeor equation, 85
migraines, 143
Miles, John C., 53
milk, 130, 176
Miller, Kevin, 151
mindfulness, 216–217, 225
minerals, 18, 130, 168, 169, 171
mitochondria, 91
monoamine oxidase inhibitor, 222
monoglycerides, 17
monosaccharides, 95, 96
Montana, Joe, 194
mood disorders, 173, 222
More, Sir Thomas, 54
Morton, Darren, 53–54
motility, 84, 87, 184, 201, 202, 203, 235, 240, 245
motion sickness, 182, 214
Mouseion of Alexandria, 14
mouth, 28; function of, 5–6
multiple sclerosis, 64
muscarinic cholinoceptor antagonists, 259 (table)
muscle: activity, 224; building, 131, 155, 168, 172; contraction, 26, 185; manipulation of, 43; mass, 162; skeletal, 134; stretch reflex, 26
music, 218–220, 225
Mutai, Emmanuel, 37
Mutai, Geoffrey, 50

N-nitroso, 129, 132
naproxen, 51
National Athletic Trainers' Association, 136
nausea, x, 48, 49, 50, 54, 60, 69, 73, 84, 113, 119, 121, 132, 138, 144, 153, 178, 183, 191; blood glucose and, 40; caffeine and, 42; causes of, 188; dehydration and, 37; development of, 33, 35, 37, 39, 83; exercise and, 30, 31, 33, 35, 41, 42, 125, 205, 215;

ginger and, 184, 188; gut symptoms and, 215; headache-induced, 34; heartburn and, 43; hormones and, 35; hypoglycemia and, 40, 41; ketones and, 187; physiology of, 32 (fig.); prevalence/ development of, 71 (table); severe, 37, 105, 182; sodium and, 152, 165; stomach emptying and, 35; stress-induced, 205, 206; vomiting and, 29–31, 32, 33–42, 205
nerves: competition-related, 193; extrinsic/intrinsic, 26; pre-competition, 221; pre-game, 191, 215
nervous system, 12, 31; autonomic, 25, 157, 204, 214, 216; central, 25, 26, 33, 191; enteric, 25–27; parasympathetic, 215, 216, 224; peripheral, 33, 203; sympathetic, 157, 215
neurons, 25, 26, 31–33, 224
Newcombe, Hoagie, 14
Newmaster, Steven G., 169
nitric oxide synthesis, 131
nitrogen, 57
noradrenaline, 33, 205
norepinephrine, 33, 205
novovirus, 60
NSAIDs, 66, 69, 183, 259 (table), 260 (table); gut and, 51–52, 253
NSF International, 172, 178, 188
nutrients, 18, 22, 28, 47, 155, 169; assortment of, 25; delivering, 107, 156; energy-dense, 113, 161; exercise and, 36; ingesting, x, 16
nutrition, 111, 136; competition, 61, 156; strategies for, 100, 140

obesity, 24, 195
Olson, Timothy, 116
omeprazole, 45
O'Neal, Shaquille, 5, 6, 7
opioids, 253, 260 (table)
organelles, fatty acids and, 91
oropharynx, 6
osmolality, 12, 19, 20, 39, 50, 99, 120; beverage, 21 (fig.); increase in, 38; serum, 149
osmosis, 19, 19 (fig.), 143
osteoarthritis, 182
oxygen, 90, 134, 155; blood and, 191; consumption, 44; delivery of, 102, 156; transporting, 66
oxytocin, 123

pain, 56; abdominal, 69; chest, 171; chronic, 197; exercise-induced, 182; gut, 183; relievers, 182; sleep deprivation and, 70; stomach, 83
pancreas, 14, 16, 19, 23, 28
pancreatitis, 62
pantoprazole, 66
paragangliomas, 35
parietal peritoneum, 53
Parkinson's disease, 64
pathophysiologies, 29
pepsin, 11, 123, 124
peptic problems, exercise and, 67
peptic ulcers, described, 241–245
peptide bonds, 10, 125

peptones, 11, 125
performance, xii, xiii, 128, 133, 176–177, 192; advantages in, 132; anxiety and, 208; better, 138, 163; caffeine and, 184; carbohydrates and, 110, 114, 120, 132, 139, 159, 161; compromising, 62; dehydration and, 140; digestive side effects and, 119; discomfort and, 145; drinking and, 139; exercise, 117, 143, 145, 156, 187; fat and, 161; gas and, 54; gut function and, 73, 112, 162; health and, 108, 136; high-fat diets and, 115–116, 121; high-intensity, 185; improving, 119, 138, 150, 177, 184, 187, 224; protein and, 125; recovery and, 109; sodium and, 148–150, 165; stress and, 195; superior, 137
peristalsis, 7, 7 (fig.), 26, 42, 44
pharmaceutical drugs, 171; anxiety and, 222–223
Phelps, Michael, 218
pheochromocytomas, 35
phospholipids, 17
physical activities, 65, 77, 79, 85, 192
physiological factors, 29, 184, 195, 224
pickle juice, 20, 151, 152, 153, 154
pituitary gland, 197
Plaschke, Bill, 193
plasma, 20, 149, 205
polypeptides, 11, 12, 121, 124
Porter, Alan, 65, 66
post-traumatic stress disorder (PTSD), 197
potassium, 149
Prefontaine, Steve, 205
probiotics, 57, 60, 172–175, 176, 188; effects of, 173, 174, 224; side effects of, 175; supplementing with, 56, 173
prosecretory drugs, 261 (table)
protein, x, 14, 15, 17, 48, 62, 78, 79, 113, 123, 129, 187; consuming, 103, 125–127, 132, 162–163; digestion of, 10–11, 11 (fig.), 14, 17, 124, 124 (fig.), 125; emptying, 162, 163; exercise and, 45, 125, 127–128, 132; gut symptoms and, 130–131; iron-containing, 66; performance and, 125; sports drinks and, 127–128; whey, 131
proton pump inhibitors, 261 (table)
psychotherapy, 220
Pugh, Jamie, 180

Radcliffe, Paula, ix, 58
ranitidine, 45
Rathe, Mathias, 176–177
rational emotive behavior therapy (REBT), 221
receptors, 43, 47, 152, 160
rectum, 24–25, 28
reflux, 42–46, 50, 60, 113, 201; prevalence/development of, 71 (table)
regurgitation, 42–46, 114; prevalence/development of, 71 (table)
relaxation, 43, 46, 220, 224
respiratory tract, 173
resting metabolic rate (RMR), 79, 80, 85, 86, 87
reticulocytes, 179
Rodgers, Bill, xiii

Rotella, Bob, 209
Rowlands, David, 50
Rupp, Galen, 37
Russell, Bill, ix, 194, 205
Ryun, Jim, ix, 34

St. Martin, Alexis, 199–200, 201
salivary glands, 28, 84
Sampras, Pete, 36
Samuelson, Joan Benoit, 49, 50
Savage, Adam, 182
Scott, Michael, 36, 114–115
secretin, 14
selective serotonin reuptake inhibitors (SSRIs), 59, 222, 223, 225, 262 (table)
Selye, Hans, 194, 195
Semple, Jock, 125, 126
serotonin-norepinephrine reuptake inhibitors (SNRIs), 223
SGLT1. See sodium-glucose linked transporter, 1
Shorter, Frank, 205
SIBO. See small intestine bacterial overgrowth
side effects, 48, 62, 152, 168, 170, 171, 213, 222, 223; digestive, 119, 131, 184; gastrointestinal, xii, 143, 175, 187, 253
side stitches, 73; described, 52–54; prevalence/development of, 72 (table)
Sims, Stacy, 143, 144
skin, 134; electrical conductivity of, 224; surges, 135
slap syndrome, 65
sleep, 198; gut function and, 70
small intestine, 12, 24, 43, 61, 66, 118, 162, 177; absorption in, 20, 28, 56; acids and, 14; adaptation by, 164; digestion in, 15 (fig.); function of, 13–20, 22; microorganisms and, 23; receptors in, 160; vitamins/minerals and, 18
small intestine bacterial overgrowth (SIBO), 245–246
sodium, 143–144; absorption of, 20; blood, 39, 142, 150; blood pressure and, 147; consuming, 147, 150; cramps and, 150–152; depletion of, 142, 165; dietary, 149–150; exercise and, 154, 165; fatigue and, 148; gut symptoms and, 148; nausea and, 152, 165; performance and, 148–150; vomiting and, 152
sodium bicarbonate, 62, 185, 186, 188
sodium chloride, 144, 148, 149, 152
sodium-glucose linked transporter 1 (SGLT1), 17, 96, 98, 158, 159, 165
somatotropin, 123
sphincters, 7, 8; anal, 25; esophageal, 42, 43, 44; pyloric, 12, 28
spinal cord, 25, 26
Spivak, Charles David, 54
sports drinks, 50, 89, 94, 95, 102, 142; carbohydrates and, 12; protein and, 127–128
sports gels, 94
Sports Medicine, 131
SSRIs. See selective serotonin reuptake inhibitors
Starling, Ernest, 26
Stenroos, Albin, 53

stimulants, 42, 168, 171, 168, 206, 208, 211

stomach, 14, 23, 28, 66, 191; adaptation by, 8, 35, 155, 164; discomfort with, 8, 138, 165, 184; environment of, 131; function of, 8–12; proteins and, 10; trainability of, 8–9

stomach emptying, 45, 101, 107, 110, 113, 118, 125, 131, 134, 144, 146, 183; delaying, 48, 63, 160; drinking and, 163; fat and, 161, 162; nausea and, 35; rate of, 139, 145; slow, 165

stomach issues, 30, 95, 201, 209

stool, 22, 24, 25, 28, 63; bloody, 64–67, 72 (table); loose, 61, 131, 174; prevalence/development of, 72 (table); watery, 59, 61

strategies, 64, 192; carbohydrate-based, 93–94; dietary, 69; feeding, 101; hydration, 138, 140, 141, 142, 143, 163; nutrition, 100, 140, 148, 164 (table)

Streep, Meryl, 5, 16

stress, 60, 68, 191, 194–199, 207, 209, 210; anxiety and, 49, 61, 194, 206, 211, 213; biological, 203; bloating and, 49; catecholamines and, 205; chronic, 197, 198; endurance races and, 203; extreme, 178; gut and, 199–206, 204 (fig.); levels of, 195, 215; managing, 209, 210, 213, 225; psychological, 51, 98, 195, 198, 199, 201, 203, 204, 206, 209, 211, 216; response, 197

sucrose, 17, 95

sugar, xi, 12, 20, 22, 147, 176; fat and, 111; nondigestible, 61; type, 95–99

supplements, 108, 183, 186; amino acid, 125; banned, 172; carbohydrate, 89; colostrum, 178; contamination of, 168, 169, 170; dietary, 62, 167, 188; electrolyte, 153; energy, 171; fiber, 64; glutamine, 180, 181; gut problems and, 131, 152–153, 184; ketone, 186, 187, 188; multivitamin-mineral, 167; nutritional, 171; probiotic, 172–175; protein, 125, 130–131; quality of, 169, 170, 172; sexual enhancement, 168; side effects of, 170–171; sodium, 148, 150, 152–153, 165; sports-enhancement, 171–172; weight-loss, 171

sweat loss, 18, 134, 136, 137, 141, 146, 164

sweat rates, 142, 146; calculating, 141, 141 (table); drinking and, 137

sweating, 37, 102, 136, 140

tachycardia, 171

Tai Chi, 217

temperature, 175, 224; body, 102, 103, 134, 148, 156; change in, 78, 149; fluid, 144–145

thoracic cavity, 44

time-to-exhaustion tests, 138

tongue, 6

training, 46, 92, 117, 178, 223; aging process and, 68; brain and, 155; carbohydrates and, 110; diet and, 156; drinking and, 164; endurance, 133, 155; energy needs and, 81; fluid loss during, 142; gut and, 156–157; high-intensity, 92; high-volume, 91; long-term, 68, 165; resistance, 155, 217; supplements and, 153

transient lower esophageal sphincter relaxation (TLESR), 43

transient receptor potential (TRP), 152, 153, 165

transporters, 17, 98, 158, 159, 165

tricyclic antidepressants, 262 (table)

Trier Social Stress Test, 204–205

triglycerides, 17, 112, 114; long-chain, 117–120, 119 (fig.), 121; medium-chain, 117–120, 119 (fig.)

trimetazidine, 168, 169

TRP. *See* transient receptor potential

trypsin, 14, 123

trypsinogen, 14

tuberculosis, 222

Turner, Martin J., 221

ulcerative colitis, 64, 249–251

ultraendurance events, 121, 148, 160, 165

ultraendurance runners, 108, 112, 115, 182–183

United States Pharmacopeia, 172, 178

upper respiratory tract infections (URTIs), 173, 174, 175, 177, 188

urine loss, 136

uvula, 6

vagal nerve, 26

van Niekerk, Wayde, 33

vanilloids, 152, 153, 165

vena cava, 10

villi, 16 (fig.), 17, 28

vitamins, 17, 18, 130, 168, 171

VO$_2$max, 44, 90, 93, 98, 110, 115, 116, 117, 121, 138, 139, 144, 163

vomiting, 73, 84, 113, 114, 153, 183, 185, 191; anxiety and, 193, 194; center, 31, 33; fear and, 193; nausea and, 29–31, 32, 33–42, 205; physiology of, 32 (fig.); poison-induced, 222; prevalence/development of, 71 (table); sodium and, 152

WADA. *See* World Anti-Doping Agency

Wadlow, Robert Pershing, 6

water, 22, 77, 79, 142; absorbing, 19, 20, 28; chugging, 156; human body and, 133; large intestine and, 23; loss of, 134, 136; low-sodium, 144; storage, 146

weight gain, 40, 164

weight lifting, 44, 85

weight loss, 84, 171, 172, 188

White, Shaun, 218

Wolf, Stuart, 200

Wolff, Harold, 200

World Anti-Doping Agency (WADA), 143, 168, 178

World Health Organization, 173

yoga, 217

yogurt, 130, 175

Young, Steve, ix, 194

ABOUT THE AUTHOR

Patrick Wilson is an assistant professor of exercise science and directs the Human Performance Laboratory at Old Dominion University. He earned a PhD in exercise physiology from the University of Minnesota and completed postdoctoral training in sports nutrition at the University of Nebraska–Lincoln. Wilson has authored more than 40 scientific articles that span the disci-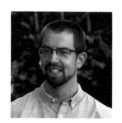plines of exercise science, sports nutrition, and health. He has spent hundreds of hours studying how dietary and psychological factors impact gut function and symptomology in exercisers and athletes, and his work has been featured in numerous national media outlets. Wilson is also a credentialed registered dietitian through the Commission on Dietetic Registration. He currently resides in Norfolk, Virginia, with his wife and son.

VISIT
VELOPRESS.COM

for more on running, cycling, triathlon,
swimming, ultrarunning,
yoga, recovery, mental training,
health and fitness, nutrition, and diet.

SAVE $10
ON YOUR FIRST ORDER

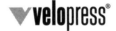